Viruses and Society

Viruses and Society is geared towards professionals and students in college-level introductory biology courses devoted to understanding viruses, vaccines, and their global impact. The beginning of the book introduces cells, DNA, and viruses themselves. There follows a review of how the immune system works and how scientists and physicians harness the immune system to protect people through vaccines. Specific chapters will focus on the 1918 influenza pandemic, the fight to eradicate polio, the HIV/AIDS pandemic, and our current COVID-19 crisis. Additionally, the book reviews the uses of viruses in genetic engineering and in gene therapy. The book will conclude by describing public health initiatives to keep emerging viruses in check and the role of scientific communication in how viruses are perceived and have an impact on our society.

Key Features:

- Employs approachable and simplified language
- Provides all the essential elements for understanding virus biology
- Includes details on how viruses affect individuals
- Describes the ways public health decisions are made in light of how viral pathogens spread
- Highlights up-to-date scientific findings on the features of emerging viruses that will always be with us

Patricia G. Melloy is a Professor in the Department of Biological Sciences at Fairleigh Dickinson University, Florham Campus. She received her undergraduate degree at Loyola University Maryland, her master's degree at Villanova University, and her PhD at the University of Pennsylvania. She was awarded the Distinguished Faculty Award for Teaching at Fairleigh Dickinson University in 2017.

Viruses and Society

Patricia G. Melloy

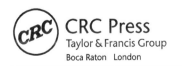

CRC Press
Taylor & Francis Group
Boca Raton   London

CRC Press is an imprint of the
Taylor & Francis Group, an **informa** business

First edition published 2023

by CRC Press
6000 Broken Sound Parkway NW, Suite 300, Boca Raton, FL 33487–2742

and by CRC Press
4 Park Square, Milton Park, Abingdon, Oxon, OX14 4RN

CRC Press is an imprint of Taylor & Francis Group, LLC

Library of Congress Cataloging-in-Publication Data
Names: Melloy, Patricia G., author.
Title: Viruses and society / Patricia G. Melloy.
Description: First edition. | Boca Raton : CRC Press, [2023] | Includes bibliographical references and index.
Identifiers: LCCN 2022005731 (print) | LCCN 2022005732 (ebook) | ISBN 9781032000091 (hardback) | ISBN 9780367771782 (paperback) | ISBN 9781003172260 (ebook)
Subjects: LCSH: Viruses. | Vaccines. | Viruses—Social aspects.
Classification: LCC QR360 .M44 2023 (print) | LCC QR360 (ebook) | DDC 579.2—dc23/eng/20220627
LC record available at https://lccn.loc.gov/2022005731
LC ebook record available at https://lccn.loc.gov/2022005732

ISBN: 978-1-03200-009-1 (hbk)
ISBN: 978-0-36777-178-2 (pbk)
ISBN: 978-1-00317-226-0 (ebk)

DOI: 10.1201/9781003172260

Typeset in Palatino
by Apex CoVantage, LLC

Contents

Contents

Acknowledgements

First, I would like to thank all the organizations that gave permission for use of photographs for figures in the textbook and their personnel who aided, including the World Health Organization; Special Collections Research Center, Temple University Libraries; National Museum of Health and Medicine, Division of Medicine and Science, National Museum of American History, Smithsonian Institution; and Johns Hopkins University and Medicine. Thanks to the National Library of Medicine for assistance in finding public domain photographs. Thanks to the Centers for Disease Control and Prevention for providing images. Thanks to Jasneet Punia for creating two original works for the figures. Thanks also to Stefan Steimle and Trevor Van Eeuwen of the University of Pennsylvania Perelman School of Medicine for assistance with the cryo-electron microscopy figure. I also need to acknowledge the librarians and personnel of the FDU library who provided encouragement and/or helped me find books and articles through interlibrary loan for over a year, especially Tracy Dante, Jason Brizzolara, Eleanor Friedl, and JR Malpere. Thank you to Katherine Dunsmore, Anthony Tasso, and Eric M. Muller who read and critiqued several chapters of the book.

In addition to those who directly assisted with the book, I want to acknowledge the scientists who have mentored me and/or inspired me in my work over the years, especially Mark Rose, Erfei Bi, Mary Desmond, Cecilia Lo, Cornelia Kurischko, and Blue Guldal. Thank you also to my former and current research students who have motivated me to keep growing, learning, and adapting over the years. Thanks also to my family and friends for their ongoing support, especially Jonathon. I dedicate this textbook to Jack, Kate, Colin, Ryan, and Conor, who I hope will help the next generation continue to value the importance of science in our society.

1

Introduction to Cells, DNA, and Viruses

Viruses and Society is a college-level textbook geared towards introductory biology students or anyone with an interest in science who wants to understand **viruses** and their impact on our world. We will begin with an introduction to **macromolecules**, **genes**, and **cells**, followed by viruses that infect cells. Then, in Chapter 2, we will cover how the immune system works and how scientists harness the immune system to enhance immunity through vaccines. Next, we will take up case studies of the 1918 influenza pandemic, the fight to eradicate polio, the HIV/AIDS pandemic, and our current coronavirus COVID-19 crisis. We will also review genetic engineering, in which deoxyribonucleic acid (**DNA**) can be manipulated to be expressed in other organisms. Viruses are also used in gene therapy, among other ways that humans have used viruses for their own productive purposes. Finally, we will end the book by talking about public health initiatives to keep emerging viruses in check and the role of science communication in how viruses are perceived and have an impact on our society.

Learning Outcomes:

1.1 Understand How Our Bodies Are Made of Cells Containing Our Genetic Material in the Form of Deoxyribonucleic Acid (DNA)

1.2 Recognize That a Virus Can Enter a Cell and Use the Host Cell's Machinery to Replicate Itself

1.3 Identify Different Types of Viruses Based on Their Properties

1.4 Understand the Impact of Certain Viruses on the Health of Human Beings and Other Organisms

1.5 Determine That There Are Many Kinds of Viruses in the World, and Not All Are Pathogens

1.6 Understand That Viruses Are Capable of Evolution

1.7 Preview Upcoming Chapters Including How Virologists Do Their Work

1.8 Recognize How Viruses Might Have an Impact on Our Society

1.1 Understand How Our Bodies Are Made of Cells Containing Our Genetic Material in the Form of Deoxyribonucleic Acid (DNA)

Before learning about viruses, it is useful to understand what they infect: our cells. It has been known for quite some time that our bodies are made of cells. Going back to the early 1800s, Matthias Schleiden and Theodor Schwann determined that all animals and plants

DOI: 10.1201/9781003172260-1

are made of cells. Cells are defined philosophically as being the fundamental units of life and are distinctive for being able to reproduce themselves to make other cells. All these ideas (animals and plants are made of cells, cells are the fundamental units of life, cells give rise to other cells) put together became what is now called the cell theory (Alberts et al. 2019). From the point of view of chemical content, one can also define cells as containing many macromolecules needed for the processes of life, protected by the **cell membrane**. Although our cells are mostly made of water, the key macromolecules present are critical for cellular function, including **nucleic acids**, carbohydrates, **proteins**, and lipids. DNA and ribonucleic acids (**RNA**) are nucleic acids, made of building blocks called nucleotides. Proteins are made of amino acids. Carbohydrates are made of sugar subunits. Lipids, also known as fats, are made of fatty acids and glycerol. See Table 1.1 for key definitions.

Our focus will be on eukaryotes, which are cells (including our cells) containing a nucleus and other organelles. However, viruses can also infect prokaryotes. The most well-known prokaryotes are bacteria. Prokaryotes lack a nucleus and membrane-bound organelles (Alberts et al. 2019). There are two prokaryotic kingdoms: Archaea and Eubacteria. Archaea includes microorganisms (or microscopic organisms) that can live in extreme environments on the planet. Eubacteria includes microorganisms also known as bacteria and cyanobacteria (Minkoff and Baker 2004d).

TABLE 1.1

Key Definitions.

Term	Definition
Allele	Different forms or versions of a gene. May arise through mutation, where they are known as variants of a gene.
Cell	The unit of life. Made of macromolecules and organelles inside a fluid-filled sac bound by a membrane. Capable of reproducing itself.
Cell membrane	Envelope enclosing a cell. Made mostly of fats. Acts as a selective wall that allows certain materials to go into the cell and certain materials to go out.
Deoxyribonucleic acid (DNA)	A type of nucleic acid making up our genes and the genes of other living organisms.
Endosome	Membrane-bound structure near the surface of the cell that is a part of the trafficking network that receives and sorts material coming into the cell. Some viruses can use endosomes to get into cells.
Evolution	Permanent genetic changes happening in a population due to random mutation.
Gene	The unit of heredity made of DNA. Each gene encodes a protein.
Genome	All the genes of an organism collectively.
Macromolecule	Building material for cells. Consists of sugars, fats, nucleic acids, and proteins.
Nucleic acid	One of the major cellular macromolecules. Includes both DNA and RNA. Made of nucleotides.
Protein	One of the major cellular macromolecules. Translated from an mRNA template. Also known as a polypeptide. Includes things like enzymes and structural components of cells that do the cell's work.
Ribonucleic acid (RNA)	A type of nucleic acid used by our cells for things like messenger RNA (mRNA), which acts as a template for translation.
Transcription	Using a DNA template to make RNA.
Translation	Using an RNA template to make protein.
Virion	Viral particle itself.
Virus	A nonliving entity that depends on cells to make copies of itself. It is capable of evolution.

Cellular macromolecules are organized into compartments called organelles (like little organs) that have an organization allowing for the work of the cell to happen. So, like organs such as the heart and lungs that have a special role in the body, organelles have a special role inside the cell. Some examples of key cellular organelles include the nucleus (where DNA is housed), mitochondria (energy generation), and ribosomes (protein production). Except for the nucleolus residing in the nucleus, organelles are found in what is known as the cytoplasm or cytosol of the eukaryotic cell. The nucleus is an important organelle because it acts as the central control point for all the activities of the cell. The nucleus houses most of the cell's DNA in the form of protein/DNA structures known as chromosomes that allow for condensation of the large amount of genetic material in each cell (Alberts et al. 2019). Cell division occurs in a process known as mitosis, in which the chromosomes are copied and separated equally between the two daughter cells. Later, we will talk about organelles that help move or traffic things around the cell, as well as into and out of the cell. Trafficking-related organelles include the endoplasmic reticulum, Golgi apparatus, and vesicles. Viruses can exploit the cellular trafficking network to move into and out of the cell.

Experiments done by scientists in the 1940s and 1950s determined that the DNA is the hereditary material in structures within the nucleus called chromosomes. Chromosomes also are made of protein, which plays a supporting structural role in the chromosomes. The DNA contains the hereditary units known as genes. The researchers Oswald Avery, Colin MacLeod, and Maclyn McCarty performed a series of experiments, an extension of experiments done by Frederick Griffith, looking at a phenomenon called bacterial transformation. Transformation in this context is the transfer of genes from one bacterium into another, with the bacterium now being transformed or changed in its heritable characteristics. They determined that DNA was responsible for the transformation (Avery, MacLeod, and McCarty 1944). Interestingly, scientists sometimes use harmless viruses as a tool in their research. In the famously elegant Hershey and Chase experiment done in 1952, researchers used a type of virus known to infect bacteria called a bacteriophage. A radioactive phosphorus label was used to track the DNA from the virus, and a radioactive sulfur label was used to track the protein of the virus. (There is no sulfur in DNA and no phosphorus in protein, so the labels are specific to those macromolecules.) These researchers discovered that the DNA was taken into the infected cells, and it encoded the genetic material needed to make copies of the bacteriophage in the host cells (Hershey and Chase 1952).

One of the biggest functions of the cell is to produce proteins to do particular jobs for cells and the body as a whole. Because humans contain so many kinds of cells, we have separation of function for different groups of cells, which are organized into tissues, organs, and organ systems. Cells duplicate themselves when they are actively dividing. Cells go through a series of steps known as the cell cycle, in which the cell prepares for DNA synthesis, then copies its DNA, then separates the DNA in the form of the chromosomes moving to opposite sides of the cell (see Figure 1.1). The cell then completes nuclear division followed by separation of the cytoplasmic contents, resulting in two cells. This process is known as mitosis. Not all cells are actively dividing, but cell division is critical during development as well as to replenish worn-out tissues in an adult organism. When cells do a particular job for the body, they need to create proteins encoded in the DNA. Cells come in many shapes and sizes, but what they all have in common is the procedure needed to convert the hereditary material to functional protein in the body.

The procedure by which cells interpret DNA to make protein is known as the central dogma. Francis Crick first coined the term "central dogma" in a lecture in the 1950s and

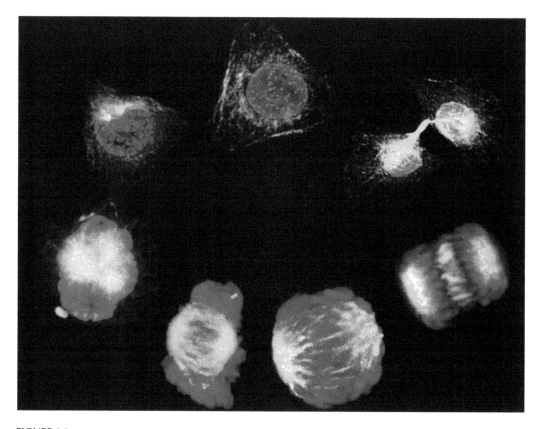

FIGURE 1.1
Fluorescence microscopy images of cell division stages.

Shown here are cells at different stages of nuclear division known as mitosis. The cells are moving through the stages in a counterclockwise manner. Cells were stained with three different fluorescence dyes (blue, green, red) and visualized using fluorescence microscopy. In this process, the cell duplicates its chromosomes containing the DNA (blue) and lines up the chromosomes in the middle of the cell using microtubules made of tubulin protein (green). A protein complex on each chromosome known as the kinetochore (pink) is used to pull the chromosomes apart. Then the cell separates the chromosomes equally for the two daughter cells. Separation of the cells is completed with cytoplasmic division known as cytokinesis.

Source: Image "Human cells showing the stages of cell division" courtesy of Matthew Daniels, Wellcome Collection, https://wellcomecollection.org/works/r8ppshar/images?id=g69v3q5m published under CC BY 4.0 https://creativecommons.org/licenses/by/4.0/

then described it later in conference proceedings and in an article for *Nature* (Crick 1958, 1970). At the beginning of the *Nature* article, Crick raises the critical question of how genetic information is transferred to what ultimately becomes protein. When Crick first articulated the central dogma, scientists were not fully aware of the details of messenger RNA (mRNA) as an intermediate between DNA and protein. In addition, scientists did not know about the role of transfer RNA (tRNA) as an adapter molecule facilitating the interpretation of the genetic code, and Crick predicted its existence (Cobb 2017). As a part of the central dogma, Crick noted that the genes encoded in the DNA could be copied in the process of replication. Then, the cell creates an RNA copy of the information, which is known as mRNA. Both DNA and RNA are the same class of macromolecule, a nucleic acid. Then, the mRNA is used to make a protein. This process is known as **translation**. The steps of the central dogma are important, as is the direction of the flow of information. Crick also speculated that the DNA sequence when translated into an amino acid sequence provided enough information to create a three-dimensional protein structure (Crick 1970; Cobb 2017). It is important to note that Crick's 1970 version of the central dogma is written in part as commentary on recent discoveries on the flow of genetic information in viruses, which can be different from that in our own cells (Cobb 2017; Temin and Mizutami 1970; Baltimore 1970). We will discuss this later in the chapter.

Not only does every eukaryotic cell interpret the genetic code in the same manner, but also all the cells of an organism, even mature, specialized cells, have the same genetic code in their nuclei. In landmark studies performed by John B. Gurdon, he determined that all cells of the body (except for sperm or egg) contain the full **genome**. Instead of losing genes as they specialize, cells vary in terms of which genes are turned "on," meaning what genes they express to make protein. In technically challenging experiments, Gurdon performed experiments using the amphibian *Xenopus laevis* indicating that an adult cell nucleus has a genome equivalent to that of a fertilized egg. As a side note, Gurdon's discoveries became an important stepping-stone towards reproductive and therapeutic cloning approaches (Gurdon 1962, 2017; Gurdon and Uehlinger 1966). These approaches are techniques that use stem cells to make new animals or tissues. The ability to replace worn-out or diseased tissues is called regenerative medicine, and we will talk more about this topic in Chapter 7.

Since viruses are using our cellular machinery for reproduction, that means that they are operating with our genetic code. Watson and Crick first published the structure of DNA, consisting of nucleotide subunits of four varieties: adenine, guanine, cytosine, and thymine (Watson and Crick 1953). In their work, Watson and Crick detailed the double-helical structure of the DNA molecule, requiring two strands of DNA in opposite orientations. Each nucleotide building block of DNA contains a nitrogenous base that would pair with a base in the opposite strand to make a "rung" of the DNA ladder, with the sugar and phosphate components of the nucleotides making up the "sides" of the ladder. Because of work done by Rosalind Franklin, Erwin Chargaff, and others, Watson and Crick were confident that the bases were turned inward as the rungs, rather than studding the sides on the outside, of the helical structure. In addition, a purine (guanine or adenine) and a pyrimidine (cytosine or thymine) aligned on each rung to create a uniform length to the ladder rung throughout the helix (Alberts et al. 2019). Rosalind Franklin made significant contributions to Watson and Crick's discovery through her X-ray crystallography work on DNA structure (Maddox 2002).

Understanding how the DNA information ultimately became protein took quite a bit of detective work before Marshall Nirenberg and Henrich Matthaei broke the code. They started on that journey performing *in vitro* experiments using cell-free extracts and long polymers of the radioactively labeled mRNA nucleotides introduced to different test tubes. It is important to note that the cell-free extracts, containing the minimum machinery for translation, provided a simple, powerful system to do their code breaking. Each test tube contained a different radiolabeled amino acid as a potential building block to be used for protein synthesis. Their experimental results were the first step towards determining how mRNA is translated into protein (Nirenberg and Matthaei 1961). In additional experiments, Nirenberg and colleagues varied the structure of the synthetic mRNA used at the start of the *in vitro* experiment, with the help of other scientists, until figuring out all the combinations that would lead to the 20 amino acids. Experiments done with Philip Leder and yet others made clear the role of the mRNA triplet brought in by tRNA to the ribosome. They also found the three mRNA options leading to no amino acid at all—the termination codons. Nirenberg's groundbreaking work is often described as the discovery of a "Rosetta stone" (a decoding method) for molecular biology (Alberts et al. 2019; Caskey and Leder 2014; Marshall 2014). It is important to also note the contributions of Har Gobind Khorana in the synthesis of synthetic mRNAs, and Robert Holley, in isolating tRNA, in building the story of how the DNA sequence is ultimately interpreted as protein (Nobel Media AB 1968).

Now that we have discussed the makeup of cells as well as the details of the genetic code and how it is interpreted, we will move into what viruses are and how they are critically dependent on cells to propagate themselves. As we talk about viruses, we will discuss their life cycle, including how they make copies of themselves and then how they move out of our cells.

1.1.1 What Is a Virus?

Before discussing "what is a virus?" it is important to introduce the idea: "what is life itself?" This topic that has fascinated scholars from an array of disciplines (e.g., philosophers, psychologists, religious figures) is decidedly a part of an introduction to the study of biology as a whole. When asked to describe the characteristics of life, most people talk about the ability to move, the consumption of fuel, and the secretion of waste products. Whenever I think of this topic, I recall my first day as a teaching assistant, sitting in on the professor's first lecture for freshman biology, and watching him walk into the room with a chainsaw! Yes, a chainsaw. He then challenged the class: does it not move, does it not consume energy, and does it not give off exhaust? Even though they were a little bit startled, the students began to challenge that the chainsaw was a living thing by listing the more complex characteristics of life, including responding to stimuli and reproducing itself. If we step away from the living thing itself for a moment, another key characteristic of life is homeostasis. This means that the living being can maintain some kind of stable balance of activities in a living system around it (Minkoff and Baker 2004a).

Now if we think about viruses for a moment, without the chainsaw, we can see that they exist in this unusual space in the world in that they do not exhibit all the characteristics of life, yet they certainly seem to be alive in their ability to enter and use cells. Upon critical examination, viruses are not organized into cells, and they cannot reproduce by themselves (Minkoff and Baker 2004a). For this reason, most scientists have settled on the idea of viruses as obligate intracellular parasites, which display many characteristics of life but are not living themselves (Summers 2009; Cossart and Helenius 2014). This definition indicates that viruses need to exist inside cells to perpetuate themselves. Virologists, scientists who study viruses, have created an even more specific list of viral characteristics based on the genes viruses must carry and how they assemble themselves. The characteristics include that a virus must have a gene with the instructions for making at least one capsomere (also called capsomer) protein that is a part of the coat protecting the viral genome (called the capsid). In addition, the virus can build itself after new viral proteins are made in the cell and the genome is copied. Finally, importantly, viruses are capable of **evolution**, like the host they infect is (Lostroh 2019).

By using this particular definition of viruses, scientists are acknowledging a virus's life-like properties—without actually calling it a living thing. This definition also establishes that viruses are in fact parasites, being dependent on host cells to keep reproducing. We will look at the complex virus-host interaction in more detail. It is important to note that some scientists point out that there is no universal standard for defining "life" (Lostroh 2019). Therefore, discussion on the boundaries between living and nonliving things will continue.

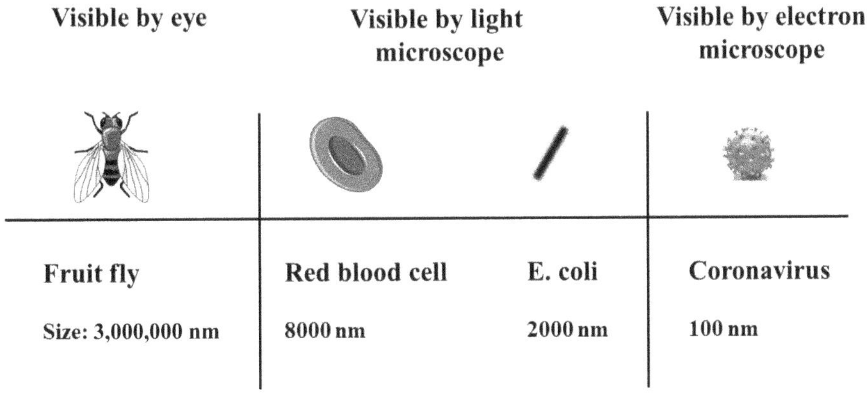

Visible by eye	Visible by light microscope		Visible by electron microscope
Fruit fly	Red blood cell	E. coli	Coronavirus
Size: 3,000,000 nm	8000 nm	2000 nm	100 nm

FIGURE 1.2
Comparison of sizes.

In this figure, one can see a typical size for a small object visible by eye like a fruit fly, but also things requiring a light microscope to view such as a red blood cell and an *E. coli* bacterium. Anything below Abbe's diffraction limit of 200 nm would require another technology such as an electron microscope to view. Please note that a large virus like a coronavirus is typically about 100 nanometers in diameter, smaller than a bacterium but larger than a protein. The fruit fly is the largest object at 3,000,000 nanometers (nm) which is 3 millimeters long and 30,000 times the size of the coronavirus.

Source: Fruit fly and red blood cell images from Servier Medical Art (CC BY3.0) https://smart.servier.com/ and the "Novel Coronavirus SARS-CoV-2" is from NIAID (CC BY 2.0) https://wordpress.org/openverse/photos/7b3b07ad-2135-4af1-bd92-7cc1cc2ee33f

So, what is a virus chemically? Typically, it is a bit of genomic material and some protein that acts like a little cell-dependent machine to make copies of itself. Critically, the virus keeps its genome light by not encoding standard genome-copying enzymes. It instead finds everything it needs in the host cell. Size-wise, a virus is typically smaller than even a bacterium and requires a special microscope to view its structure (Figure 1.2).

1.2 Recognize That a Virus Can Enter a Cell and Use the Host Cell's Machinery to Replicate Itself

Viruses typically contain a bit of nucleic acid (DNA or RNA) containing its small genome, have a protein coat, and may or may not be covered in an envelope or membrane made of lipids like the phospholipids that make up our own cell membrane. When the virus is fully assembled with its nucleic acid in its protective coat, it is called either a **virion** or a viral particle (Lostroh 2019). Assembly of new virions depends on the host cell's raw materials to make the new nucleic acid, protein, and lipids, as well as the machinery for **transcription** of mRNA and translation of proteins. Viruses can typically exist in one of two states: lytic or lysogenic. Viruses may go through a period when they are in the cell and get passed from cell to cell as they divide, but the virus has actually inserted its genome into the host cell's genome. The virus is said to be in a latent or lysogenic state. Some viruses may exist as "persistent infections" where virions are not actively being made for years (Lostroh 2019).

When the virus does start reproducing, it will assemble everything it needs to make many copies of itself, like enzymes to copy its genome, and then will leave the cell through lysis when the cell bursts open. This is the lytic state of the virus (Summers 2009). When virions first enter a cell, there is typically a unique stage to viral replication in which the virions seemingly go under the radar and cannot be detected, although they are replicating. This is known as the eclipse period. When lysis does occur, it typically occurs in a "burst" that may release thousands of virions to go on to infect more cells (Lostroh 2019; Summers 2009).

We know that viruses can infect many kinds of host cells and can therefore have a range of effects on the host. We call the different species infected by a virus the "host range," while the "tissue tropism" of a virus indicates the different tissues within a host that can become infected. These characteristics have a lot to do with how the virus gets inside the cells (Lostroh 2019). Sometimes the virus has no noticeable effect; sometimes it kills the host. However, all viruses have a mechanism to get their genome into the host cell and make many copies of the virus, and then eventually the new viral particles leave the host. The effect on the host in this process can be anticipated based on the virus's virulence that is often expressed in adjective form as virulent. Virulence has to do with the ability to cause disease or its symptoms (Summers 2009). One might say that virulence tells you what the collateral damage might be to the host upon viral infection. However, many factors like the health of the patient prior to infection contribute to the disease outcome as well.

To get into a cell, the virus latches onto some type of cellular structure like a receptor on the outside of the cell. Receptors are ordinarily used to receive signals from other cells. Sometimes not even the entire virus enters the cell, just the genome (Summers 2009). In the case of SARS-CoV-2, the receptor for the virus is the ACE2 receptor (Lu et al. 2020; Zhou et al. 2020). Typically, the virus displays a protein spike or similar protein allowing it to bind to the receptor and get inside the cell. A virus might actually have more than one kind of receptor it can bind to (Cossart and Helenius 2014). If the virus has an envelope or membrane around it, this can act as convenient "transport vesicle" to move the virus into the host cell. If the virus does not have an envelope, it can break the membrane, bore through, or hitch a ride with part of the cell that naturally crosses the envelope. Most viruses depend on the cells' own process of moving things into the cell known as endocytosis to get into the cell. There is a specific kind of endocytosis called receptor-mediated endocytosis in which the "cargo" coming into the cell binds to a receptor and then the receptor and cargo are engulfed together into a transport vesicle coming into the cell (Cossart and Helenius 2014). Receptor-mediated endocytosis is critical for moving cholesterol from the blood into the cells in the form of low-density lipoprotein (LDL) particles (Alberts et al. 2019). Actually, the LDL receptor itself is known as a target for some viruses to get into cells (Cossart and Helenius 2014). Besides receptor-mediated endocytosis, a virus might enter a cell through "micropinocytosis," which is like a type of "cell drinking" to bring things into the cell, or by concentrating bound receptors into special regions of the cell membrane (Cossart and Helenius 2014). Interestingly, going into the cell through the cell's natural trafficking mechanism is a way to evade the immune system—at least temporarily. In addition, the low pH environment (acidic) of parts of the trafficking network, such as structures known as **endosomes**, can actually activate the viruses (Cossart and Helenius 2014).

If we return to the central dogma for a moment, it is important to note that all cells obey the central dogma, but viruses do not. This became completely clear when the first viruses were discovered that did not have a DNA-based genome, and the central dogma had to be revisited because of these discoveries (Baltimore 1970; Temin and Mizutami 1970). Viruses can house their genetic material in the form of either DNA or RNA, single-stranded or double-stranded. There are actually many RNA viruses. A eukaryotic cell will carry its genetic material in the form of double-stranded DNA in the nucleus and make a single-stranded messenger RNA copy of any genes that are expressed. Viruses evolved to consist of all different kinds of genomes, but in the end, each template is adapted or converted in some way to fit in almost seamlessly to use the eukaryotic host cell's transcriptional and translational mechanisms to make its necessary viral proteins and copy its genome. If the viral genome can somehow be converted to an mRNA transcript to be read by the host cell's ribosomes, the virus can reproduce in that cell. In addition, because viruses are using the cell's machinery, even though a virus may start out with different genetic material, viruses still follow the genetic code language of cells where mRNA is translated into certain amino acids that make up proteins (Lostroh 2019).

Virologists know a tremendous amount of detail on the synthesis of viral proteins in cells. Typically, for its replication, the virus first has the cell make "early proteins" that help with the expression of other viral genes and may block proteins from the host cell from being made. Then "late proteins" are made, including proteins needed for the structure of the infectious viral particle (Lostroh 2019).

1.3 Identify Different Types of Viruses Based on Their Properties

Viruses can be classified in many ways. Viruses come in a variety of shapes and sizes (Figure 1.3). One initial way to classify a virus is just by type of genome: whether the genome is DNA or RNA. You can also classify viruses based on the hosts that they infect. The International Committee on the Taxonomy of Viruses (ICTV) has subcommittees formed based on viral host as well as genome type. As of 2021, there are three committees devoted to animal viruses of different genome types, one committee for archaeal viruses, one for bacterial viruses, and one for fungal and protist viruses. There is also a committee for plant viruses. ICTV has an online database available to the public (Lefkowitz et al. 2018). David Baltimore, a scientist who has worked on viruses for over 50 years, came up with an initial classification system designating categories of animal viruses based on the type of viral genome that is still used to this day (Baltimore 1971). This classification will be described in more detail later. Dr. Baltimore also has articulated another way to classify viruses, calling them either "equilibrium" or "non-equilibrium" viruses (Baltimore 2017). An equilibrium virus has most likely been infecting the host for a long time and does not cause severe disease in the host. One example would be a rhinovirus causing the common cold in humans. However, a non-equilibrium virus has recently jumped or spilled over from one species to another and tends to be more lethal. An example of a non-equilibrium virus would be HIV causing AIDS in humans (Baltimore 2017).

When it comes to the classifications of animal viruses, all roads lead to a functional mRNA product. The initial classes were labeled I–VI, with a seventh category added later (Baltimore 1971; Summers 2009; Lostroh 2019). Class I contains viruses with a double-stranded DNA viral genome. Class II contains viruses with a single-stranded DNA genome. This single strand happens to be a "+ strand" of DNA, meaning that it is the "sense" strand, equivalent to the mRNA product except for thymidine being replaced with uracil. Class III has viruses with a double-stranded RNA genome. Class IV contains viruses with a + strand, single-stranded RNA genome. Class V contains viruses with a single-stranded RNA genome that

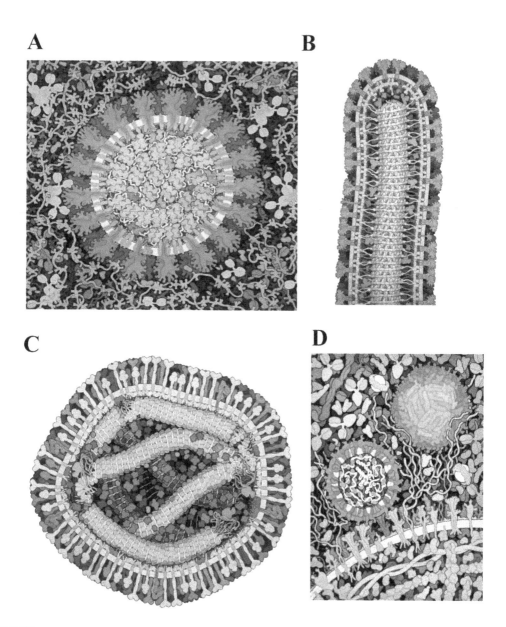

FIGURE 1.3
Viral diversity.

Shown here are an artist's color illustrations of four different kinds of viruses, based on structural features visualized through biological imaging techniques. A coronavirus is shown in (A). A cross section of Ebola virus is shown in (B). Panel (C) is a cross section of a measles virus, and (D) are two Zika virus particles.

Sources and acknowledgements: Illustrations by David S. Goodsell, RCSB Protein Data Bank: doi: 10.2210/rcsb_pdb/goodsell-gallery-013 (*cross section of Ebola virus, 2014*), doi: 10.2210/rcsb_pdb/goodsell-gallery-018 (*cross section through measles virus, 2019*), doi: 10.2210/rcsb_pdb/goodsell-gallery-019 (*Coronavirus, 2020*); https://doi.org/10.2210/rcsb_pdb/goodsell-gallery-015 (*Zika virus*, 2016) for additional information, please see D.S. Goodsell, M. Voigt, C. Zardecki, and S.K. Burley (2020) Integrative illustration for coronavirus outreach. PLoS Biol 18(8): e3000815. https://doi.org/10.1371/journal.pbio.3000815. Published under CC BY 4.0.

is the "– strand," or antisense strand, being the opposite polarity of the mRNA. Class VI and VII are related in that a nucleic acid intermediate has been found between the viral genome and the mRNA product. In Class VI, there is a DNA intermediate for a single-stranded RNA genome of the sense orientation. In Class VII, there is a DNA intermediate for a double-stranded DNA genome (Summers 2009; Baltimore 1971).

Classification of viruses can also focus on comparisons of genomic sequences showing the evolutionary relatedness of viruses. The ICTV conducts their work based on outward or structural characteristics of the viruses like shape and type of genome, which are elements of classical taxonomy, as well as type of host infected and gene-based compari-sons. Members of the ICTV emphasize that taxonomy is fluid and not fixed (Siddell 2018). However, some scientists have called on a greater emphasis on genomic comparisons of viruses to classify them. Recently, one group conducted a metagenomics analysis of viral genomes available in public databases (Mahmoudabadi and Phillips 2018). A metagenom-ics approach involves looking at the entire genes of the virus but also looking at many types of viruses all at the same time. They performed an analysis of characteristics like gene length and functional categories of viral genes present. They found some interesting results, including that RNA viruses tend to have longer genes than DNA viruses. In addi-tion, eukaryotic viruses as a group have longer genes than bacterial viruses in the same category based on Dr. Baltimore's classification system (Mahmoudabadi and Phillips 2018). Future studies will include ongoing refinement of viral classifications based on many characteristics, but for the purposes in this book, we will use the major established clas-sification system to identify viruses relevant to society.

On another note, an even more complicated entity to define is a prion. Prions are even smaller than viruses, being defined as infectious proteins. Prions have been associated with neurodegenerative diseases in humans and other animals such as scrapie and Creutzfeldt-Jakob syndrome (Alberts et al. 2019; Nobel Media AB 1997).

1.4 Understand the Impact of Certain Viruses on the Health of Human Beings and Other Organisms

Viruses that are most heavily studied tend to be the ones with the biggest impacts on human lives. Viruses causing diseases are known as pathogens. A scientist named Robert Koch working in the 1800s helped establish a universally accepted scientific process to estab-lish the connection between a microbe and a disease. His guidelines were called Koch's postulates. These four rules or assumptions proposed by Koch have become the standard for assessing if a microbe, like a virus, causes a disease. They include find the microbe in almost all people with the disease, do not find the microbe in unaffected people, isolate the microbe on its own (the tricky part), and then reintroduce the single microbe into an animal to cause the same disease (Minkoff and Baker 2004e). It is important to note that some people are calling for a readjustment of these postulates, especially in the context of the communities of microorganisms living together, dependent on one another, inside the body that may affect susceptibility to a pathogen (Byrd and Segre 2016).

A few key terms are associated with describing a disease caused by a pathogen that has taken hold in a community. For example, if a pathogen were creating disease at low but consistent levels in a geographic area, the disease would be called endemic. If there is a sudden increase in the number of cases of a disease, and the disease begins to spread in new ways, the disease would be called an epidemic. Finally, a disease that becomes prevalent worldwide is known as a pandemic (Minkoff and Baker 2004f). Pathogens also typically have some kind of vector contributing to the spread of the disease to humans. The vector is a living thing, like an animal, interacting with humans while remaining unimpacted by the disease. I consider it like the "bagman" for the virus. The abundance of the vector itself is affected by one of the key characteristics affecting the spread of a pathogen—weather and environment as well as travel and trade.

Other characteristics affecting pathogen spread include the susceptibility of the host to the virus, balanced with the virus's competence in causing disease (virulence), route of transmission, and herd immunity (Minkoff and Baker 2004f). Herd immunity refers to the amount of non-susceptible individuals who either have had the disease or have had a vaccine against the disease (Fine 1993). For many years, scientists have been trying to understand the balance between pathogen virulence and transmission. A famous hypothesis known as the "virulence-transmission trade-off hypothesis" indicates that as virulence increases, so does transmission. At some point, the cost of damaging the host for virus transmission, to the point of killing the host, affects the ability of the virus to move from person to person (Anderson and May 1982; Ewald 1991). However, a recent large-scale statistical analysis of previously published studies did not find a direct relationship between virulence and transmission, so more research needs to be done in this area (Acevedo et al. 2019; Hector and Booksmythe 2019). Achieving a high percent of non-susceptible individuals in the population is one of the goals of disease eradication programs and is a way to fight epidemics and pandemics. Herd immunity also gains attention because of the way it creates an invisible wall of protection for those in the population who cannot be vaccinated in certain circumstances, such as infants and pregnant women. Vaccination stops the "chain of transmission" and builds herd immunity in a community (Piot et al. 2019).

Achieving high herd immunity in a community is particularly important when the virus is very efficient at causing disease. Scientists track a reproductive rate (commonly known as R_0) for each virus. This value indicates the average number of cases arising from each individual case. It is quite a large number with a virus like measles, ranging from 12 to 18 additional people arising from a single case (Piot et al. 2019). The R_0 acts as an indicator of contagiousness and is a critical factor in terms of how a pathogen spreads. The virus's ability to spread is also linked to the susceptibility of the host. The average age of the human population and the prevalence of other diseases or conditions in a community can affect how the virus spreads as well. For example, in the case of SARS-CoV-2 (the cause of COVID-19), which is a respiratory virus, a smoking habit could make a person more susceptible to the virus (Purkayastha et al. 2020).

Speaking of respiratory viruses, how the virus enters the body, the route of transmission, is critical to understanding how to stop it. For example, precautions like masks and social distancing would be appropriate for a respiratory virus that is spread when someone carrying the virus coughs or sneezes. However, some pathogens enter the body in other ways, such as the digestive system or the blood. Something as simple as an insect bite could introduce a pathogen into the bloodstream (Summers 2009). Viruses can also enter the body through the reproductive or urinary system, the eyes, and lesions in the skin. Typically, viruses take one particular path as the means of transmission, although a virus entering through the blood may enter the body through other bodily fluids as well (Lostroh 2019). Understanding how a pathogen enters the body can help prevent infection.

Returning to viral vectors, how the virus encounters humans in the first place often has a lot to do with our environment. One group of scientists analyzed the emerging infectious diseases (EID) cataloged globally between 1904 and 2004 and found that 60.3% came from animals to humans (zoonosis) (Jones et al. 2008). How humans interact with animals, including wildlife and livestock, in our daily lives and while traveling can have a huge impact on the spread of a pathogen.

West Nile virus (WNV) transmission in North America has been studied closely since cases were diagnosed in New York City in 1999. Its vector, the mosquito, transmits WNV, and may have arrived in New York through passenger or cargo air travel. Within four years, scientists reported that WNV had made it to the West Coast. Most people recover quickly from infection and may not actually fall ill. Over a million human infections in the first 11 years in the U.S. resulted in about 1,300 deaths. However, millions of birds have died of West Nile virus because of infected mosquito bites. The ability of WNV to spread to new species of mosquitoes and to the birds thriving in urban and agricultural areas has contributed to the spread of the disease among humans (Kilpatrick 2011; Minkoff and Baker 2004f; Zimmer 2011). In terms of its spread as a pathogen, first travel and then the environment cultivated by humans to promote mosquito population growth have been critical to the spread of West Nile virus in the United States. In addition, the effects of climate change, including warmer temperatures and higher humidity for a sustained period in the summer months, will promote a larger mosquito population in the future, potentially promoting spread of WNV (Zimmer 2011). The many factors contributing to the spread of an emerging virus like WNV are illustrated in Figure 1.4.

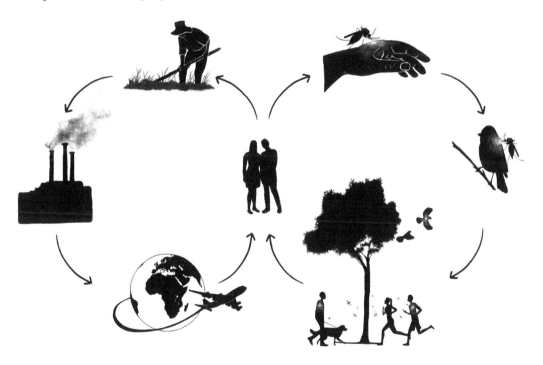

FIGURE 1.4
Contributing factors to spread of West Nile virus (WNV).

West Nile virus thrives for several reasons. First, changes to habitat like industrialization and clearing land for farming (far left and upper left) affect the abundance of mosquito vectors carrying WNV. The mosquitoes can infect people and birds (upper right and far right) in their environment (lower right). Then, travel and trade also contribute to the introduction of WNV through mosquitoes into new areas (lower left).

Source: Created by Jasneet Punia, used with permission.

1.4.1 Tumor Viruses

Some of the most heavily studied viruses in the 20th century were ones that caused cancer called tumor viruses. Tumor viruses have had an interesting history in terms of their connection to the launch of the first major cancer genetics studies done in the 1970s. Back in 1909, Peyton Rous started studying a sarcoma, muscle cancer, found in a chicken. He removed the sarcoma from the chicken, ground up the sarcoma, passed it through a filter, and then injected the filtrate into a new healthy chicken, which soon also developed a sarcoma. Rous's experimental procedure, including passing the sarcoma contents through a filter, led Rous to believe that he had found an infectious agent causing the cancer. The agent turned out to be Rous sarcoma virus (RSV). He won the Nobel Prize in 1966 for this work (Weinberg 2014; Nobel Media AB 1966). At the time, scientists had not yet observed the structure of viruses, but they knew that they were working with some type of "infectious material" that could pass through a filter with pores narrow enough to stop bacteria (Lostroh 2019). We will talk later about the tools that virologists use to observe viruses now, as well as the results of viral infection.

It took a while for researchers to understand how RSV perpetuated its genetic material in infected cells, since it turned out to be an RNA-based virus. Researchers discovered that the virus could integrate a DNA copy of its genome in the host cell genome. This DNA copy is called a provirus, and an enzyme called reverse transcriptase makes the DNA copy for the virus. (Backwards regarding the central dogma.) David Baltimore and Howard Temin received the Nobel Prize in 1975 for their work on RNA tumor viruses, along with Renato Dulbecco who had been researching DNA tumor viruses (Nobel Media AB 1975; Weinberg 2014). In the 1970s, scientists began studying the genetic causes behind the cancer-causing capability of RSV. Researchers including Michael Bishop and Harold Varmus discovered that the virus had actually "kidnapped" a gene called *SRC* from the host human cells and that this gene was responsible for the cancer-inducing power of the virus. *SRC* was found to be an enzyme, which, when expressed by the tumor virus, stimulated uncontrolled cell growth in the patient's cells. This work took on even greater importance when researchers found out that *SRC* is activated in nonviral related cancers, thus becoming the first oncogene (cancer-causing gene). Bishop and Varmus won the Nobel Prize in 1989 for their work (Nobel Media AB 1989; Weinberg 2014).

As you can see, three Nobel Prizes over a 30-year period were devoted to groundbreaking research on viruses. In addition to learning about viruses in their research, scientists learned much about human cell biology through their studies of cellular interactions with viruses. Scientists eventually found out that viruses only cause a small number of cancer types. Most cancers are caused by genetic or environmental factors like diet and occupational environment. However, certain cancers caused by viruses, such as cervical cancer, are still a scourge to the planet and need to be eliminated.

1.5 Determine That There Are Many Kinds of Viruses in the World, and Not All Are Pathogens

Some scientists have noted that there are at least one million viruses on the planet (that we have the capability of identifying as viruses). However, there may be millions and millions more viruses out there, in all corners of the earth (Baltimore 2017). Notably, recent work by marine biologists indicates that there may be billions of viruses in the ocean alone (Zimmer 2011). The first virus to be discovered was the tobacco mosaic virus in the late 1800s, and the first virus infecting people, the yellow fever virus, was found in 1901 (Woolhouse et al. 2012).

Researchers created a human virus discovery curve based on published data from 1901 to 2005. They found that three to four human viral pathogens were typically described every year in that timeframe, although that trend appears to be slowing down. They also reported that two-thirds of the human viral pathogens also have nonhuman host species, typically other mammals or birds. However, importantly, these researchers confirmed what many suggest in that the discovery of new viruses will be an ongoing process for humans (Woolhouse et al. 2012). At the time of the first human viral pathogen discovery, viruses were described as infectious particles captured by filtration, but the infectious agent structure itself could not be seen with existing technology. Technology has improved ever since then and new tools aided the discovery of new viruses (Woolhouse et al. 2012; Zimmer 2011). In 1931, Ernst Ruska, working with Max Knoll, developed the first electron microscope, which broke through the 200 nm size limit of light microscopy. With the invention of the electron microscope, viruses could be visualized for the first time, including the tobacco mosaic virus (Zimmer 2011). Ruska eventually went on to share the 1986 Nobel Prize in Physics for his invention. Ernst Ruska even included an electron micrograph of a bacteriophage, a bacteria-infecting virus, in his Nobel lecture (Nobel Media AB 1986). Consistent with the link between new technology and virus species discovery, the scientists who completed the viral discovery curve noted an upward trend of new viral pathogen discovery around 1930 (Woolhouse et al. 2012). Transmission electron microscopy (TEM) is still one of the most common techniques used today to visualize viruses and is useful when potentially an unknown virus or more than one viral species may be present in a sample and identifying viral structure may be important. TEM can also be used to check biological products or cell lines for viral contamination (Roingeard et al. 2019). Other techniques used by virologists to study viruses will be described at the end of the chapter.

More recently, giant viruses, called megaviruses, that are comparable to the size ranges seen with cells (see Figure 1.2), were discovered. One example includes the mimivirus that was discovered in 1992 but was not recognized as a virus until 11 years later. Megaviruses have been found to be common in aqueous environments (Lostroh 2019; Zimmer 2011).

The remnants of viruses integrated into host genomes, called endogenous viral elements (EVEs), have been found in many different prokaryotic and eukaryotic genomes, including ours. Although typically small, extremely large EVEs, over a million nucleotide base pairs in length, have recently been identified in green algae. Scientists believe that these integrated viral genes may play a larger role in eukaryotic genome evolution than once thought (Moniruzzaman et al. 2020).

In addition, scientists are trying to harness viruses to treat cancer. Oncolytic viruses have been known for over a hundred years but are not well understood. These viruses can attack cancer cells as well as mobilize other parts of the immune system by their presence, leading to immune cells going after the cancer cells as well. Studies are underway on the use of "virotherapy" as an additional treatment option for cancers like multiple myeloma (Brown 2020).

1.6 Understand That Viruses Are Capable of Evolution

As mentioned earlier, viruses are capable of evolution like the host cells they infect. Some say that viruses and their hosts even coevolve together. Before discussing virus evolution, let us briefly review the principles of evolution dating back to the seminal work of Charles Darwin in the 1800s. Evolution can be defined as "the process of lasting change among biological populations" (Minkoff and Baker 2004c). It is important to note that unlike the casual use of the word "evolve" to indicate a change that an individual might go through after a major life event, evolutionary change is based on changes within a population, happening over a period usually related to the time it takes to produce the next generation of offspring. Two of the main points of evolution first hypothesized by Darwin include "descent with modification" and "natural selection." Descent with modification refers to our relatedness in the tree of life, as evidenced by fossils, bones, embryos, and genetic sequence similarities. Natural selection refers to the idea that certain "genotypes" or particular **alleles** within the population confer a selective advantage in terms of reproduction and other characteristics like the ability to avoid predators. These genotypes make an individual more "fit" and more likely to have more offspring in the next generation, leading to a potential shift in the allele distribution in the population toward certain genotypes (Minkoff and Baker 2004c). If you are unfamiliar with the idea of natural selection, the Howard Hughes Medical Institute has put together interactive materials including a short film on the topic, using the rock pocket mouse as a model for natural selection (Interactive 2021).

So where do viruses fit into the idea of evolution? Well, viruses do undergo allelic changes (changes in the particular version of a gene) even in their small genome. These changes can happen quite rapidly given that viruses have a short generation time if they quickly enter the lytic phase of growth upon host entry, and they do not have the same proofreading mechanisms in many cases as eukaryotic cells (like our cells) do to protect the integrity of the genome. Therefore, random mutations occur as viruses replicate, and there is always the potential that an allele will give the virus an advantage over previous iterations, leading to a viral variant. Another source of variation is recombination or DNA rearrangements. Recombination can occur if two or more different virus strains infect a host cell at the same time. The viruses can exchange some genetic material through a process known as horizontal gene transfer, resulting in viruses with some genomic segments from the original parent virus and some segments from the other virus. Recombination events are common with different types of influenza A viruses (Lostroh 2019). We will return to this idea when we discuss the 1918 influenza pandemic. There actually is evidence from bacteriophage and simian immunodeficiency virus (SIV) that the virus and the host it infects can coevolve (Lostroh 2019).

1.7 Preview Upcoming Chapters Including How Virologists Do Their Work

Virologists are scientists who study viruses. They typically conduct their work in laboratory settings, although they occasionally conduct their research outside the laboratory and engage in more field work. A virologist might conduct experiments using live animal models (*in vivo* research) or work with mammalian or other animal cells grown in culture in the laboratory (*in vitro* research). One commonly used technique to study viral growth in the lab is known as a plaque assay. In this technique, host cells are added to media in a petri dish, and then the cells are infected with virus for several days. Scientists then monitor the clearings in the cell layer created by the virus killing cells in that local area. The clearing is known as a plaque. The number of plaques can be counted to quantify the amount of virus present (Lostroh 2019). The virologist uses all the tools that a typical cell and molecular biologist might use to analyze genes and gene expression into a protein. DNA sequencing is used to compare one virus to another. A powerful technique used to amplify DNA sequences is known as polymerase chain reaction (PCR), and this tool can be used for medical diagnostics to look for viral nucleic acid as well (Nobel Media AB 1993). Techniques such as northern blot and western blot are used to study RNA and protein expression respectively. Scientists may also use online databases or tools to study viral DNA sequences or protein structure.

Finally, virologists who observe viral particles in tissues might turn to microscopy techniques such as electron microscopy and fluorescence microscopy to study viral protein structure and their interaction with cells. Because of the high magnification and resolution capability of electron microscopy, this microscopy technique has historically been used most often to visualize viruses (Figure 1.5) (Alberts et al. 2019; Lostroh 2019). The techniques of atomic force microscopy and a specialized type of electron microscopy called cryo-electron microscopy are often used as well. Superresolution microscopy has increased the capabilities of light microscopy as well (Nobel Prize Outreach AB 2014). However, cellular changes resulting from viral infection can be observed using conventional light microscopy and have been used even before the viral particles themselves could be visualized (Lostroh 2019).

In the next few chapters, we will cover some of the most famous viruses that have affected societies in the past century. First, we will talk about the 1918 influenza pandemic and its impact on the United States and the world. Then, we will talk about polio and the race to create a vaccine against poliovirus in the early 20th century. Next, we will cover a pandemic that has been with us for almost 40 years, the HIV/AIDS pandemic. Finally, we will move to the story of SARS-CoV-2, the novel coronavirus that may or may not have taken the world by surprise in 2019 when it was linked to the disease COVID-19.

In the next part of the book, we will shift to other ways that viruses influence our society. Although we may think immediately of disease when we think of viruses, not all viruses are pathogens. Scientists have found ways to use viruses to correct monogenic diseases such as severe combined immune deficiency (SCID) using a method called gene therapy (Minkoff and Baker 2004b). In this technique, typically a virus like an adenovirus is modified to contain the normal gene of interest. Then the patient's own cells are infected with the modified adenovirus, correcting the error, and putting the cells back in the patient. Gene therapy will be described in more detail in Chapter 7. Besides using viruses for gene therapy, scientists have also engineered viruses to fight cancer. Viruses have become a powerful synthetic biology tool for scientists.

As we near the end of the book, in Chapter 8 we will talk about how the public health system works to inform the public about threats to their health (including viruses), manages our local communities to protect against disease outbreaks, and mobilizes if a new public health threat emerges. Finally, the book ends with the topic of scientific communication and how all members of society, scientists and nonscientists alike, can work together so that everyone can benefit from scientific innovation.

A.

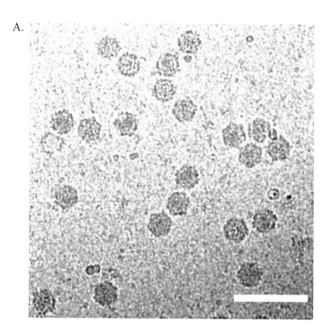

B.

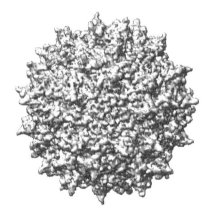

FIGURE 1.5

Cryo-electron microscopy of adeno-associated virus (AAV) particles and AAV structure.

Shown in (A) is a micrograph obtained using cryo-electron microscopy. About 22 AAV particles are shown in the image (scale bar is 100 nm). Thanks to Stefan Steimle of the University of Pennsylvania Perelman School of Medicine for the cryo-electron microscopy slice. Used with permission.

Shown in (B) is a molecular surface map for a single adeno-associated virus derived from the 1LP3.pdb file from the Protein Data Bank. The map was created using UCSF chimera by Trevor van Eeuwen. AAV-2 is shown in the map (www.rcsb.org/structure/1LP3). Used with permission.

UCSF Chimera was developed by the Resource for Biocomputing, Visualization, and Informatics at the University of California, San Francisco, with support from NIH P41-GM103311. UCSF Chimera—a visualization system for exploratory research and analysis. Pettersen EF, Goddard TD, Huang CC, Couch GS, Greenblatt DM, Meng EC, Ferrin TE. *J Comput Chem.* 2004 Oct; 25(13):1605–12.

1.8 Recognize How Viruses Might Have an Impact on Our Society

If you did not recognize how viruses had an impact on your life in the past, you do now after living through the COVID-19 pandemic. I still remember when a small group of students approached me just before spring break 2020, asking if I thought we would be back in the classroom after the break. I assumed that we would do remote learning for part of the semester, but little did I know how quickly things would change and how unprepared many people would feel for the days ahead. During this difficult time, individuals have begun to reevaluate many of our institutions and what role they should play in our society. In addition, how much of our day-to-day lives should be managed solely by individuals themselves, and how many decisions need to be tempered by their impact on those around us? How truly interdependent are we, and what does that mean for the future of our society?

Our society consists of all the institutions and organizations of people within our country, including neighborhood communities, houses of worship, schools, civic groups, community service organizations, government, and the individuals within all those organizations. Our society is influenced by the products of human achievement such as art, music, literature, scientific and technological innovation, as well as communication within our society through popular culture, TV, the internet, and social media. Viruses have affected the way we interact with each other since the start of human civilization, although we may not have recognized it until now. I hope that by the end of this book you will have a better understanding of viruses and how they can affect our lives.

1.9 Summary

Viruses are obligate intracellular parasites that can be found all over the natural world. Viruses are typically considered nonliving, consisting of some genetic material and protein, which may or may not be covered by a membrane. Viruses enter cells and use all the host cell's machinery, like an unwanted houseguest, to make many copies of itself and eventually leave the cell. Many viruses known as pathogens cause disease and many factors govern the impact of the pathogen on a host cell. Viruses come in many different types, and can be classified in numerous ways, including based on their genome using a method known as the Baltimore classification system. Viruses may have a DNA or an RNA genome. Viruses can evolve, one of the reasons that they can be so difficult to stop if they are pathogens. Virologists study viruses, using tools like microscopy and other assays used by other cell and molecular biologists.

Discussion Questions and Activities:

1. In your own words, describe the relationship between DNA, cells, and genes.
2. What are the general stages of the viral life cycle? What stage do you think is the most important for determining how a virus gets into the host and which host it uses?

3. Describe two alternative ways to classify viruses.

4. Microbiologists typically test for the connection between a pathogen and a disease using Koch's postulates. Go to the History of Vaccines website and follow the interactive describing the steps of Koch's postulates: www.historyofvaccines.org/content/koch%E2%80%99s-postulates

    a. Summarize the major steps of Koch's test of his postulates using the bacterial pathogen anthrax.

    b. What would you call a person who has the pathogen in their system but does not have the disease?

5. As described in the chapter, there are four major factors governing the spread of pathogens. One of them is herd immunity. Please go to the History of Vaccines website, and follow the interactive on Herd Immunity: www.historyofvaccines.org/content/herd-immunity-0

    a. How does the number of people vaccinated affect the spread of the pathogen in the simulation?

    b. What is the value of vaccination to the greater community?

6. Is experiencing a pandemic just a part of the human condition? Is interacting with viruses in our world something to come to terms with, or should we attempt to eradicate viruses from our world?

7. Choose a scientific topic from this chapter. Your objective will be to communicate a scientific concept or idea to a general audience—for example, your grandmother, neighbor, or roommate. Possible projects include a review article that could appear in a magazine or newspaper, science educational brochure, piece of creative writing like a short story or a series of poems, short video with transcript, cartoon, digital work of art, etc.

8. Create an analytic memo (Angelo and Cross 1993) to explain one of the following issues or problems for the relevant stakeholders:

    a. What is the best way to understand and contain a new viral pathogen in a local community?

    b. You would like to see if there are any unknown types of viruses infecting plants in a local botanical garden. What types of studies would you propose to the botanical garden's board of directors?

    c. Why is including the biology of viruses critical to a high school science education curriculum?

References

AB, Nobel Media. 2021a. "The Nobel prize in physiology or medicine 1966." Accessed 4 February 2021. www.nobelprize.org/prizes/medicine/1966/summary/.

———. 2021b. "The Nobel prize in physiology or medicine 1968." Accessed 30 January 2021. www.nobelprize.org/prizes/medicine/1968/summary/.

———. 2021c. "The Nobel prize in physiology or medicine 1975." Accessed 4 February 2021. www.nobelprize.org/prizes/medicine/1975/press-release/.

———. 2021d. "Ernst Ruska-Nobel lecture." Accessed 3 April 2021. www.nobelprize.org/prizes/physics/1986/ruska/lecture/.

———. 2021e. "The Nobel prize in physiology or medicine 1989." Accessed 4 February 2021. www.nobelprize.org/prizes/medicine/1989/summary/.

———. 2021f. "The Nobel prize in chemistry 1993." Accessed 30 January 2021. www.nobelprize.org/prizes/chemistry/1993/summary/.

———. 2021g. "The Nobel prize in physiology or medicine 1997." Accessed 30 January 2021. www.nobelprize.org/prizes/medicine/1997/summary/.

AB, Nobel Prize Outreach. 2014. "The Nobel prize in chemistry 2014." Accessed 30 January 2021. https://www.nobelprize.org/prizes/chemistry/2014/summary/.

Acevedo, M.A., F.P. Dillemuth, A.J. Flick, M.J. Faldyn, and B.D. Elderd. 2019. "Virulence-driven trade-offs in disease transmission: A meta-analysis*." *Evolution* 73 (4):636–47. doi: 10.1111/evo.13692.

Alberts, B., K. Hopkin, A.D. Johnson, D. Morgan, M. Raff, K. Roberts, and P. Walter. 2019. *Essential Cell Biology*. 5th ed. New York, NY: W.W. Norton & Company, Inc.

Anderson, R.M., and R.M. May. 1982. "Coevolution of hosts and parasites." *Parasitology* 85 (2):411–26. doi: 10.1017/S0031182000055360.

Angelo, T.A., and K.P. Cross. 1993. *Classroom Assessment Techniques: A Handbook for College Teachers.* New York, NY: Wiley.

Avery, O.T., C.M. MacLeod, and M. McCarty. 1944. "Studies on the chemical nature of the substance inducing transformation of pneumococcal types: Induction of transformation by a desoxyribonucleic acid fraction isolated from pneumococcus type III." *The Journal of Experimental Medicine* 79 (2):137–58.

Baltimore, D. 1970. "Viral RNA-dependent DNA polymerase: RNA-dependent DNA polymerase in virions of RNA tumour viruses." *Nature* 226 (5252):1209–11.

———. 1971. "Expression of animal virus genomes." *Bacteriological Reviews* 35 (3):235.

———. 2017. "Part One: Introduction to viruses." Accessed 16 February 2021. www.ibiology.org/human-disease/reverse-transcriptase/#part-1.

Brown, C. 2020. "Scientists are harnessing viruses to treat tumours." *Nature* 587 (7835):S60-S2.

Byrd, A.L., and J.A. Segre. 2016. "Adapting Koch's postulates." *Science* 351 (6270):224–6. doi: 10.1126/science.aad6753.

Caskey, C.T., and P. Leder. 2014. "The RNA code: Nature's Rosetta stone." *Proceedings of the National Academy of Sciences* 111 (16):5758–9.

Cobb, M. 2017. "60 years ago, Francis Crick changed the logic of biology." *PLoS Biology* 15 (9):e2003243.

Cossart, P., and A. Helenius. 2014. "Endocytosis of viruses and bacteria." *Cold Spring Harbor Perspectives in Biology* 6 (8). doi: 10.1101/cshperspect.a016972.

Crick, F. 1970. "Central dogma of molecular biology." *Nature* 227 (5258):561–3.

Crick, F.H. 1958. "On protein synthesis." *Symposia of the Society for Experimental Biology* 12:138–63.

Ewald, P.W. 1991. "Transmission modes and the evolution of virulence." *Human Nature* 2 (1):1–30. doi: 10.1007/BF02692179.

Fine, P.E. 1993. "Herd immunity: History, theory, practice." *Epidemiologic Reviews* 15 (2):265–302. doi: 10.1093/oxfordjournals.epirev.a036121.

Gurdon, J. 2017. "Nuclear transplantation, the conservation of the genome, and prospects for cell replacement." *The FEBS Journal* 284 (2):211–7.

Gurdon, J.B. 1962. "The developmental capacity of nuclei taken from intestinal epithelium cells of feeding tadpoles." *Development* 10 (4):622–40.

Gurdon, J.B., and V. Uehlinger. 1966. " 'Fertile' intestine nuclei." *Nature* 210 (5042):1240–1.

Hector, T.E., and I. Booksmythe. 2019. "Digest: Little evidence exists for a virulence-transmission trade-off*." *Evolution* 73 (4):858–9. doi: 10.1111/evo.13724.

Hershey, A.D., and M. Chase. 1952. "Independent functions of viral protein and nucleic acid in growth of bacteriophage." *Journal of General Physiology* 36 (1):39–56.

Interactive, HHMI. 2021. "The making of the fittest: Natural selection and adaptation." *Howard Hughes Medical Institute.* Accessed 2 March 2021. https://media.hhmi.org/biointeractive/interactivevideo/pocketmousequiz/.

Jones, K.E., N.G. Patel, M.A. Levy, A. Storeygard, D. Balk, J.L. Gittleman, and P. Daszak. 2008. "Global trends in emerging infectious diseases." *Nature* 451 (7181):990–3. doi: 10.1038/nature06536.

Kilpatrick, A.M. 2011. "Globalization, land use, and the invasion of West Nile virus." *Science* 334 (6054):323–7. doi: 10.1126/science.1201010.

Lefkowitz, E.J., D.M. Dempsey, R.C. Hendrickson, R.J. Orton, S.G. Siddell, and D.B. Smith. 2018. "Virus taxonomy: The database of the International Committee on Taxonomy of Viruses (ICTV)." *Nucleic Acids Research* 46 (D1):D708-d17. doi: 10.1093/nar/gkx932.

Lostroh, P. 2019. *Molecular and Cellular Biology of Viruses.* 1st ed. Boca Raton, FL: Taylor & Francis Group, LLC.

Lu, R., X. Zhao, J. Li, P. Niu, B. Yang, H. Wu, W. Wang, H. Song, B. Huang, and N. Zhu. 2020. "Genomic characterisation and epidemiology of 2019 novel coronavirus: Implications for virus origins and receptor binding." *The Lancet* 395 (10224):565–74.

Maddox, B. 2002. *Rosalind Franklin: The Dark Lady of DNA.* New York, NY: HarperCollins.

Mahmoudabadi, G., and R. Phillips. 2018. "A comprehensive and quantitative exploration of thousands of viral genomes." *eLife* 7:e31955. doi: 10.7554/eLife.31955.

Marshall, J. 2014. "The genetic code." *Proceedings of the National Academy of Sciences* 111 (16):5760-.

Minkoff, E.C., and P.J. Baker. 2004a. "Chapter 1: Biology: Science and ethics." In *Biology Today: An Issues Approach*, 1–32. New York, NY: Garland Science.

———. 2004b. "Chapter 4: Genetic engineering and genomics." In *Biology Today*, 95–122. New York, NY: Garland Science.

———. 2004c. "Chapter 5: Evolution." In *Biology Today: An Issues Approach*, 123–57. New York, NY: Garland Publishing.

———. 2004d. "Chapter 6: Classifying nature." In *Biology Today: An Issues Approach*, 159–202. New York, NY: Garland Publishing.

———. 2004e. "Chapter 16: HIV and AIDS." In *Biology Today: An Issues Approach*, 573–609. New York, NY: Garland Science.

———. 2004f. "Chapter 17: New infectious threats." In *Biology Today: An Issues Approach*, 611–40. New York, NY: Garland Press.

Moniruzzaman, M., A.R. Weinheimer, C.A. Martinez-Gutierrez, and F.O. Aylward. 2020. "Widespread endogenization of giant viruses shapes genomes of green algae." *Nature* 588 (7836):141–5.

Nirenberg, M.W., and J.H. Matthaei. 1961. "The dependence of cell-free protein synthesis in E. coli upon naturally occurring or synthetic polyribonucleotides." *Proceedings of the National Academy of Sciences* 47 (10):1588–602.

Piot, P., H.J. Larson, K.L. O'Brien, J. N'kengasong, E. Ng, S. Sow, and B. Kampmann. 2019. "Immunization: Vital progress, unfinished agenda." *Nature* 575 (7781):119–29. doi: 10.1038/s41586-019-1656-7.

Purkayastha, A., C. Sen, G. Garcia Jr, J. Langerman, D.W. Shia, L.K. Meneses, P. Vijayaraj, A. Durra, C.R. Koloff, and D.R. Freund. 2020. "Direct exposure to SARS-CoV-2 and cigarette smoke increases infection severity and alters the stem cell-derived airway repair response." *Cell Stem Cell* 27 (6):869–75.e4.

Roingeard, P., P.-I. Raynal, S. Eymieux, and E. Blanchard. 2019. "Virus detection by transmission electron microscopy: Still useful for diagnosis and a plus for biosafety." *Reviews in Medical Virology* 29 (1):e2019-e. doi: 10.1002/rmv.2019.

Siddell, S.G. 2018. "Why virus taxonomy is important." In *Microbiology Today*. London: Microbiology Society.

Summers, W.C. 2009. "Virus infection." *Encyclopedia of Microbiology*:546–52. doi: 10.1016/B978-012373944-5.00323-0.

Temin, H.M., and S. Mizutami. 1970. "RNA-dependent DNA polymerase in virions of Rous sarcoma virus." *Nature* 226:1211–3.

Watson, J.D., and F.H. Crick. 1953. "Molecular structure of nucleic acids: A structure for deoxyribose nucleic acid." *Nature* 171 (4356):737–8.

Weinberg, R.A. 2014. *Biology of Cancer.* 2nd ed. New York, NY: Garland Science, Taylor & Francis Group.

Woolhouse, M., F. Scott, Z. Hudson, R. Howey, and M. Chase-Topping. 2012. "Human viruses: Discovery and emergence." *Philosophical Transactions of the Royal Society of London. Series B, Biological Sciences* 367 (1604):2864–71. doi: 10.1098/rstb.2011.0354.

Zhou, P., X.-L. Yang, X.-G. Wang, B. Hu, L. Zhang, W. Zhang, H.-R. Si, et al. 2020. "A pneumonia outbreak associated with a new coronavirus of probable bat origin." *Nature* 579 (7798):270–3. doi: 10.1038/s41586-020-2012-7.

Zimmer, C. 2011. *A Planet of Viruses*. 2nd ed. Chicago, IL: University of Chicago Press.

2

An Introduction to the Immune System and Vaccines

In this chapter, we will first examine the basic principles of how the immune system works in the human body. Then, we will talk about the body's response to a foreign invader, such as a virus. We will consider how antiviral therapies work to block the ability of the virus to either replicate or infect new cells, as well as how vaccines specifically prime the immune system to be better prepared for a viral attack.

Learning Outcomes:

2.1 Describe the Major Parts of the Immune System, Including Understanding the Difference between the Innate and Adaptive Aspects of the Immune System

2.2 Discover How Professionals Test for Viral Infection

2.3 Understand the Body's Response to Viral Infection, and How Some Pathogens Avoid the Immune System

2.4 Describe Immunity and How It Is Achieved in Human Beings

2.5 Examine the History of Antiviral Measures Such as Vaccines

2.6 Understand the Key Aspects of Vaccine Development and the Different Types of Vaccines

2.7 Explain New Directions in Vaccination Research

2.8 Discuss Other Types of Antiviral Therapies besides Vaccines

2.9 Explain the Impact of Vaccines on Our Society

2.1 Describe the Major Parts of the Immune System, Including Understanding the Difference between the Innate and Adaptive Aspects of the Immune System

In the human body, we have two major branches to the immune system, the innate branch and the adaptive (acquired) branch. The two branches can communicate. Scientists refer to the two aspects of adaptive immune response as humoral immunity (older term referring to bodily fluids) and cell-mediated immunity. Humoral immunity involves two kinds of white blood cells: the B cells that make antibodies and the T cells that are responsible for cell-mediated immunity. Many good reviews or books of the immune system are available (Lostroh 2019; Coico and Sunshine 2015; Nicholson 2016; Marshall et al. 2018; Chaplin 2010).

The timing of the response for the two branches of the immune system is different. The innate branch of the immune system mobilizes within minutes to hours but does not retain a "memory" of the response. In contrast, the adaptive immune branch acts within hours

DOI: 10.1201/9781003172260-2

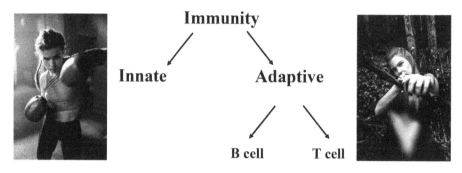

FIGURE 2.1
The parts of the immune system.

The two main branches of the immune system are the innate branch, which is nonspecific, and the adaptive branch, which is specific and acquired. Both B cells and T cells can be mobilized as a part of the adaptive branch, among other cell types. The innate branch is like a boxer punching at whatever threats come forward into their space, whereas the adaptive branch is like an archer, targeting a threat directly.

Source: Archer photo by Thiago Schlemper from Pexels; boxer photo by cottonbro from Pexels. All photos and videos on Pexels are free to use: www.pexels.com/license/

to days in a delayed response that is specific to that particular pathogen threat and has a "memory" of the response because of the information retained in the antibody-producing B cells (Marshall et al. 2018).

One could say that the innate branch reacts the same way to all viruses. An everyday example is if you were a boxer and lashed out with all your might against a new opponent in the boxing ring in a way dependent on your existing skills and your reach, not specific to the opponent (Figure 2.1). During the innate response, cells release signaling molecules such as cytokines like interferon (IFN) Type I and II that tell cells to prepare for a fight (Lostroh 2019). Cytokines have been described as "biological response modifiers" (Cruse and Lewis 2009). Also, special white blood cells called neutrophils can move into an area of the tissue to engulf foreign invaders through phagocytosis "cell eating" (Lostroh 2019). Typical side effects of this early response are fever and inflammation.

In the acquired response, also known as the adaptive response, a particular reaction by the immune system is triggered in a way that is specific to a particular type of foreign material entering the body, which can be recognized again at another point. I would describe this part of the immune system as being like a skilled archer, who can aim at a specific target and take it out in one shot (Figure 2.1). All living things on earth have some way of monitoring their surroundings to defend themselves. The immune system is critical for survival of an individual and a population, so many of the organism's resources are devoted to this type of protection (Nicholson 2016).

The cells, tissues, organs, and vessels of the immune system of the human body are physically known as the lymphatic system. Lymphatic tissue can also be found in other body systems, including the digestive system and the respiratory system. Lymph, a fluid that circulates in the body independent of blood, flows into lymph nodes (glands) that are connected by lymphatic vessels. Organs such as the spleen, thymus, and bone marrow are all networked with the lymph nodes through the lymphatic system (Ross and Pawlina 2011). Lymph nodes can filter lymph and are major sites where immune reactions take place (Cruse and Lewis 2009). The major parts of the lymphatic system are shown in Figure 2.2.

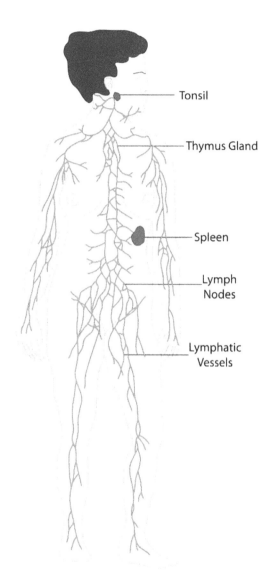

Tonsil

Thymus Gland

Spleen

Lymph Nodes

Lymphatic Vessels

FIGURE 2.2
The lymphatic system of the human body.

Shown here are some of the major structures of the lymphatic system, connected by lymphatic vessels.

Source: Courtesy of Wikimedia Commons, published under CC BY 3.0 (not modified) https://creativecommons.org/licenses/by/3.0/deed.en. Wikimedia site: https://commons.wikimedia.org/w/index.php?curid=10212847

Many kinds of cells participate in immunity. One kind is the white blood cell, which is produced in the bone marrow of adults and can be divided into five major categories. These categories include neutrophils, monocytes, basophils, eosinophils, and lymphocytes. Neutrophils and monocytes (which become macrophages) are a part of the innate immune response. For example, macrophages can engulf foreign material using phagocytosis. Basophils and eosinophils are kinds of white blood cells known for the special granules in their cytoplasm. They participate in the response to parasites as well as the allergy response. Lymphocytes include the B and T cells that are a part of adaptive immunity (Nicholson 2016).

Scientists can get even more specific in the classification of these lymphocytes based on the types of proteins displayed on the cell surface of the white blood cell (Nicholson 2016). Lymphocytes can be found concentrated in lymph nodes as well as moving around the body using lymphatic or blood vessels (Ross and Pawlina 2011). Two major T cell types include CD4+ helper T and CD8+ cytotoxic T lymphocytes (Lostroh 2019). The name "T cell" comes from the word "thymus," a major site where T cells mature. The name "B cell" comes from "bursa of Fabricius," a type of lymphatic tissue in birds like the bone marrow and gut-associated lymphatic tissue in humans. Studies in chicken embryos indicated that the bursa of Fabricius was critical for B cell formation and humoral immunity (Ross and Pawlina 2011). Another special type of white blood cell, the natural killer (NK) cell, is relevant for the response to viral infection (Coico and Sunshine 2015).

Many immunologists have spent their careers trying to figure out the critical question in immunology: how the body recognizes "self" versus "nonself" (Nicholson 2016). More specifically, scientists wonder what the body is recognizing when the immune cells identify something as nonself. How does the body know a foreign invader is present? It turns out that immune cells can recognize viral proteins, like proteins that coat the outside of the virus, as well as viral DNA or RNA. These molecules, when identified in a virus, are called pathogen associated molecular patterns (PAMPs). Certain immune cells can display pattern recognition receptors (PRRs) on their cell membranes or internal endosomal membranes that can detect PAMPs and stimulate the release of cytokines. In addition, other immune cells can actually recognize if damage has occurred from a viral infection. This is a way that the body can detect the virus in a secondary manner through signs of a viral presence, not the virus itself (Mueller and Rouse 2008; Amarante-Mendes et al. 2018). Interestingly, the cells of the immune system are said to be surveying the environment and putting proteins that they find in the body in particular categories. They are "continuously sampling these proteins" in the form of short peptides (protein fragments) to ensure the security of the body (Nicholson 2016). Scientists note that about 70% of lymphocytes in the body are circulating, checking for signs of foreign invaders (Ross and Pawlina 2011).

Another critical immunology question is understanding how reinfection by the same pathogen is "remembered" by the adaptive immune system. A strong memory response is necessary to protect the body if a pathogen presents itself in the future. Antibodies are a part of that memory bank. There are five major kinds of antibodies in the body, also known as immunoglobulins (Ig). They include IgM, IgA, IgD, IgG, and IgE (MADGE acronym to remember) (Nicholson 2016). A molecule that is foreign to the body that can react with an antibody is known as an antigen. Immunologists also use the more specific term of "immunogen" as a molecule that reacts with an antibody and causes an immune response (Cruse and Lewis 2009). However, antigen is more commonly used. Any of the four major macromolecules in nature—carbohydrate, nucleic acid, protein, or lipid—could be an antigen (Coico and Sunshine 2015). These macromolecules can be quite large, however, so it is not the entire macromolecule involved in the antigen-antibody interaction. A short region of the antigen, known as an epitope, is considered the "antigenic determinant" (Cruse and Lewis 2009).

An elaborate process is in place in the body to set off antibody production to protect the body. Cells called antigen-presenting cells (APCs) help prop up an antigen, presenting it at the cell surface so it can be recognized as foreign, along with the assistance of a T cell. Then, the B cell can start making antibodies against the antigen. Some B cells will continue

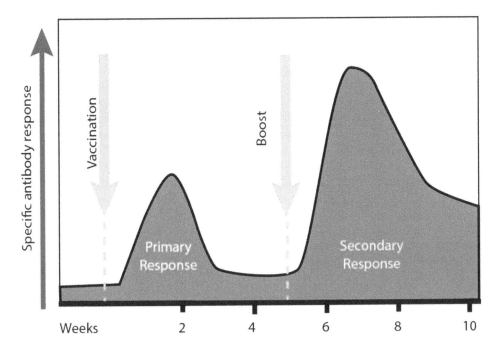

FIGURE 2.3
Antibody response to immune challenge.

Shown here is a general depiction of the response after vaccination. A couple weeks after the vaccination, a primary response in the form of antibody production is seen but then levels off. Following a second challenge to the immune system, a boost, antibody production occurs faster and there is a larger response. The difference in the secondary response versus the primary response is an indication of immune memory.

Source: "Figure 8. Antibody responses to vaccination" from Nicholson, L.B. 2016. The Immune System. Essays in Biochemistry 60: 275–301. Published under CC BY 4.0 (https://portlandpress.com/essaysbiochem/ article/60/3/275/78223/The-immune-system).

to make antibodies for a long time, while others will retain that memory, but only make antibodies if needed. Often, more than one challenge is needed to the immune system to boost antibody production over time (Nicholson 2016). B cells can be converted to specialized antibody-producing cells called plasma cells in lymph nodes (Cruse and Lewis 2009). Scientists have found that T cells have a memory as well, based on particular T cell receptors that are retained (Nicholson 2016). Antibody production is not the only option for the immune system adaptive response if the early response of the innate branch of the immune system fails. Certain cells called cytotoxic killer cells can kill off the infected cell, so the infection does not spread (Nicholson 2016).

2.2 Discover How Professionals Test for Viral Infection

There are a few ways to test for a viral infection. Scientists have found that antibody-antigen reactions can work *in vivo* (in the body) or *in vitro* (in a test tube). The interaction itself may cause a precipitation or clumping of the reacting material out of solution, which can be picked up by several tests. Scientists often do a type of test known as an enzyme-linked immunosorbent assay (ELISA), in which an antigen/antibody interaction can be quantified (Coico and Sunshine 2015). The test relies on a fluorescent tag on the antibody or an enzymatic reaction with a substrate that changes color to detect the antigen-antibody interaction. In an ELISA test, an interaction between an antigen (foreign material) and an antibody (protein made in response to a particular antigen) is detected using a plastic welled plate to perform the binding reactions. Plates can be examined by eye for a positive test or can be read in a machine to quantify the strength of the antigen-antibody interaction. Another more labor-intensive test, known as a western blot, involves separating proteins using agarose gel electrophoresis, transferring them to a membrane, and then probing for a particular antigen using an antibody (Coico and Sunshine 2015; Alberts et al. 2019). Antibody testing has become a powerful laboratory tool for the detection of viral infection.

We now have more sensitive techniques that can detect a viral infection earlier or when less virus is present. Scientists can use a test known as polymerase chain reaction (PCR) to find the viral RNA or DNA from the pathogen in a patient sample. The PCR technique, a type of "gene copier machine," was developed by Kary Mullis, for which he won the Nobel Prize (Nobel Media AB 1993). Mullis addressed the fundamental question of how one could identify and amplify a target DNA sequence of interest, among all the other nucleic acid sequences present in cells. Like finding a needle in a haystack, the nucleic acid sequence of interest is amplified many, many times using a pair of "primer" or "oligonucleotide" sequences. The primers are short stretches of nucleotides specific to the target sequence of interest, in this case the viral sequence. DNA from the patient and primers, free nucleotides, buffering solution, and an enzyme capable of replicating the target DNA are combined in a tube or well of a plastic plate for a PCR reaction. The tube is put through many cycles in a thermocycler machine repeating three major events: using a high temperature to separate the DNA strands, lowering the temperature a bit to allow the binding of the primers (finding the target DNA sequence), and then lowering the temperature a bit again to allow for extension of a new DNA copy. The steps of the cycle mimic what happens naturally in the cell during DNA replication. With each cycle, copies of the copies of DNA can be used as templates for duplication in the next cycle, resulting in an exponential increase in the number of DNA copies of the target sequence. At the end of the PCR program, one has millions and millions of copies of the DNA of interest, if the primers recognize its target in the original DNA sample (Alberts et al. 2019; Minkoff and Baker 2004a). Once amplified, the DNA is now present in usable amounts for other applications, including in the use of DNA profiling in forensic science (Houck and Siegel 2009).

2.3 Understand the Body's Response to Viral Infection, and How Some Pathogens Avoid the Immune System

What are the specific events in or layers to the development of an immune response? Our skin and mucous membranes act as a natural anatomical barrier to infection (Marshall et al. 2018). If a pathogen breaches that barrier to enter the body, the body does have ways of preventing a pathogen from getting into cells. For example, an enzyme found in tears and mucus called lysozyme can break down bacteria. Stomach acid can break down some pathogens as well. If a pathogen gets past the initial defenses into cells, the body can set off the alarm in the form of signaling molecules such as interferons and other cytokines that are a part of the innate response (Nicholson 2016). A chemical arsenal of proteins to respond to the pathogen can be mobilized (Marshall et al. 2018). However, the alarm reaction itself may cause quite a bit of damage to the body if the response is prolonged. If the body cannot recover from the side effects of the immune response or defeat the virus, serious illness or death can result. The body can also react abnormally to its own macromolecules in an autoimmune response (Coico and Sunshine 2015).

After the initial steps, the cellular immune response begins, as does antibody production. Antibodies can do things like block viral enzymes and coat viral particles to make them more easily phagocytosed in a process known as "opsonization." Certain types of T cells can induce more cytokines and activate macrophages. If needed, natural killer cells can be mobilized to kill infected cells (Coico and Sunshine 2015). Some people will find it comforting to know that the immune system in humans has evolved to be highly redundant in the sense that more than one type can do phagocytosis, more than one cell type can act as an antigen-presenting cell, and several different cell types can make cytokines sounding the alarm on viral infection (Coico and Sunshine 2015).

The incubation period for viruses varies tremendously, ranging from a few days to years. Viruses can also induce other longer-term responses, such as when a tumor virus causes infected cells to deregulate their cell division cycle, leading to uncontrolled cell growth and potentially cancer (Summers 2009). An example of a tumor virus is the human papilloma virus (HPV). Certain strains of HPV can cause cancer (Nobel Media AB 2008). Sometimes after an initial recovery from illness, a virus such as a herpesvirus stays latent in the body. The virus could be reactivated to replicate later if the person's immune system is weakened. For example, the same virus, varicella-zoster (VZV), causes both chicken pox and shingles. Other viruses like hepatitis B virus (HBV) and hepatitis C virus (HCV) persist in chronic infections that can go on for years (Summers 2009; Lostroh 2019).

Viruses and other pathogens have ways of avoiding the immune system. Some bacteria, for example, have evolved ways of surviving inside cells, evading the immune system. Some viruses can suppress the immune system, by acting upon certain immune cells to disrupt their function. Finally, viruses like influenza are capable of something known as "antigenic variation," in which the virus can alter two major surface antigens, hemagglutinin "H" and neuraminidase "N," through the reassortment of the RNA segments into the genome encoding the proteins. These changes to the proteins displayed on the viral particle surface make the virus more difficult to recognize by the immune system. HIV is also capable of this antigenic variation, mainly because of the lack of proofreading (like a spellcheck program) of its reverse transcriptase enzyme that makes a DNA copy of the RNA genome. Errors in the genome conveying a selective advantage are retained (Coico and Sunshine 2015).

The term "antigenic drift" is used to describe changes in the shape of these key antigen proteins of the virus as the strain evolves, and "antigenic shift" refers specifically to changes in these antigens through the combination of new nucleic acid segments, such as what occurs with the influenza virus (Minkoff and Baker 2004b). One could say these changes to viral surface antigens are analogous to a wanted criminal putting on a new disguise to avoid capture by the police. In a similar analogy, Professor Sunetra Gupta described a pathogen as slightly changing its wardrobe over time to avoid detection, in a series of cartoons presented as a part of her Royal Society lecture in 2009 (Society 2009). Finally, insidiously, some viruses like Epstein-Barr virus and herpes simplex virus can affect the function of immune cells and their proteins, cutting the immune system off at its knees (Coico and Sunshine 2015).

2.4 Describe Immunity and How It Is Achieved in Human Beings

There are several ways to become immune to a particular pathogen. In the process of passive immunization, antibodies themselves can be passed from mother to child in breast milk, for example, or through direct introduction of antibodies to an ill patient. Passive immunization usually offers temporary protection against a pathogen. In active immunization, getting the disease itself or a vaccination can create a long-lasting immunity (Marshall et al. 2018; Coico and Sunshine 2015). Vaccination can also reduce the number of susceptible individuals in the population, reducing the ability of the pathogen to spread (four factors governing spread of a pathogen from Chapter 1). Therefore, vaccination can protect others in the population who cannot be vaccinated (Piot et al. 2019).

Vaccines work against a pathogen because the vaccine mobilizes the immune system to fight off the pathogen without actually causing the person to get sick. So how does a vaccine protect a person? Well, it is thanks to what scientists call "memory" cells. Upon first exposure to an antigen, the adaptive branch of the immune system will mobilize both B and T cells after a lag period. However, the second exposure, inducing a secondary or "anamnestic response," is quicker (see Figure 2.3). The B and T cells respond faster this time, with more antibodies being made, because of the immune system's previous exposure to the antigen through actual disease or vaccination (Coico and Sunshine 2015; Cruse and Lewis 2009). Most of the research focus on vaccine response has involved looking at antibody production, but the T cell response to a vaccine can also be critical.

It is almost as if the vaccine creates a dress rehearsal for the immune system to prepare for the pathogen. Just like real actors doing a dress rehearsal before a play, all the key immune system actors are prepared to play their role, ready to go, but the actual production does not take place. However, if the real actors were called upon to do the play, just like the waiting immune cells ready to fight the infection, the actors would be ready to give a flawless performance on stage. In the next part of the chapter, we will talk about how vaccines were first developed, how they have been used to prevent disease, and their impact on our society.

2.5 Examine the History of Antiviral Measures Such as Vaccines

Many good reviews are available that discuss the history of vaccines and how they work (Graham and Sullivan 2018; Piot et al. 2019; Plotkin 2005). However, to understand the history of vaccines, one must go back to an earlier process known as variolation. In variolation, pus or scabs from a person who has had smallpox (variola) were ground up and placed under the skin or inhaled by another individual, thus protecting the new individual from smallpox. Variolation has been documented as early as AD 1000 in India while additional data suggest the practice could have originated in Central Asia or China as well. Legend has it that Lady Mary Montague witnessed the practice of variolation while living in Turkey and brought that variolation to England (Pemberton 2014; Plotkin 2005; Zimmer 2011; Plotkin and Plotkin 2017). It is also worth noting that George Washington had his Continental Army undergo variolation against smallpox in the 1770s (Plotkin and Plotkin 2017; NPS, 2022). However, there were risks associated with variolation, and it is estimated that 1%–2% of people who underwent variolation died (Medicine 2021).

Edward Jenner in England is credited with a technique that soon replaced variolation called vaccination, published in 1798. It was known at the time that milkmaids did not get smallpox like other members of the population. They seemed to be protected from smallpox because of exposure to a related virus, cowpox. Jenner famously gave pus from the lesion of a milkmaid with cowpox to a boy and found that the boy was protected from smallpox. The word vaccination comes from the Latin word *"vacca"* for cow (Coico and Sunshine 2015; Plotkin 2005; Zimmer 2011; Piot et al. 2019). Vaccination is sometimes used interchangeably with immunization. The term inoculation is often used as well, although it has a broader use as a general term for exposing an animal to some type of immunogen to produce immunity (Cruse and Lewis 2009).

What was novel about Jenner's approach is the idea that exposure to a virus related to smallpox, cowpox, could cross-protect against the more dangerous human pathogen, smallpox (Plotkin 2005). Some sources also note the work of Benjamin Jesty, a layperson who noticed the cowpox/smallpox connection as well, who vaccinated his family but then did not publish his findings or popularize the practice like Jenner did (Plotkin and Plotkin 2017). Jenner initially met some opposition to his approach, including people protesting the use of cow material in the procedure. At the same time, others who profited from conducting variolation feared being put out of business. Eventually, vaccination became an accepted and widely used practice (Laboratories, 2021). Jenner dedicated his life to helping others carry out vaccinations and was widely acknowledged for saving many, many lives, even catching the attention of Thomas Jefferson (Trust 2021). Many others came after Jenner, including Louis Pasteur, whose numerous accomplishments in microbiology including developing vaccines that did not require one to transfer human material from one person to another, making vaccines safer (Plotkin and Plotkin 2017).

2.6 Understand the Key Aspects of Vaccine Development and the Different Types of Vaccines

Vaccine development is a long process with four major steps. The first step involves the initial discovery period in which promising approaches are first worked out by conducting studies with cells grown in petri dishes in the lab or in animal models. The second step, typically taking at least 3–10 years and being the most expensive hurdle, involves getting the vaccine into clinical trials to test its safety and efficacy in people. The third step involves getting permission to market the vaccine and then scaling up so that the vaccination can be given to many people. Finally, the fourth step involves supply issues so that the vaccine is available when needed long term (Piot et al. 2019). Some sources note that the quality control aspects of vaccine development alone could take two years or more, with the entire timeline of vaccine development lasting 10 to 30 years. Although most of the public interest is focused on the innovation of the vaccine itself, practical issues, such as scaling up the vaccine and quality control, can take a lot of time. However, in a public health emergency, agencies do have the ability to come together and work faster (Preiss et al. 2016). We will discuss how the COVID-19 vaccine was fast-tracked, including the use of preexisting vaccine technology, knowledge from research on other coronaviruses, and other details, in Chapter 6.

After a vaccine is released, monitoring vaccine safety is an ongoing process. Adverse events following immunization (AEFI) such as pain, redness, or swelling at the vaccination site may occur. People who have received a vaccine are encouraged to report any other events or symptoms to their physician. Unlike when someone is given a drug to treat a disease, vaccines are typically given to healthy people, so it is said that people have high expectations for how they feel after the vaccine. People do not expect to have any adverse effects making them feel temporarily unwell in any way after a vaccination. However, the benefits of the vaccination could be measured against any potential risks of side effects to the patient in consultation with a physician (Di Pasquale et al. 2016).

There are many kinds of vaccines, including those made from live, attenuated (disabled) pathogens, those made from dead pathogens, and those made from parts of the pathogen itself, which can be made in a cellular system using recombinant DNA technology (Coico and Sunshine 2015). Typically, the vaccines made from part of a pathogen, such as a virus, are nucleic acid–based (Ahmed, Ellis, and Rappuoli 2017). Louis Pasteur initially developed the attenuation technique using a chemical process to weaken rabies virus as well as the bacterial pathogen anthrax. Others subsequently used a technique called "passaging," in which the virus is grown in cell culture for a period, selecting for weaker strains of the virus (Plotkin 2005). Other methods used in live vaccines include taking a related virus from another species and using it, such as the case with the smallpox vaccine using cowpox. Temperature-sensitive viral variants are also available in some cases. These are viruses that behave normally at one temperature, but then can be disabled at another temperature, usually a higher temperature. For an inactivated vaccine, scientists have created a variety of approaches, including using whole inactivated virus or just parts of it such as a viral protein, part of a viral protein, or a viral carbohydrate (Ahmed, Ellis, and Rappuoli 2017). Some of the latest vaccines, including vaccines used against SARS-CoV-2, are based on mRNA technology (Pardi et al. 2018). We will discuss the details of these vaccines in Chapter 6.

Genetic engineering has dramatically contributed to the options available when designing a vaccine. In genetic engineering, a gene from one source, such as a virus or an organism, can be expressed in another biological system. We also use the term recombinant DNA technology to refer to a practice in which DNA from different sources is combined. In this way, a viral protein can be expressed in a simple organism like budding yeast, and then used as a vaccine component (Plotkin 2005). We will talk more about genetic engineering and viruses in Chapter 7.

The use of sequencing techniques (ways to read the genetic code) and genome-wide analysis has greatly aided the process of finding an antibody that would work to block a pathogen, as well as candidate antigens that might work well in a vaccine. The approach of starting with a candidate structure or sequence first and then testing for the ability to induce an immune response is known as "reverse vaccinology" (Ahmed, Ellis, and Rappuoli 2017). One can examine all the potential antigens of the pathogen first, in a large-scale study, and select which antigens to test for vaccine development. Researchers emphasize that you may not even need to culture the pathogen in the lab with this approach, starting with computational analysis instead and then moving to working with recombinant pathogen proteins for testing in animal models (Del Tordello, Rappuoli, and Delany 2017). In addition, high throughput approaches have been used to identify all the antibodies produced in an immune response, "the antibody repertoire" (Ahmed, Ellis, and Rappuoli 2017). Not only has antibody repertoire analysis been used in vaccine development, but this approach has also been useful in studies of autoimmune diseases. One can identify potential "autoantigens," which are proteins from one's own body that are recognized abnormally by the immune system, and also the "auto-antibodies" created by the immune system to treat and screen for autoimmune diseases (Robinson 2015).

A technique known as "rational vaccine design" is also used to develop vaccines like a potential universal flu vaccine. This means that researchers look at the immune response and try to find the best antigen to use in the vaccine. Because there is a lot of antigenic variation in certain parts of the influenza A virus, such as the hemagglutinin and neur-aminidase proteins, researchers are testing other components of the virus, such as the stalk protein, to see if it will work well in a flu vaccine (Lostroh 2019).

There are a few critical components to the vaccine besides the part inducing the immune response. Something known as an "adjuvant" is critical in helping to boost the immune response. Aluminum salts are the most widely used. Vaccines may also include something known as a "delivery system" to make sure the immune system is properly exposed to the antigen in the vaccine. For example, lipid might be used to help with delivery of a nucleic acid–based vaccine. The vaccine formulation typically might contain preservatives or anti-biotics, so the vaccine is not contaminated with bacteria, something to stabilize the vaccine if it has an extended shelf life (Ahmed, Ellis, and Rappuoli 2017). It is important to note that not only the antigen itself is critical in a vaccine, but also the other parts of the formulation ensure that a safe, effective, contamination-free vaccine is delivered to the patient.

2.7 Explain New Directions in Vaccination Research

There are many exciting new directions in vaccine research. Different combination vac-cines are being developed to fight more than one pathogen with a single vaccine. New ways to deliver vaccines are also being explored, such as intranasal delivery of a vaccine against a respiratory virus. Outside of an epidemic or pandemic, vaccination campaigns have tended to focus on childhood vaccination. Scientists and physicians are now looking at the benefits of certain vaccinations in adults. Finally, immunizations to help chronic infections and to fight drug addiction are being developed (Plotkin 2005). Anti-drug vac-cines, for example against cocaine, are under development using animal models. These vaccines work largely by activating production of anti-cocaine antibodies that bind to cocaine and prevent it from reaching its targets in the brain. However, some issues have arisen related to the variability of the number of antibodies being produced in the ani-mal model, as well as the stability of the antibody response (Havlicek et al. 2020; Kinsey, Kosten, and Orson 2010).

Some cancer vaccines are available, and many are being tested right now to treat such cancers as ovarian cancer, melanoma, colorectal cancer, and breast cancer. Scientists know that T cells can identify antigens from cancer cells and recognize the cancer as "nonself." In addition, if a virus causes the cancer, the virus could be recognized and blocked before it could infect a person. For example, there is a vaccine against human papilloma virus (HPV) and against hepatitis B virus (HBV). These vaccines can not only prevent infec-tion, but also potentially prevent cancer caused by the virus. Other cancer vaccines are being tested for administration during a course of treatment, to slow disease progression or help other treatments work better (Bot, Berinstein, and Berinstein 2017; Plotkin and Plotkin 2017).

2.8 Discuss Other Types of Antiviral Therapies Besides Vaccines

It is important to note that antibiotics do not work against viral infection since they only specifically stop bacterial pathogens by preventing new cell wall synthesis or blocking a bacterial enzyme, for example. So, what drugs or tools are available if there is no vaccine against a viral pathogen? Scientists seek antiviral therapies that go after viral proteins, rather than the cellular proteins of the host itself. If the therapy is specific to the virus, there will be fewer side effects. For example, some antiviral therapies are available that compete with or interfere with viral enzymes. We have drugs available that can be used to affect viral replication in influenza A, for example. Other treatments, like interferon, can be introduced to complement the immune response (Lostroh 2019). One of the most successful anti-viral regiments out there is a combination therapy to treat and cure hepatitis C infection. However, it is a very expensive treatment (Lostroh 2019). This treatment for hepatitis C was created only about 30 years after this particular hepatitis virus was discovered (Houghton 2019). Combination therapies to treat and prevent HIV infection have been widely used too, since a vaccine has not yet been developed. In addition to treating HIV-positive individuals, one combination therapy known as pre-exposure prophylaxis or PrEP is being recommended for HIV-negative individuals at high risk for infection (Gulick and Flexner 2019). Combination therapy means that more than one viral protein is targeted at the same time in the drug cocktail, and this strategy seems to reduce the chance of the virus developing resistance to the drug. These drugs will be explained in more detail in Chapter 5.

Considering the COVID-19 pandemic, scientists have revisited the idea of creating more antiviral therapies acting against a variety of viruses to keep on hand in the event of another pandemic. For example, remdesivir, an antiviral drug that was developed to treat Ebola, was used to treat COVID-19 patients as well. However, we are not yet sure how effective it was as a treatment (Dolgin 2021).

Antibody therapy as a treatment for viral infection was in the news during the COVID-19 pandemic. Famously, then-president Trump was given monoclonal antibody therapy to treat SARS-CoV-2 infection (Cohen 2020). Some form of antibody therapy has been around for 100 years, and antibodies can be purified from the blood plasma of disease survivors and then used to treat other patients (Coico and Sunshine 2015). There are two major kinds of antibodies derived from the body that are used by scientists. Antibodies taken directly from the blood of a person or an animal, which are not identical and may recognize different epitopes (particular parts) of the antigen, are known as polyclonal antibodies. However, in a more involved process, a single kind of B cell making a single kind of antibody, against one epitope, can be isolated and fused with another cell line in culture so the B cell line will grow and divide virtually forever if maintained in a petri dish. The fusion cell line created is known as a hybridoma, and the name of the kind of antibody being generated by this hybridoma is monoclonal antibody. Cell and molecular biologists use monoclonal antibodies for several different laboratory procedures, including western blotting, to identify proteins in a specific way (Alberts et al. 2019). Kohler and Milstein famously developed the technique to use hybridomas to produce monoclonal antibodies consistently in 1975. It is considered a major breakthrough in scientific research (Rajewsky 2019). Clinically, monoclonal antibodies can also be used for therapeutic purposes to block a particular pathogen or protein. In fact, monoclonal antibody therapies, such as Herceptin, are used to block cancerous proteins and treat the cancer (Coico and Sunshine 2015). New ways of using monoclonal antibodies are continually being developed.

2.9 Explain the Impact of Vaccines on Our Society

Vaccines have a huge impact on our society. They can change how people go about their days, including doing activities they enjoy, places they travel, and personal interactions. Many have lived in fear in the past when word reached them of an outbreak of some kind in their community. Scientists are working hard to eradicate diseases that cause pain and suffering around the world. Many people have indicated that vaccinations, along with clean water and sanitation, are the two most important human interventions for improving health worldwide (Greenwood 2014).

Vaccination campaigns may happen nationally or internationally when people are faced with a pathogen threat. In the 20th century in the United States, for example, mass vaccination campaigns took place in 1947 against smallpox, 1955 against polio, 1976 against the swine flu, and 2009 against H1N1 influenza (Gross 2021). These campaigns were organized by the government to quickly stop a pathogen threat and reduce the number of people being affected by the disease, although not all the pathogens ended up being such a threat as anticipated, as in the case of the swine flu in 1976. Success or failure of these campaigns had much to do with public buy-in to the need for vaccination, so science communication was critical for making them work. We will discuss more about science communication in Chapter 9.

Many other groups besides the government need to be involved in a successful vaccination campaign, including policy makers, healthcare workers, and institutions like health systems partnered with academic research centers. An adequately funded local healthcare system is essential for carrying out vaccinations and monitoring patient health. Members of the local community need to be included in communicating the need for vaccination as well (Hardt et al. 2016). Equitable distribution of vaccine is also required for a successful vaccination campaign, and public health approaches have not always distributed vaccines in this way, at least initially, as we will discuss in our public health chapter. These other recent vaccination campaigns will be compared to the COVID-19 vaccination campaign later in the book, too.

The ultimate goal of any vaccination campaign is to remove the pathogen from the human population. Smallpox was eradicated in 1980 after approximately 3,000 years of being a scourge of the planet (WHO 2021c). It is rare to find a physician on the planet who has seen a case of smallpox at this point. There were two versions of smallpox: variola major, which caused a severe rash that led to disfigurement and killed 30% of those it infected, and variola minor, which was caused by a different strain and produced a milder form of the disease (Cruse and Lewis 2009). Two physicians who worked in the field in the 1970s have spoken publicly about their observations in a "Jenner Conversation" webinar recorded by the Jenner Museum during the COVID-19 pandemic. These physicians described their use of a smallpox recognition card to help identify any individuals in a household with smallpox during canvassing from home to home in an affected area (Figure 2.4) (Fine and Heymann 2020). They then used a "ring vaccination" approach to vaccinate individuals in a community, once they found either an individual who had smallpox or someone they had contacted (CDC 2021). As is the case with other public health issues, community-based efforts to tackle a disease are critical, and governments and institutions depend on these "on the ground" efforts for a successful vaccination campaign.

Another disease, polio (poliomyelitis), has nearly been eradicated (Piot et al. 2019). In 2020, Africa was declared free of wild poliovirus, after going four years without a case. (We will explain what is meant by "wild" poliovirus in Chapter 4.) Now that Africa is polio-free, Afghanistan and Pakistan are the only countries left in the world with wild poliovirus (WHO 2021a). On the other hand, in the United States and a few other countries, several childhood

A.

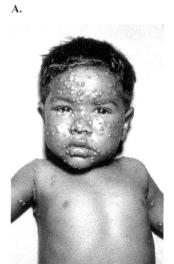

B.

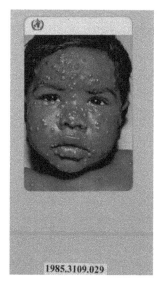

FIGURE 2.4
Smallpox recognition field card.

(A) Here is the original photograph taken by the World Health Organization of a child with smallpox lesions on his face and torso. Copyright World Health Organization, 1971 (internal ID: 38147). Used with permission.

(B) Shown here is a smallpox recognition card developed by the World Health Organization (WHO), which was used by physicians and public health officials in the field for identification of individuals with smallpox. Note that there are no words on the card, so it can be used for communication universally without knowledge of the local language.

Source: Used with permission from Division of Medicine and Science, National Museum of American History, Smithsonian Institution, catalog number: 1985.3109.029 (www.si.edu/object/world-health-organization-field-card-smallpox-identification%3Anmah_1450765).

diseases that were virtually eliminated in the 20th century because of vaccination are now occurring more often in case clusters due to low vaccination rates in certain communities. The WHO has set up a vaccine-preventable diseases monitoring system, where one can click on any country providing vaccination data to see how that country is doing in terms of coverage of its citizens (WHO 2021b). A sampling of these data is shown in Figure 2.5.

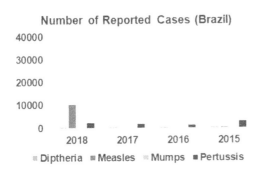

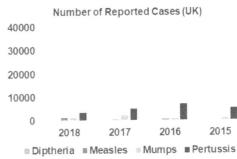

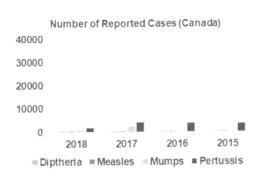

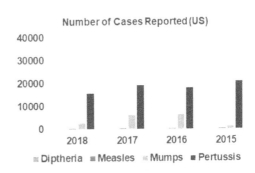

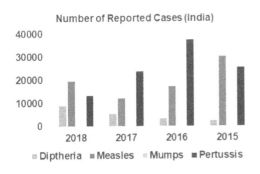

FIGURE 2.5
Vaccine-preventable disease comparison.

Shown here is the number of reported cases of select vaccine-preventable diseases from five countries: Brazil, Canada, India, United Kingdom, and the United States for the period of 2015–2018 as reported to the World Health Organization (WHO).

Source: Graphs generated from data from WHO vaccine-preventable diseases monitoring system. 2020 global summary (last updated July 15, 2020, data as of October 12, 2020). No bar indicates no data were reported or there were no cases reported (https://apps.who.int/immunization_monitoring/globalsummary/countries?cou ntrycriteria%5Bcountry%5D%5B%5D=USA&commit=OK).

In fact, vaccine hesitancy is a threat to global health (Piot et al. 2019). In Chapter 9, we will discuss the role of science communication in helping to communicate effectively the benefits of vaccination to parents. Despite the setbacks, the world has overwhelmingly benefited from vaccination campaigns from both an economic and a health point of view. The World Health Organization indicates that at least "2–3 million deaths" are prevented every year because of immunizations, boldly stating that immunization is "an indisputable human right" (WHO 2021d). Fourteen diseases have been effectively controlled using vaccination: "smallpox, diphtheria, tetanus, yellow fever, pertussis, *Haemophilus influenzae* type b disease, poliomyelitis, measles, mumps, rubella, typhoid, rabies, rotavirus, and hepatitis B" (Plotkin and Plotkin 2017).

2.10 Summary

The major branches of the immune system include the innate and adaptive branches. If someone has a viral infection, there are ways of detecting that infection, including testing for antibodies against the pathogen and doing a PCR test to detect viral nucleic acid. The body responds to viral infection in a number of ways, including its early responding cells called neutrophils causing inflammation, as well as by releasing signaling molecules such as cytokines to help the body quickly respond. Production of antibodies can be an effective way to inactivate a pathogen, and it creates an active immunity for the future. Vaccines have been developed to prevent certain viral diseases, and usually take many years to develop. New ways of creating vaccines as well as new uses of vaccines for noninfectious diseases such as addiction and cancer are being developed. If a vaccine is not available against a pathogen, other antiviral therapies such as interferon or drugs targeting viral proteins may be employed. Many diseases caused by viruses are either treatable or can be prevented using vaccines. Scientists will prepare for new potential viral pathogen threats in the future by creating new antivirals and potentially certain universal vaccines.

Discussion Questions and Activities:

1. The Howard Hughes Medical Institute (HHMI) developed a virtual immunology laboratory where one can follow the steps of doing an ELISA experiment. A link to the lab can be found here: www.biointeractive.org/classroom-resources/immunology-virtual-lab. Please summarize the major steps of an ELISA procedure.

2. The development of PCR has revolutionized many aspects of science involving detection of small amounts of any specific DNA or RNA, not just viral DNA or RNA. Describe three major applications of PCR besides viral testing. You can use the interactive website on PCR applications created by the LabXChange group affiliated with Harvard University: www.labxchange.org/library/items/lb:LabXchange:bc4846e2:lx_simulation:1

3. Go to the website, Bite Sized Immunology: www.immunology.org/public-information/bitesized-immunology. Search one of the topics listed on the site such as: immune development, pathogens and disease (select a pathogen to research), experimental techniques (ELISA).

4. We should celebrate vaccines! Go to the website of the same name: www. immunology.org/celebrate-vaccines

   a. Record three reasons to celebrate vaccines.

   b. What are three ways that we can do better?

5. To celebrate 60 years of the British Society for Immunology, the society created a webpage on the history of immunology in 60 objects (www.immunology.org/days). Look at some of the items on the webpage or explore them using other online resources. Why were the following items, for example, critical for the development of the field of immunology?

   a. A microscope

   b. A culture plate

   c. Alum

   Students can present what they found to the class.

6. Go to the History of Vaccines webpage on vaccine development: www. historyofvaccines.org/content/articles/vaccine-development-testing-and-regulation. Watch Dr. Paul Offit's brief video on making vaccines. What is the main way that all vaccines work, according to Dr. Offit?

References

AB, Nobel Media. 2021a. "Nobel prize in chemistry 1993." Accessed 12 June 2021. www.nobelprize.org/prizes/chemistry/1993/summary/.

———. 2021b. "The Nobel prize in physiology or medicine 2008." Accessed 11 June 2021. www.nobelprize.org/prizes/medicine/2008/summary.

Ahmed, S.S., R.W. Ellis, and R. Rappuoli. 2017. "Technologies for making new vaccines." In *Vaccines E-Book*, edited by S.A. Plotkin, W. Orenstein, P.A. Offit and K.M. Edwards, 1283–304.e7. Saint Louis, MO: Elsevier.

Alberts, B., K. Hopkin, A.D. Johnson, D. Morgan, M. Raff, K. Roberts, and P. Walter. 2019. *Essential Cell Biology*. 5th ed. New York, NY: W.W. Norton & Company, Inc.

Amarante-Mendes, G.P., S. Adjemian, L.M. Branco, L.C. Zanetti, R. Weinlich, and K.R. Bortoluci. 2018. "Pattern recognition receptors and the host cell death molecular machinery." *Frontiers in Immunology* 9 (2379). doi: 10.3389/fimmu.2018.02379.

Bot, A., E.M. Berinstein, and N.L. Berinstein. 2017. "Cancer vaccines." In *Vaccines E-Book*, edited by S.A. Plotkin, W. Orenstein, P.A. Offit and K.M. Edwards, 161–84.e5. Saint Louis, MO: Elsevier.

CDC, Centers for Disease Control and Prevention. 2021. "Ring vaccination." Accessed 6 July 2021. www.cdc.gov/smallpox/bioterrorism-response-planning/public-health/ring-vaccination.html.

Chaplin, D.D. 2010. "Overview of the immune response." *The Journal of Allergy and Clinical Immunology* 125 (2 Suppl 2):S3–S23. doi: 10.1016/j.jaci.2009.12.980.

Cohen, J. 2020. "Update: Here's what is known about Trump's COVID-19 treatment." *Science* 372:abf0974.

Coico, R., and G. Sunshine. 2015. *Immunology: A Short Course*. 7th ed. Hoboken, NJ: John Wiley & Sons, Incorporated.

Cruse, J.M., and R.E. Lewis. 2009. *Illustrated Dictionary of Immunology*. Boca Raton, FL: CRC Press, Taylor & Francis Group.

Del Tordello, E., R. Rappuoli, and I. Delany. 2017. "Chapter 3—Reverse vaccinology: Exploiting genomes for vaccine design." In *Human Vaccines*, edited by K. Modjarrad and W.C. Koff, 65–86. New York, NY: Academic Press, an Imprint of Elsevier.

Di Pasquale, A., P. Bonanni, N. Garçon, L.R. Stanberry, M. El-Hodhod, and F. Tavares Da Silva. 2016. "Vaccine safety evaluation: Practical aspects in assessing benefits and risks." *Vaccine* 34 (52):6672–80. doi: 10.1016/j.vaccine.2016.10.039.

Dolgin, E. 2021. "The race for antiviral drugs to beat COVID—and the next pandemic." *Nature* 592 (7854):340–3. doi: 10.1038/d41586-021-00958-4.

Fine, P., and D. Heymann. 2020. "Smallpox: Lessons from eradication." In *Jenner Conversations*, edited by G. Williams. Berkeley, England: Jenner Museum.

Graham, B.S., and N.J. Sullivan. 2018. "Emerging viral diseases from a vaccinology perspective: Preparing for the next pandemic." *Nature Immunology* 19 (1):20–8.

Greenwood, B. 2014. "The contribution of vaccination to global health: Past, present and future." *Philosophical Transactions of the Royal Society of London. Series B, Biological Sciences* 369 (1645):20130433. doi: 10.1098/rstb.2013.0433.

Gross, J. 2021. "Five past vaccine drives and how they worked." In *The New York Times*. New York, NY: The New York Times Company.

Gulick, R.M., and C. Flexner. 2019. "Long-Acting HIV drugs for treatment and prevention." *Annual Review of Medicine* 70:137–50. doi: 10.1146/annurev-med-041217-013717.

Hardt, K., P. Bonanni, S. King, J.I. Santos, M. El-Hodhod, G.D. Zimet, and S. Preiss. 2016. "Vaccine strategies: Optimising outcomes." *Vaccine* 34 (52):6691–9. doi: 10.1016/j.vaccine.2016.10.078.

Havlicek, D.F., J.B. Rosenberg, B.P. De, M.J. Hicks, D. Sondhi, S.M. Kaminsky, and R.G. Crystal. 2020. "Cocaine vaccine dAd5GNE protects against moderate daily and high-dose 'binge' cocaine use." *PLoS One* 15 (11):e0239780. doi: 10.1371/journal.pone.0239780.

Houck, M.M., and J.A. Siegel. 2009. *Fundamentals of Forensic Science*. New York, NY: Academic Press, an Imprint of Elsevier.

Houghton, M. 2019. "Hepatitis C virus: 30 years after its discovery." *Cold Spring Harbor Perspectives in Medicine* 9 (12). doi: 10.1101/cshperspect.a037069.

Kinsey, B.M., T.R. Kosten, and F.M. Orson. 2010. "Anti-cocaine vaccine development." *Expert Review of Vaccines* 9 (9):1109–14. doi: 10.1586/erv.10.102.

Laboratories, Jenner Institute 2021. "About Edward Jenner." Accessed 30 June 2021. www.jenner.ac.uk/about/edward-jenner.

Lostroh, P. 2019. *Molecular and Cellular Biology of Viruses*. 1st ed. Boca Raton, FL: Taylor & Francis Group, LLC.

Marshall, J.S., R. Warrington, W. Watson, and H.L. Kim. 2018. "An introduction to immunology and immunopathology." *Allergy, Asthma, and Clinical Immunology: Official Journal of the Canadian Society of Allergy and Clinical Immunology* 14 (Suppl 2):49. doi: 10.1186/s13223-018-0278-1.

Medicine, National Library of. 2021. "Smallpox a great and terrible scourge." Accessed 30 June 2021. www.nlm.nih.gov/exhibition/smallpox/sp_variolation.html.

Minkoff, E.C., and P.J. Baker. 2004a. "Chapter 3: Human genetics "In *Biology Today: An Issues Approach*, edited by E.C. Minkoff and P.J. Baker, 64–93. New York, NY: Garland Science

———. 2004b. "Chapter 17: New infectious threats." In *Biology Today: An Issues Approach*, 611–40. New York, NY: Garland Press.

Mueller, S.N., and B.T. Rouse. 2008. "Immune responses to viruses." *Clinical Immunology*:421–31. doi: 10.1016/B978-0-323-04404-2.10027-2.

National Park Service (NPS). 2022. "Smallpox, inoculation, and the revolutionary war." Accessed 4 Apr 2022. https://www.nps.gov/articles/000/smallpox-inoculation-revolutionary-war.htm.

Nicholson, L.B. 2016. "The immune system." *Essays in Biochemistry* 60 (3):275–301. doi: 10.1042/EBC20160017.

Pardi, N., M.J. Hogan, F.W. Porter, and D. Weissman. 2018. "mRNA vaccines—a new era in vaccinology." *Nature Reviews Drug Discovery* 17 (4):261–79. doi: 10.1038/nrd.2017.243.

Pemberton, S. 2014. "NOVA: Vaccines-calling the shots." In *NOVA*, 53:10. Boston, MA: WGBH Boston (Public Broadcasting System).

Piot, P., H.J. Larson, K.L. O'Brien, J. N'kengasong, E. Ng, S. Sow, and B. Kampmann. 2019. "Immunization: Vital progress, unfinished agenda." *Nature* 575 (7781):119–29. doi: 10.1038/s41586-019-1656-7.

Plotkin, S.A. 2005. "Vaccines: Past, present and future." *Nature Medicine* 11 (4):S5–S11.

Plotkin, S.L., and S.A. Plotkin. 2017. "A short history of vaccination." In *Vaccines E-Book*, edited by S.A. Plotkin, W. Orenstein, P.A. Offit and K.M. Edwards, 1–15.e8. Saint Louis, MO: Elsevier.

Preiss, S., N. Garçon, A.L. Cunningham, R. Strugnell, and L.R. Friedland. 2016. "Vaccine provision: Delivering sustained & widespread use." *Vaccine* 34 (52):6665–71. doi: 10.1016/j.vaccine.2016.10.079.

Rajewsky, K. 2019. "The advent and rise of monoclonal antibodies." *Nature* 575 (7781): 47–49.

Robinson, W.H. 2015. "Sequencing the functional antibody repertoire—diagnostic and therapeutic discovery." *Nature Reviews Rheumatology* 11 (3):171–82. doi: 10.1038/nrrheum.2014.220.

Ross, M.H., and W. Pawlina. 2011. *Histology*. New York, NY: Lippincott Williams & Wilkins.

Society, The Royal. 2009. "Royal society Rosalind Franklin prize lecture 2009." In *LabXchange*. Cambridge, MA: President and Fellows of Harvard College.

Summers, W.C. 2009. "Virus infection." *Encyclopedia of Microbiology*:546–52. doi: 10.1016/B978-012373944-5.00323-0.

Trust, Jenner. 2021. "Jenner museum learning history." Accessed 20 June 2021. https://jennermuseum.com/learning/history.

WHO, World Health Organization. 2021a. "Global polio eradication initiative applauds WHO African region for wild polio-free certification." Accessed 21 June 2021. www.who.int/news/item/25-08-2020-global-polio-eradication-initiative-applauds-who-african-region-for-wild-polio-free-certification.

———. 2021b. "WHO vaccine-preventable diseases: Monitoring system. 2020 global summary." Accessed 6 July 2021. https://apps.who.int/immunization_monitoring/globalsummary/countries?countrycriteria%5Bcountry%5D%5B%5D=USA&commit=OK.

———. 2021c. "Smallpox overview." Accessed 21 June 2021. www.who.int/health-topics/smallpox#tab=tab_1.

———. 2021d. "Vaccines and immunization." Accessed 21 June 2021. www.who.int/health-topics/vaccines-and-immunization#tab=tab_1.

Zimmer, C. 2011. *A Planet of Viruses*. 2nd ed. Chicago, IL: University of Chicago Press.

3

The 1918 Influenza A Pandemic

Learning Outcomes:

3.1 Describe the Details of the Influenza Virus behind the 1918 Influenza Pandemic

3.2 Compare the 1918 Influenza A Virus to the Characteristics of Other Well-Studied Viruses

3.3 Interpret the Historical Factors That Contributed to the Spread of the Influenza A Virus Worldwide in 1918

3.4 Treatments for Influenza in 1918

3.5 Understand How Scientists Raced to Find the Cause of the 1918 Pandemic, and What They Found Using Koch's Postulates

3.6 Examine Modern Analysis of the 1918 Pandemic and the Influenza A Virus Itself

3.7 Understand the Impact of the 1918 Pandemic Including How Our Society Handles Pandemics in General and Seasonal Influenza Specifically Today

In this chapter, we will explore the influenza A virus, the cause of the worst pandemic in recorded history, taking into account the number of people who died in a short period of time (Crosby 1989; Barry 2018). It is estimated that 50–100 million people died in the pandemic, and 500 million became ill, in about a two-year period. Please keep in mind that the population of the world at the time was 1.5 billion, so that meant that one-third of the planet became ill (Crosby 1989; Barry 2018; Zimmer 2011; Spinney 2017; Kolata 1999; Brown 2018).

We will look at the molecular biology behind the virus and some properties that make this virus unique among other viruses. In addition, we will explore the historical context of the 1918 influenza pandemic, since human activity affects the transmission of human pathogens and the influenza virus is no exception. In fact, the human activity happening on the planet at the time in 1918 may have created an ideal environment for the spread of such a pathogen. Finally, we will examine the relationship between the 1918 pandemic and other flu pandemics.

There are many good historical accounts of the 1918 pandemic that I used as sources for this section of the book (Kolata 1999; Spinney 2017; Crosby 1989; Barry 2018; Brown 2018). Certain texts emphasized particular aspects of the story over others, as indicated by particular citations. One of the first breakthrough books retelling the story specifically of the 1918 pandemic, apart from World War I (WWI) itself, was published in 1989 (Crosby 1989). In 2019, the Mütter Museum of the College of Physicians of Philadelphia commemorated the 1918 pandemic with an exhibit called "Spit Spreads Death: The Influenza Pandemic of 1918–19 in Philadelphia," and a virtual tour is available online (Philadelphia 2020). However, before getting into the historical timeline of the pandemic, I would like to start with the biological details of the virus.

3.1 Describe the Details of the Influenza Virus behind the 1918 Influenza Pandemic

Influenza belongs to the family of viruses known as Orthomyxoviridae (Orthomyxoviruses). Members of this viral family are characterized by a segmented genome made of negative-sense single-stranded RNA. (A negative-sense RNA strand is the antisense strand, the opposite of what would code for mRNA.) Orthomyxoviruses can infect a wide range of species (Lostroh 2019; Couch 1996; Ackermann, Berthiaume, and Tremblay 1998). Influenza viruses have been found in birds, pigs, horses, seals, mink, and whales, in addition to humans (Webster et al. 1992). A translation of the term "orthomyxoviruses" indicates that this is a "straight-mucus family of viruses" (Brown 2018). Using the Baltimore classification system, influenza A would be a member of Class V, based on its genome type (Baltimore 1971).

Influenza virus is a classic example of a lytic virus as described in Chapter 1. This type of virus will invade host cells, use the host cell machinery to make copies of itself, and then get out. Influenza uses the host cell as if it owns the place. First, the virus binds to a host cellular receptor. Then the virus enters through the cellular trafficking network, sneaking into endosomes that normally bring in materials needed by the cell. Next, the viral genome is pushed into the cytoplasm of the cell, where it can be moved into the nucleus to make an RNA copy of the genome that can be recognized by the workings of the cell for genome replication. It is important to note that the influenza virus uses the cell's own receptors, membranes, cytoskeleton, and ribosomes to complete its life cycle (Figure 3.1) (Lostroh 2019).

If one examines the structure of an influenza virus, one will see two major kinds of spike proteins coming out of the envelope: the hemagglutinin (H) and neuraminidase (N) proteins. The hemagglutinin spike proteins attach to sialic acid, a type of sugar or carbohydrate, displayed on respiratory cells. The neuraminidase proteins later clear sialic acid molecules out of the way, preventing any obstacles to catch the influenza viral particles as they bud back out of the cell, thousands of viral particles at a time (Barry 2018; Brown 2018; Lostroh 2019). There are sugars bound to proteins and lipids on cell surfaces as well as on secreted molecules. Sialic acid is a type of sugar attached to the "outermost part" of the sugar chain in certain cell types. Sialic acid has a normal role in cell interactions as well as affecting protein stability. However, viral, bacterial, and parasitic pathogens can use sialic acid as a way to gain entry into cells (Varki 2008).

Influenza A, B, and C strains exist, but only influenza A has been associated with epidemics or pandemics (Barry 2018; Brown 2018). A fourth type, influenza D, has been added to the list as a type found mainly in cattle, with no illnesses reported in people (CDC 2021c). Influenza B and C are only able to infect humans, but influenza A can thrive in animal hosts, for example. The risk of an emerging new virus spilling over from animals to people through reassortment occurs with influenza A specifically (Clancy 2008). The particular version of hemagglutinin protein in the subtype of the virus and the kind of sialic acid it recognizes play a big role in the host range for the virus and help define the subtype of the influenza virus (within the A, B, or C types) (Webster et al. 1992). For example, the 1918 flu pandemic was caused by an H1N1 subtype of influenza A. Influenza A causes a type of avian flu, meaning that one of its major vectors is birds. It can also be carried by pigs (Spinney 2017; Barry 2018; Crosby 1989; Zimmer 2011; Brown 2018). There are many different versions of hemagglutinin and neuraminidase. Antibodies generated by the body in an immune response specifically recognize one version of the protein but

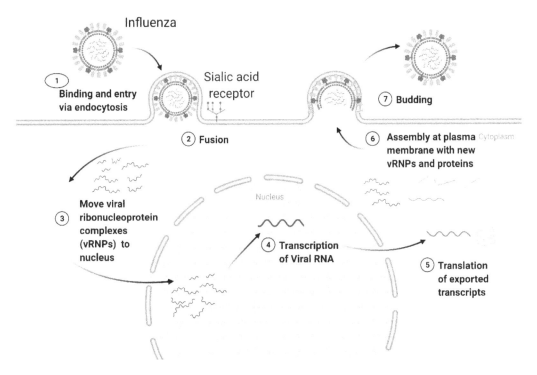

FIGURE 3.1
Influenza Life Cycle

Shown here are the major steps of the viral replication cycle for the influenza virus. First, the virus binds to the sialic acid receptor and enters the cells. Then, it releases the viral ribonucleoprotein complexes (vRNPs) into the cytoplasm, which then move into the nucleus. Then the viral RNA is transcribed. The transcripts are then exported, and the translated proteins assemble at the plasma membrane with the new vRNPs to make new viral particles that then bud out of the plasma membrane.

Created using Biorender.com.

not another (Lostroh 2019). The Centers for Disease Control and Prevention indicate that there are currently 18 different versions of hemagglutinin and 11 different versions of neuraminidase known in nature (CDC 2021c).

Looking inside the virus's spherical or filamentous-shaped envelope, the viral genome is eight separate genome segments (seven in type C), about 10,000–15,000 base pairs of RNA in total. Each segment is packaged in a viral ribonucleoprotein (vRNP) made of protein and RNA. Once new vRNPs are made using the host cell, then the whole viral particles are assembled, thousands of copies of them, and move out to infect a new cell. The viral particles are typically 80–120 nanometers in diameter (Lostroh 2019; Couch 1996). By retaining its genome on eight different RNA segments, these segments can undergo an independent reassortment inside the host cell. Many rearrangements are possible, especially if the host cell has been infected by another strain of the virus (Lostroh 2019; Barry 2018; Zimmer 2011; Brown 2018). This means that if other strains of the virus are in the same cell, they can combine and then sort out again the genome segments to make a new strain of the influenza A virus (Lostroh 2019; Clancy 2008). John Barry in *The Great Influenza* (2018, p. 112) likens reassortment to "shuffling two different decks of cards together, then making up a new deck with cards from each one." Influenza also has error-prone RNA polymerases that copy the influenza genome, leading to many muta-tions that can be retained if they give the virus a selective advantage. Therefore, one can see both antigenic drift through mutation and antigenic shift through reassortment in influenza viruses (Lostroh 2019; Clancy 2008).

The influenza virus is transmitted from person to person through respiratory droplets dispersed with sneezing or coughing by the infected individual. Symptoms of influenza can vary, but classic symptoms include headache, chills, fever, pain, sneezing, runny nose, and "nonproductive" cough, among others. However, not everyone with influenza viral infection will show these symptoms (Couch 1996; Krammer et al. 2018). The symptoms last from one to five days before the body can fight off the infection. Full recovery from influ-enza may take weeks even without major complications, resulting in reduced productivity in school for children and work for adults (Krammer et al. 2018).

Interferon is one of the major cytokines mobilized in the innate immune system response to the influenza virus (Couch 1996). Researchers studying influenza have found that certain influenza viral proteins can reduce gene expression in the host cell, affecting the timing and level of interferon expression (Krammer et al. 2018). The adaptive immune system also kicks in to make antibodies against the influenza virus, specific to the subtype. Scientists have found that there is something important about the first antibody response to an influ-enza virus subtype, and that this response may affect all future responses to influenza virus subtypes encountered later in life. Influenza antibodies made in childhood can be detected in the elderly (Krammer et al. 2018; Couch 1996; Dhakal and Klein 2019). If the body cannot fight off the infection, it can lead to a viral pneumonia. In addition, the patient could suffer from secondary bacterial infections like bacterial pneumonia (Couch 1996).

3.2 Compare the 1918 Influenza A Virus to the Characteristics of Other Well-Studied Viruses

When comparing pathogens, it is important to go back to the four major factors governing the transmission of a pathogen as mentioned in Chapter 1 (Minkoff and Baker 2004b). The vector, if there is one known for the pathogen, is critical to understanding how the virus is transmitted. Weather and environment, including human activity such as travel and trade, are also important.

As mentioned earlier, the vector for influenza A is birds, meaning that this animal har-bors the virus but does not actually get sick from it. One can look at sequence data to compare the influenza A virus affecting people to viruses found in birds and see their relatedness (Spinney 2017). However, once the 1918 influenza pandemic virus made the leap to people and then displayed sustained transmission from person to person, human activity became critical to the success of the virus. The human migrations and troop move-ments that were a part of WWI contributed to spread of the influenza virus (Barry 2018; Spinney 2017; Crosby 1989; Brown 2018; Kolata 1999). The 1918 influenza pandemic was propelled by human activity. Since influenza is a respiratory virus, people living in close quarters, especially in large cities and military installations, were at great risk. Some have labeled influenza as one of those diseases that thrive in crowded environments, rather than dispersed farming communities, along with measles, tuberculosis, and smallpox (Spinney 2017).

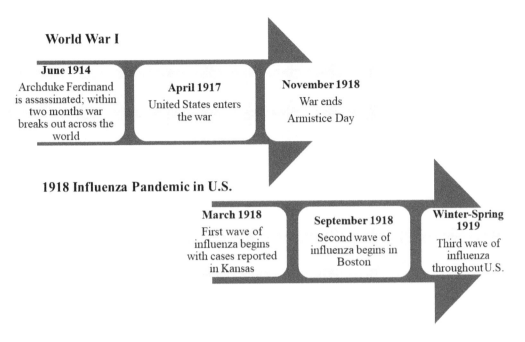

FIGURE 3.2
Timeline of key events in World War I relative to the 1918 pandemic.

Shown here is a timeline of World War I side by side with a timeline of the 1918 influenza pandemic in the United States.

Sources: Dates for World War I key events were based on the website entitled "Interactive WWI timeline" (www. theworldwar.org/explore/interactive-wwi-timeline). Key events in the pandemic were based on the website "1918 Pandemic Influenza Historic Timeline" (www.cdc.gov/flu/pandemic-resources/1918-commemoration/pandemic-timeline-1918.htm).

One must also consider host susceptibility, the pathogen's virulence, and herd immunity in the population when talking about the spread of a pathogen (Minkoff and Baker 2004b). As the virus mutates, it can become more virulent. At least three waves of the pandemic occurred in the United States (Figure 3.2). As described in detail later, it was the second wave of the 1918 influenza pandemic that was the most virulent (Crosby 1989; Barry 2018; Spinney 2017).

Who was most susceptible to the virus, and did anyone have immunity against it? When looking back at the main details of the 1918 pandemic, some of the most striking features include descriptions of how many young people (in their 20s, 30s, and 40s) became ill because they had not been exposed to a virus like this before. For seasonal influenza, typically a U-shaped death curve is seen, where the peak deaths occur in the very young and the very old. However, in the case of the 1918 influenza pandemic, even in the spring 1918, there was a W-shaped death curve, with a third middle peak of deaths among those people 20–40 years old (Barry 2018; Crosby 1989; Spinney 2017; Brown 2018; Short, Kedzierska, and van de Sandt 2018; Ahmed, Oldstone, and Palese 2007; Taubenberger and Morens 2006) (Figure 3.3).

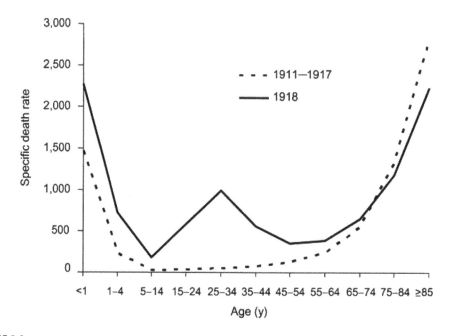

FIGURE 3.3

Influenza and pneumonia deaths combined, deaths per 100,000 individuals, as reported in each age range for the year 1918 (solid line) versus 1911–1917 (dashed line) in the United States.

In this graph, one can see the typical "U-shaped" death curve for seasonal influenza, with a higher death rate in the very young and very old (dashed line). In contrast, the death rate for influenza in 1918 also had a third peak, creating a "W-shaped" death curve, in the middle age range (solid line).

Sources: Reprinted from Taubenberger, JK and Morens, DM. 2006. 1918 Influenza: The Mother of All Pandemics. *Emerging Infectious Diseases*: 12 (1): 15–22. [Figure 2, open source].
Emerging Infectious Diseases is an open access journal: https://wwwnc.cdc.gov/eid/about/general

Taubenberger and Morens cite two studies for the data used in this figure:
Grove RD, Hetzel AM Vital statistics rates in the United States: 1940–1960. Washington: U.S. Government Printing Office, 1968
Linder FE, Grove RD Vital statistics rates in the United States: 1900–1940. Washington: U.S. Government Printing Office, 1943

Some people think that individuals with healthier, fully developed immune systems may have been more vulnerable to the 1918 pandemic influenza virus because of an overreaction by their immune systems to fight the virus, leading to something known as "cytokine storm." This "cytokine storm" ended up damaging the body in the process of fighting the infection (Spinney 2017; Zimmer 2011; Brown 2018; Short, Kedzierska, and van de Sandt 2018). Now that we have more information on the particular strain of the virus, studies seem to indicate that this virus was also capable of blocking interferon production, affecting the initial activation of the immune response in the body (Brown 2018; Spinney 2017; Kolata 1999). In addition, older people may have encountered a similar strain of influenza circulating in Europe 20 years earlier, originating in Russia in 1889. This exposure could have provided some protection to older individuals (Spinney 2017; Zimmer 2011; Brown 2018; Short, Kedzierska, and van de Sandt 2018; Ahmed, Oldstone, and Palese 2007).

3.3 Interpret the Historical Factors That Contributed to the Spread of the Influenza A Virus Worldwide in 1918

One cannot tell the story of the 1918 pandemic without telling the story of World War I. These stories are forever intertwined, part of the reason that we know so few specifics about the pandemic. World War I, known as the Great War before World War II, started in June 1914 when Archduke Ferdinand of Austria-Hungary was assassinated. Since Austria-Hungary blamed Serbia for the assassination, they declared war on Serbia, and this set off a chain of events that culminated in a huge war being fought in Europe, the Middle East, Asia, and Africa. The Allied Forces and those on their side included Britain and France (and the parts of their empires as well), Russia, Serbia, and Japan, among others. The Central Powers on the opposite side included Germany, Austria-Hungary, Bulgaria, and the Ottoman Empire. The United States was initially neutral, but then entered the war in April 1917. The war ended on November 11, 1918, because of the negotiations that occurred at the Paris Peace Conference (Memorial 2021). It was estimated that just over 20 million people died during WWI: 8.5 million soldiers and 13 million civilians (Britannica 2021).

3.3.1 First Wave of the 1918 Influenza Pandemic

Although the 1918 influenza pandemic became "a national catastrophe in autumn 1918," a first wave of mild influenza had occurred in spring 1918 in the United States (Crosby 1989). Any deaths that happened would have typically been noted as pneumonia and were not required to be reported to national public health officials, so a clear connection to a particular pathogen was not discovered at that time (Barry 2018; Crosby 1989). However, large numbers of Ford Motor Company workers and prisoners at San Quentin Prison (California) became sick with the flu that spring. In addition, the Metropolitan Life Insurance Company found a higher-than-expected number of deaths due to pneumonia, as well as cases noted specifically as influenza, in spring 1918 (Crosby 1989).

It is believed that the first cases that led to the pandemic appeared in Kansas at or near a military base (Barry 2018; Spinney 2017). Severe cases of the flu had been reported in Haskell County, Kansas, and many soldiers at Camp Funston in Kansas nearby had flu or flu-like symptoms (Crosby 1989). A Haskell County physician, Dr. Loring Miner, took the initiative to contact the Public Health Service because of the severity of the influenza cases that he had seen in his practice in spring 1918. We do not know for sure if the virus moved from Haskell County, Kansas, to the army base, but many believe that was the case. However, others suggested that the virus responsible for the 1918 influenza pandemic could have originated in another country all together, such as France, Vietnam, or China, so we will most likely never known the answer. However, it was not disputed that the movement of U.S. troops as a part of WWI did contribute to the spread of the virus (Barry 2018; Spinney 2017; Brown 2018). By May 1918, a pneumonia epidemic was happening among U.S. troops at bases around the country and among the troops shipped to France (Crosby 1989). The German soldiers called it "Flanders Fever" (Crosby 1989).

Some people speculated that a German ship had brought influenza to Boston. In her short novel *Pale Horse, Pale Rider*, Katherine Anne Porter wrote a work of fiction using characters set in the time of the 1918 pandemic. One character states "they think the germs were sprayed over the city—it started in Boston, you know—and somebody reported seeing a strange, thick, greasy-looking cloud float up out of Boston Harbor and spread slowly all over that end of town" (Porter 1967, pp. 162–163).

For our purposes, I will refer to the influenza pandemic of 1918 as the "1918 influenza pandemic" or the "1918 pandemic," but at the time, the pandemic was known as "Spanish influenza." How did the pandemic get such a name? Well, news reporting of widespread pneumonia and/or influenza was not censored in Spain, many say because Spain was neutral in World War I and did not need to suppress a potential impact on its adversaries. The King of Spain and about 8 million people in Spain got the flu in spring 1918 (Crosby 1989; Barry 2018).

Although a major infectious disease problem was brewing at this point in several places in the world, a lack of national and international health bureaucracy and the will to figure out was happening amid World War I led to the influenza epidemic occurring unchecked, and the problem was about to explode. As Alfred Crosby wrote in *America's Forgotten Pandemic* (p. 46): "The interweaving of the war and the pandemic make what from a distance of a half-century seems to be a pattern of complete insanity."

3.3.2 Second Wave

Although not many cases of the flu occurred during the summer months in North America, influenza was raging in other parts of the world. As we know, the more times the influenza A virus replicates itself, the more opportunities it has for a mutation to occur allowing a more virulent form of the virus to emerge. Troop movements meant that people from all different parts of the world were coming together. Scholars have noted that the severity and timing of influenza cases indicate that the flu spread from the armed services to civilians (Crosby 1989).

The second wave of the 1918 influenza pandemic in the United States began in August 1918. Many people note flu epidemics broke out in three major port cities around the world at the same time in August 1918: Freetown, Sierra Leone; Brest, France; and Boston, Massachusetts, U.S.A. (Crosby 1989; Bristow 2021). Freetown was a major port for the British Empire at the time. Brest, France, was a major landing site for the American Expeditionary Forces coming to Europe to fight in World War I. Although New York was the major site from which U.S. troops embarked to Europe, Boston still was a key port for troop and supply movements (Crosby 1989).

Unlike the cases of influenza seen in the spring, doctors began seeing very severe illness, sometime to the point where the person turned blue due to lack of oxygen (Barry 2018). In cases where death occurs after two to three days, what we now call acute respiratory distress syndrome (ARDS) was happening, where the immune response itself causes destruction of lung tissue. If a patient survived ARDS, there was also the risk of secondary pathogens like bacteria infecting the patient as well (Barry 2018; Spinney 2017). The respiratory system includes two major sections: the section including the nasal cavity, pharynx, larynx, trachea, bronchi, and bronchioles that conditions and conducts air to the lungs, and the section that participates in the gas exchange, taking in oxygen to be used by the body, made of the respiratory bronchioles, alveolar ducts, alveolar sacs, and alveoli. If you were to look at a normal lung tissue section, one prominent feature would be the large air spaces in the alveoli, critical for efficient gas exchange. In pneumonia, the tissue is inflamed, capillaries can become enlarged, and the air spaces fill with fluid containing white blood cells trying to fight the infection (Ross and Pawlina 2011; Pritt and Aubry 2017). Researchers have looked at autopsies in patients who died during the 1918 influenza pandemic, confirming "massive infiltration of neutrophils" into air spaces in the lungs. Severe damage to alveoli was seen along with secondary bacterial infections (Figure 3.4) (Sheng et al. 2011).

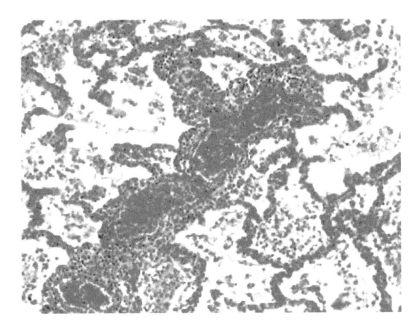

FIGURE 3.4
Effects of influenza A on the lung.

Shown in this image is an example of the early alveolar damage done by the influenza A virus to the lungs. In this tissue section, the air sacs of the lung, known as alveoli, appear as an open meshwork with short, flat cells lining the alveoli and open space for air. In the middle of the image, one can see what the authors describe as "hyperemic alveolar septa," where one observes an increase in blood flow to the walls separating the air sacs and inflammatory cells such as white blood cells beginning to fill in the area. (Hematoxylin and eosin staining, 200X magnification)

Source: Reprinted with permission from Bobbi S. Pritt and Marie Christine Aubry. 2017. "Histopathology of viral infections of the lung." *Seminars in Diagnostic Pathology,* 34 (6):510–7. (Permission obtained through RightsLink.)

As mentioned earlier, WWI had a compounding effect on the ability of the pathogen to spread, as well as the ability of institutions to respond. There was a shortage of doctors and nurses who had gone oversees for the war effort (Crosby 1989; Barry 2018). In general, there was much confusion and panic amid strained social conditions in big cities when the pandemic hit. Still, different cities in the United States had their own unique trajectories in terms of the number of cases and deaths with the 1918 flu pandemic. Philadelphia had one large wave of an epidemic, while San Francisco had two waves (Crosby 1989). When Philadelphia was compared to a city like St. Louis, one saw a huge spike in the death rate during fall 1918 in Philadelphia, but a similar spike was not seen in St. Louis. Instead, a steady but lower rise in the death rate was observed through the fall 1918 and into the winter in that city (for Figure 3.5) (Hatchett, Mecher, and Lipsitch 2007).

3.3.3 Philadelphia

Most scholars acknowledge that Philadelphia, Pennsylvania, U.S.A., was one of the hardest hit cities in the world due to the severity of the pandemic in a short period. For example, 700 people died in one day in Philadelphia (Crosby 1989). The series of events leading to

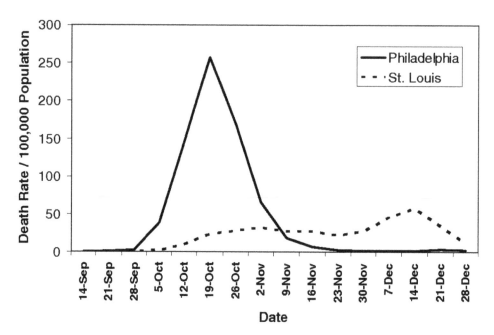

FIGURE 3.5

Death rate for second wave of the 1918 pandemic in Philadelphia (solid line) versus St. Louis (dashed line).

Shown here is the death rate per 100,000 people in Philadelphia versus St. Louis for the fall and winter 1918.

Source: From Figure 1 on page 7583 of Hatchett, R.J., C.E. Mecher, and M. Lipsitch. 2007. "Public health interventions and epidemic intensity during the 1918 influenza pandemic." Proceedings of the National Academy of Sciences of the United States of America, 104 (18):7582–7. doi: 10.1073/pnas.0610941104. Hatchett, et al., cites this study as the source material for the data used in the graph: Sattenspiel L., Herring D.A. 2003. Bulletin of Mathematical Biology 65:1–26. Copyright (2007) National Academy of Sciences, U.S.A. Reprinted with permission.

this severe outcome were first set in motion by troop movements. On September 7, 1918, sailors from Camp Devens in Boston arrived at the Philadelphia Naval Yard. Cases of severe influenza at Camp Devens had just started to be reported at that time (Crosby 1989; Barry 2018; Brown 2018; Kolata 1999). Then, on September 28, 1918, Philadelphia held a Liberty Loan parade, with 200,000 people in attendance, despite warnings from national public officials to cancel major public events during fall 1918. The parade went on as scheduled, to sell war bonds (Crosby 1989; Barry 2018; Spinney 2017; Brown 2018).

Within two to three days, people were sick and dying. The State of Pennsylvania did react to close public places like schools and churches, but it was too late. Many medical personnel like doctors and nurses were abroad for World War I, and so there were not enough personnel to treat patients, nor were there enough of other essential workers like cleaners and orderlies. Undertakers were overwhelmed, and dead bodies were piled up at the morgue (Crosby 1989). Many workers were absent from work in a range of industries, and the Baltimore and Ohio Railroad went so far as to set up emergency hospitals for employees (Barry 2018). Public health messages were posted everywhere, including "spit spreads death" (Figure 3.6).

Political, social, and religious organizations mobilized to step in to care for the sick, even using private vehicles to drive people to the hospital. These groups also distributed food to keep the well from going hungry. Finally, they organized efforts to bury the dead in the

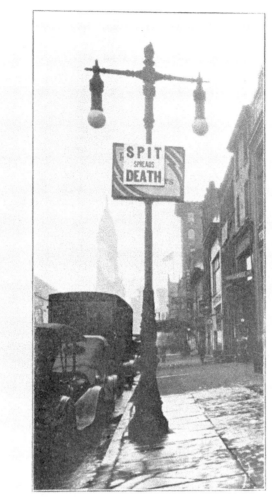

Spitters were arrested and fined

FIGURE 3.6
Spit spreads death.

Picture of "spit spreads death" poster displayed in Philadelphia 1918. City Hall is visible in the distance.

Photo credit: George D. McDowell Philadelphia Evening Tribune Collection, SCRC170, "Spitters were arrested and fined." Courtesy of the Special Collections Research Center. Temple University Libraries. Philadelphia, PA.

city. By the end of October 1918, schools were reopened, and Philadelphians emerged to celebrate Armistice Day in November (Crosby 1989).

3.3.4 Third Wave

Woodrow Wilson became ill at the Paris Peace Conference, most likely due to the 1918 flu pandemic (Barry 2018; Spinney 2017). World War I ended on November 11, 1918. However, a third wave of the 1918 influenza pandemic in the United States took place between

December 1918 and January 1919. This version of influenza was considered milder than the first two waves (Crosby 1989). Some mention that the influenza pandemic "rallied" in January and February 1920, but due to herd immunity and other factors, it did not have a significant impact (Crosby 1989). We do not know exactly why the 1918 influenza A virus went away. It may have been because of the level of herd immunity in the population, or through mutation the virus became unrecognizable from a seasonal flu.

3.4 Treatments for Influenza in 1918

So what treatments were available to help the sick? If you were lucky enough to be under the care of a nurse, treatment at the time was geared towards keeping people comfortable and clean (Philadelphia 2020). Others tried home remedies like garlic and whisky (Barry 2018; Philadelphia 2020). Scientists tried experimental treatments using blood and blood derivatives to help patients (Barry 2018). Experimental trials were conducted using candidate vaccines, but these were bacterial vaccines developed under the mistaken premise that bacteria were responsible for the 1918 pandemic (see next section) (Eyler 2009).

Antibiotics had not yet been discovered, so they were not available to people with secondary infections as they are now (Barry 2018). The lack of treatment for secondary infections may have been one of the reasons for the high mortality rate of the virus (Brown 2018). However, aspirin was available to treat pain to a certain degree, but was often overprescribed resulting in toxic side effects (Spinney 2017; Brown 2018). Other physicians, like Arthur Hopkirk, became famous for their influenza treatment recommendations, including herbal treatments and large doses of laxatives (Brown 2018). Just as a malarial treatment was advocated for treatment of COVID-19 for a time, doctors also tried the anti-malarial drug quinine to treat influenza as well (Brown 2018; Spinney 2017). In the end, not one effective universal treatment for influenza was developed, other than the rest and supportive environment that a good nurse could provide. Among those who survived, it was reported that some people suffered long-term effects from the influenza infection or its treatments, affecting balance or hearing in some people (Spinney 2017). In addition, certain factors like malnutrition and co-infection with another pathogen may have made recovery more difficult (Short, Kedzierska, and van de Sandt 2018).

3.5 Understand How Scientists Raced to Find the Cause of the 1918 Pandemic, and What They Found Using Koch's Postulates

Microbiologists working in the 19th century had established strict criteria for linking a pathogen to a disease. These rules are known as Koch's postulates, as mentioned in Chapter 1 (Minkoff and Baker 2004a). Following Koch's postulates, a scientist or group of scientists would first determine that the pathogen of interest is found in all or nearly all of the cases of the disease and is not harbored in those individuals without the disease.

Then, the scientists must isolate the pathogen away from other organisms, and then typically using an animal model, reintroduce the isolated pathogen into a new organism and recreate the original disease. These standards are still used today.

Many scientists, including scientists from American institutions like the Rockefeller Institute for Medical Research, the New York City Department of Public Health, and University of Pennsylvania, were working hard to identify the pathogen causing the 1918 flu pandemic. Scientists were much better at managing bacterial than viral pathogens in the laboratory. (Since the electron microscope had not yet been invented, scientists could not see viruses, only the impact of viral infection or whether the infectious material could pass through a filter, as described in Chapter 1.) Some scientists began to culture consistently one type of bacterium, Pfeiffer's bacillus, from material taken from influenza patients. This bacterium, also known as *Bacillus influenzae* and now known as *Hemophilus influenzae*, had been isolated from flu patients during the 1889–90 pandemic in Europe by a German scientist named Richard Pfeiffer. Pfeiffer was convinced that this was the pathogen responsible for influenza (Crosby 1989; Barry 2018; Kolata 1999; Spinney 2017).

However, Pfeiffer's bacterium was not found in all 1918 influenza patients. For example, scientists working at the New York City Department of Public Health found another kind of bacterium, *Streptococci*, among others, but not *Bacilli* in samples taken from the lungs of those who died from the pandemic. In addition, in rigorous experimental examination following Koch's postulates, Pfeiffer's bacterium did not pass the test as the causative agent of influenza (Barry 2018; Spinney 2017; Kolata 1999).

The scientist Richard Shope, working with pigs in the 1930s, discovered that a virus was responsible for swine flu, long after the 1918 flu pandemic was long over (Crosby 1989; Barry 2018; Spinney 2017; Kolata 1999; Van Epps 2006). Shope and Paul Lewis were able to isolate Pfeiffer's bacillus from the pigs that were sick with swine flu, but when these bacteria were introduced back into healthy pigs, it did not cause the flu. However, there was a filterable infectious agent isolated from the sick pig samples that could recreate the flu. In addition, Shope and colleagues went back to Pfeiffer's bacillus, and demonstrated that introducing this bacterium into the pigs after swine flu infection could be deadly, mimicking what happened to the victims of the 1918 pandemic (Barry 2018; Kolata 1999; Van Epps 2006). The researchers Smith, Andrewes, and Laidlaw began using ferrets as a model organism for flu. They found that they could give the ferrets the flu either using a filtered infectious agent taken from people with the flu or taken from other ferrets. The ferrets could also be protected against flu using serum from patients who recovered from the flu. Both teams of researchers found that the human and swine flu viruses were very similar, and that people who survived the 1918 flu pandemic carried antibodies capable of blocking the swine flu (Kolata 1999; Van Epps 2006). These studies indicated that the 1918 flu pandemic was a very close relative of swine flu. The studies also supported the idea that pigs are an intermediary organism between birds and humans for perpetuating the virus (Spinney 2017). However, others believed that the 1918 pandemic virus most likely passed directly from birds to humans. Some research studies indicated that transmission from human to swine was more common than swine to human. In addition, the levels and type of sialic acid receptors (the receptor for the influenza A virus) were more similar in swine and humans than expected, so an avian virus would not necessarily get a foothold in pigs before moving to humans. The possibility of reassortment of the viral genome in pigs is still a part of the ongoing debate (Nelson and Worobey 2018; Lostroh 2019; Short, Kedzierska, and van de Sandt 2018).

3.6 Examine Modern Analysis of the 1918 Pandemic and the Influenza A Virus Itself

In the 1990s with the improvement in DNA technology, including the development of polymerase chain reaction (PCR), researchers began to seek out samples to study the 1918 influenza viral genetic code. As mentioned in Chapter 2, the use of PCR allows for small amounts of nucleic acid, like viral DNA or RNA, to be amplified for further study like sequence analysis. Researchers were able to obtain partial sequence data for the 1918 influenza pandemic virus from a tissue sample preserved in the U.S. Armed Forces Institute of Pathology, taken from a soldier who died in the pandemic named Roscoe Vaughn. In the study, parts of the hemagglutinin and neuraminidase genes, along with three other genes, were amplified using reverse transcriptase polymerase chain reaction (RT-PCR) and sequenced. With this information, the researchers were able to determine that the 1918 influenza virus was a new H1N1 influenza A virus (Taubenberger et al. 1997; Spinney 2017; Kolata 1999) (Figure 3.7).

Another researcher, Johan Hultin, read Taubenberger's 1997 publication. Hultin had been interested in this topic for his entire career, so he returned to Alaska where he had once attempted to recover samples for analysis from a mass grave of 1918 pandemic victims before sequencing were possible. Hultin identified new well-preserved biological material to send to Taubenberger for PCR. Taubenberger and members of his team, including Ann Reid, were able to use Hultin's sample that had been preserved in the Alaskan permafrost, along with their original sample and one other sample, to sequence the entire hemagglutinin gene from the 1918 influenza viral genome. Their findings indicated that the 1918 influenza viral sequence had strong similarities to the avian version of the virus, although the number of mutations in the hemagglutinin gene indicated that the virus would be grouped as a mammalian virus when compared to other similar viruses (Spinney 2017; Kolata 1999; Reid et al. 1999).

Taubenberger and his research team continued their sequence analysis, eventually sequencing the entire 1918 influenza viral genome (Tumpey et al. 2005). Once the 1918 viral sequence was known, researchers designed antibody tests against viral proteins in the blood. Using a genetically engineered version of the HA protein found in that subtype of the virus, scientists tested the blood of 1918 pandemic survivors. The results indicated that survivors still carried antibodies that specifically recognize the 1918 influenza A virus in their blood, almost 90 years after the pandemic occurred (Yu et al. 2008).

Taubenberger and his colleagues also carried out animal studies using genetically engineered versions of the influenza A virus. These synthetic viruses incorporated some of the specific influenza genes found in the 1918 pandemic viral subtype and became a valuable model for testing the effects of influenza in laboratory studies. In the animal models, the scientists looked at tissues to see the effects of the immune response to the virus, tested the effectiveness of antiviral drugs, and tried out H1N1 vaccines against the synthetic viruses. Taubenberger and colleagues have summarized their prolific work in a series of review articles, and some representative articles are mentioned here (Taubenberger, Hultin, and Morens 2007; Taubenberger and Morens 2006; Taubenberger, Kash, and Morens 2019; Taubenberger and Morens 2020). Other groups also performed similar studies using recombinant influenza viruses in animal models (Kobasa et al. 2004; Kobasa et al. 2007). Recombinant or synthetic viruses were developed to better understand other viruses as well, such as poliovirus. Taubenberger and colleagues have presented the benefits of synthetic virus research, but also have emphasized the importance

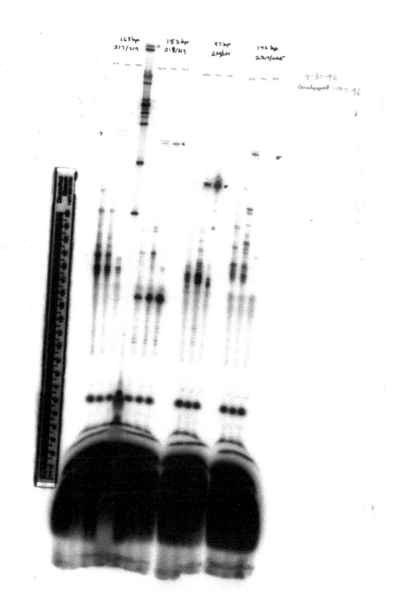

FIGURE 3.7
Using modern molecular biology techniques to uncover the 1918 influenza pandemic viral genetic code from "1918 case 1."

Shown here is an X-ray film displaying the autoradiogram produced by a sequencing gel. This sequencing gel was used to separate out the largest viral genomic fragments amplified using PCR (indicated by small arrows) in each of the four sample sets. These fragments were used to identify the 1918 influenza genetic code by Dr. Taubenberger and colleagues.

Photo credit: "X-ray film; x-ray plate used to locate influenza DNA," (M-722.10195–002). Historical Division, National Museum of Health and Medicine. Used with permission (www.medicalmuseum.mil/index. cfm?p=visit.exhibits.virtual.1918killerflu.page_01).

More information on this research study can be found at Taubenberger, J.K., A.H. Reid, A.E. Krafft, K.E. Bijwaard, and T.G. Fanning. 1997. "Initial genetic characterization of the 1918 "Spanish" influenza virus." *Science* 275 (5307):1793–6. doi: 10.1126/science.275.5307.1793. PMID: 9065404.

of science communication in explaining why this kind of research is valuable to the public (Wimmer et al. 2009).

Other influenza research has been more controversial due to what might be seen as higher-risk experiments, taking an influenza pathogen to the next level—purposely selecting for a more virulent version of an influenza virus in animal studies. In 2012, two research groups published data on NIH-funded studies looking at transmission of an H5N1 influenza A virus among ferrets (Herfst et al. 2012; Imai et al. 2012). In one study, researchers took the original H5N1 strain, mutated it, and then let it replicate in ferrets, moving the virus from one ferret to another, until they were able to obtain a version of the virus that could be transmitted from ferret to ferret through the air (Herfst et al. 2012). The other study involved more characterization of mutated versions of the H5N1 virus first *in vitro* using cell culture and receptor-binding assays, but then the altered virus was ultimately introduced into ferrets, and then ferret-to-ferret airborne transmission was tested and confirmed. The publications also contain the particular amino acid changes that conferred ferret-to-ferret transmission of the virus, allowing this airborne transmission to happen. Some people questioned whether these studies should have been done at all, and if these data should have been published. The experiments were controversial because they represented a type of "Dual Use Research of Concern (DURC)." This label indicates that the research could be used to learn more about influenza A virus and how to prevent an epidemic or pandemic, or the research could be used in an unethical way to purposely attempt to harm others (Office of Intramural Research 2021).

The journal *Science* published a special issue on the H5N1 topic. In the end, *Science* chose to publish one of the original research articles, as well as a follow-up study, after the research was reviewed by the U.S. National Science Advisory Board for Biosecurity (NSABB) (Alberts 2012; Herfst et al. 2012; Russell et al. 2012). The second breakthrough study by a different research group was published in *Nature* (Imai et al. 2012). The follow-up study in *Science* actually looked at the influenza virus genetic changes reported in the two original studies, to see if the mutations were already naturally existing in influenza A. Some but not all of the genetic changes in the H5N1 virus were detected in human isolates, and the group used mathematical modeling to assess the risk that the other genetic changes could occur naturally in the virus as well (Russell et al. 2012). Two leading scientists at the NIH, Dr. Anthony Fauci and Dr. Francis Collins, supported the decision to publish the H5N1 transmission research, citing the valuable lessons that could be learned from such studies, including what changes in the virus to look out for that may lead to human-to-human transmission, and if existing antiviral therapies would work against the virus. They mentioned that H5N1 is a "highly pathogenic avian influenza virus" and that researchers have been concerned about this influenza A subtype for some time. H5N1 had been detected in chickens and had crossed over into humans who worked closely with the birds. The subtype exhibited a high mortality rate in the infected humans but had not yet spread from person to person. Nevertheless, Fauci and Collins did cite the importance of a new national oversight committee to evaluate potential DURC-related projects before they reach the publication stage (Fauci and Collins 2012). In a related commentary Dr. Fauci remarks, "The game has changed for influenza virus scientists and the agencies that support them" (Fauci 2012). The H5N1 virus continues to be an influenza A subtype of concern. So far, Indonesia, Vietnam, and Egypt have the most reports of human sporadic cases, but H5N1 human infection in the United States was first reported in 2014 (CDC 2021b).

Aside from publishing the H5N1 research, others wanted to revisit if the H5N1 transmission research should have been conducted at all. A voluntary 60-day moratorium on H5N1 transmission research, as well as similar research on other avian influenza viruses, was extended to a full year at the time in 2012–13 (Fouchier et al. 2012). Some scientists called for additional training for those researchers conducting experiments considered DURC. In addition, some thought the moratorium should go on until a major scientific confer- ence could be organized to discuss the ethics of conducting research on highly pathogenic viruses, such as was done with the advent of recombinant DNA technology (Falkow 2012). In the end, the moratorium went on for only a year, and then was lifted, being announced with a letter to *Science*, including the original researchers among the authors of the letter (Fouchier et al. 2013).

The H5N1 studies and similar studies using synthetic viruses represent what are known as "gain of function" studies, where an existing virus is manipulated or allowed to evolve in the laboratory to see if it gains new properties like changes in transmission (Lostroh 2019). In Chapter 9, we will talk about science communication and the responsibilities of scientists to communicate their work to the public. What rights do the public have in terms of being informed of controversial influenza research, and what are the responsibilities of scientists to report it and have it vetted? Who vets the research? Are any scientific topics off limits because of national or international concerns? If a society wants to place limits on influenza research, what then is the best way to anticipate the next pandemic, trying to be at least one step ahead of an emerging virus?

3.7 Understand the Impact of the 1918 Pandemic Including How Our Society Handles Pandemics in General and Seasonal Influenza Specifically Today

The impact of the 1918 influenza pandemic is hard to sort out independently of the impact of WWI. It is difficult to find many specific social impacts from the 1918 influenza pan- demic documented separately from those of WWI, although some have noted an increase in orphans during the time of the pandemic, such as those orphans seeking admission to a special school in Philadelphia known as Girard College (Philadelphia 2020). The Red Cross indicated in 1919 that the pandemic left many widows and orphans throughout the United States, as well as more people struggling in poverty (Barry 2018). However, the indigenous peoples of Alaska in isolated villages, where the virus was brought in by outsiders, were particularly hard hit by the virus, leaving behind many flu orphans (Barry 2018; Spinney 2017; Ahmed, Oldstone, and Palese 2007; Gray 2021; Reid et al. 1999; Crosby 1989). It has been estimated that one in 20 people in Alaska died during 1918 flu pandemic, with 80% of them being native Alaskans (Carney 2020). At the same time, a very small number of places where people successfully isolated themselves, such as Princeton University, were spared from the 1918 flu pandemic (Gray 2021; Bernstein 2008; Wright 2021). Overall, the horror of the trench warfare endured by the soldiers in Europe, and the millions of deaths from the war alone, overshadowed the pandemic suffering, or some might say merged with the pandemic suffering, for the people of the world at that time.

We can look for the cultural impact of the pandemic among the works of artists who sur- vived or avoided the pandemic. For example, the artist Gustav Klimt died in the pandemic, while the artist Edvard Munch got influenza and recovered (Outka 2020). Several scholars cite *Pale Horse, Pale Rider* by Katherine Anne Porter as a major work inspired by the pan- demic (Outka 2020; Barry 2018; Crosby 1989; Spinney 2017). In the story, one witnesses a woman's suffering and recovery from the 1918 influenza pandemic, only to discover that the man she loves has died from influenza (Porter 1967). The story makes one wonder how close it is to Porter's own story of survival after getting influenza (Barry 2018; Crosby 1989; Spinney 2017; Outka 2020). The realities of the pandemic and the war are an integral part of the story. One witnesses the confusion and pain as the main character suffers with influenza, as well as details of the war experience for civilians such as the peer pressure to buy Liberty Bonds (Outka 2020).

Other than the imprint that the 1918 influenza pandemic left in works of art and in stories quietly passed down in families, it does not seem like the 1918 influenza pandemic left a lasting impact on how people in general prepare for pandemics or react to them. When one reads accounts of everyday people's reactions to the 1918 influenza pandemic, they seem eerily like what was experienced with the COVID-19 pandemic. First, workers started staying home out of fear at the height of the wave of influenza cases in Philadelphia, such as workers at the Bell Telephone Company of Pennsylvania, just as was seen with the COVID-19 pandemic. In addition, immigrants were at greater risk of getting sick, as well as anyone living at high densities in bigger cities. Many people living in cities like Philadelphia had boarders/lodgers in their homes (Crosby 1989). A housing shortage meant that many people were crammed together, living in tenement housing as well in major cities (Barry 2018). At times, public officials had to close churches, schools, and other institutions, like the conditions experienced with the COVID-19 pandemic. Instead of using social media and television to spread public health messages like "mask up," "wash your hands," and "practice social distancing," cities put up "no spitting" signs and used mottos such as "spit spreads death" in their attempts to convey a public health message to the people (Philadelphia 2020; Brown 2018). The surgeon general advised people to avoid crowds, seek out fresh air, and wash their hands (Barry 2018). As was the case with the COVID-19 pandemic, those messages were often ignored. Other people were looking for someone to blame for the pandemic, but everyone around them seemed to be affected, especially in densely populated cities (Barry 2018).

Researchers have gone back and looked at "nonpharmaceutical interventions (NPIs)" like closing churches, schools, and theaters and making funerals private in 17 cities at the time of the 1918 influenza pandemic. These interventions were typically in place for two to eight weeks at a time just as the influenza epidemic was starting to grow in that city, critically being implemented before cases started to rapidly increase. The researchers found that if more than one NPI was used, the city had a lower peak death rate when compared to other cities (Philadelphia versus St. Louis). They concluded that NPIs were quite valuable in slowing the spread of the influenza virus, although cities were at risk again for another wave when the interventions were taken away. These data indicated that the timing and execution of interventions were powerful, yet difficult to time (Hatchett, Mecher, and Lipsitch 2007).

In some ways, one can liken the September 1918 Liberty Loan Parade in Philadelphia to the August 2020 Sturgis Motorcycle Rally in South Dakota, since both were large events reportedly linked to large numbers of disease cases after the event. As mentioned earlier, many people got sick and died after the Liberty Loan Parade in 1918. In 2020, months after the Sturgis rally, it is known that hundreds of people got sick from COVID-19 and some did die, although cases were difficult to track since people came to the event from multiple states (Walker and Healy 2020). If troop ships were incubators of disease for the 1918 pandemic, one might take note of the outbreaks of COVID-19 on cruise ships in early 2020 (Apuzzo, Rich, and Yaffe-Bellany 2020). In the case of both respiratory virus pandemics, human activity in large gatherings within close quarters was directly connected to cases of the disease. These respiratory viruses thrive on the human need for social interaction, especially when humans balk at the idea of isolating themselves from an invisible threat.

Although flu pandemics are rare, others occurred in 1957, 1968, and 2009, each from a virus carrying a slightly different version of the hemagglutinin gene (Spinney 2017). None of these pandemics caused anywhere near the number of cases or fatalities as the 1918 influenza pandemic. Researchers have studied the last five influenza pandemics: 1889, 1918, 1957, 1968, and 2009 and found major characteristics that all these pandemics had in common. They all happened in waves, and each wave had different characteristics in terms of pathogen virulence (Barry 2018).

In 1976, a soldier at Fort Dix, New Jersey, came down with a severe case of swine flu and died. Because the virus was an H1N1 version of the virus, national officials were afraid that they might have another 1918 pandemic on their hands. The government mobilized quickly to make a vaccine, but it turns out that the flu never left Fort Dix. In addition, a small percentage of people who received the vaccine came down with Guillain-Barre syndrome after getting the shot, and many believed there was an association with the vaccine, although how close an association is not completely known. The response to the 1976 swine flu is often cited as an overreaction in terms of pandemic preparedness (Kolata 1999).

Seasonal influenza still occurs every year, primarily in the winter months in temperate zones of the world. The Centers for Disease Control and Prevention (CDC) have an influenza surveillance system that can help the agency predict the trajectory of each flu season. The CDC gathers local and national data weekly, working with clinical laboratories, public health officials, and healthcare providers in hospitals and outpatient facilities. The CDC not only looks at the number of cases and deaths, but also characterizes the virus itself, keeping an eye out for new versions of the influenza A virus (CDC 2021d). Companies like Google have also gotten involved in influenza surveillance. Google created a website called "Google Flu Trends," but retired the website in 2015 when it was found that it could not reliably be used to predict flu cases (Brown 2018). The overprediction of flu cases by Google Flu Trends may have been due to "big data hubris" and changes in the Google algorithm that occurred over time during the flu season, adjustments that may improve Google searches but also affect the strength of the forecasting (Lazer et al. 2014). To try to get ahead of the game, the CDC tries to predict the patterns of season influenza, including how long the season will last and how bad it will be, in a program known as FluSight. The program directors also invite academic and private industry researchers to participate in their annual challenge to forecast the flu season, allowing the CDC to develop external research partners for their efforts (CDC 2021a). Effective modeling approaches tend to consider many different kinds of data, including social media posts, web search data, and information such as weather and humidity, analyzed using either a "statistical" or "mechanistic" model (Ali and Cowling 2021). We also must not forget about surveilling wild birds to figure out what subtypes of influenza A are circulating among the birds, in addition to conducting whole genome analysis. Scientists have called for greater coordination and standardization of practices among countries for monitoring of birds long term (Machalaba et al. 2015). Aside from U.S. flu surveillance efforts, over 100 research centers around the world communicate with the WHO, so that the WHO can make recommendations on the composition of the seasonal flu vaccine (Krammer et al. 2018).

Even if our surveillance systems for influenza A were not able to stop an epidemic or pandemic, more treatment options are available to those who have influenza in the 21st century than in 1918. However, if no complications develop, managing fever, staying hydrated, and treating symptoms still works well in treating the flu (Krammer et al.

2018). There are drugs called "neuraminidase inhibitors" like Tamiflu (oseltamivir) that can reduce the length of influenza in patients as well, if given early in the course of the illness (Brown 2018; Ison 2017; Krammer et al. 2018). Drugs like amantadine and rimantadine were used for a time to block the M2 protein of influenza A, but more recent articles indicate that existing influenza A strains are resistant to these drugs (Couch 1996; Ison 2017; Krammer et al. 2018). Antibiotics are available to treat secondary, nonviral infections. Modern testing also makes an influenza viral infection diagnosis much easier than in 1918. Influenza can be diagnosed using antibody tests like an ELISA (Couch 1996). Newer technologies such as RT-PCR, a rapid antigen test, a rapid molecular test looking at viral nucleic acid, and a viral culture test can be employed to identify influenza virus infection as well (Krammer et al. 2018). Also, every year a new flu vaccine is developed to help cut down on the number of cases and fatalities from the flu.

Will we ever have a universal flu vaccine? In the past, a universal flu vaccine which can be used every flu season has been hard to develop because of how rapidly influenza mutates into different strains (Brown 2018; Lostroh 2019). Researchers have explored using other proteins of the virus such as a stalk protein or an ion channel protein as the immunogen in a universal flu vaccine, since these genes may not mutate as quickly as the genes encoding hemagglutinin and neuraminidase. However, getting these other parts of the virus to invoke a strong immune response with vaccination has been challenging, but different recombinant protein vaccines are being explored (Lostroh 2019). Other scientists are looking at what contributing factors might make a seasonal flu vaccine less effective in one person versus another. Characteristics like age, biological sex, obesity, and even perhaps one's microbiome may have an effect, in addition to previous exposures to influenza virus as mentioned earlier (Dhakal and Klein 2019). In addition to finding the best possible vaccine to elicit a sufficient universal immune response, physicians will need to look at these other aspects of the patient profile to help improve the effectiveness of a universal flu vaccine.

3.8 Summary

The 1918 influenza pandemic affected millions of people's lives right in the middle of World War I. The outbreak of an H1N1 influenza A avian flu most likely started in Kansas in spring 1918 and spread rapidly through troop movements, becoming a pandemic. A second, more virulent, wave of the 1918 flu pandemic swept through the United States in fall 1918, causing much suffering, disease, and death in a short period of time in the major cities. Influenza A is an enveloped virus of the Orthomyxovirus family causing respiratory disease that spreads from person to person through coughing and sneezing. Through antigenic drift caused by mutation, and antigenic shift caused by genome reassortment, new strains of influenza A arise quite often. This is one reason that influenza recurs every year in the winter months of temperate climates. More treatment options are available for influenza now than in 1918, but certain interventions not requiring drugs, like limiting large gatherings and vaccinating vulnerable populations, can help slow or stop an influenza epidemic or pandemic. Researchers are working hard to study how influenza is transmitted using animal models, in sometimes controversial studies. At the same time, international and national flu surveillance efforts are helping to prevent the next epidemic. Hopefully, in the future, we will have a universal flu vaccine that will prevent future epidemics from happening at all.

Discussion Questions:

1. Please answer the following questions on World War I related to those appearing on the website: "The Influenza Pandemic: Educator Resource" https://www.theworldwar.org/learn/educator-resource/influenza-epidemic-educator-resource

   a. Describe the connection between the spread of the 1918 influenza pandemic virus and the events of WWI.

   b. How did the name "Spanish Flu" come about and what are the risks of using the name of a place for a virus?

2. As mentioned in the chapter, many scientists convinced themselves that bacteria were causing the 1918 pandemic instead of a virus. Was there a system in place to prevent a scientist from misleading the public with such an idea?

3. What are the similarities and what are the differences between the 1918 pandemic and the COVID-19 pandemic?

4. In 2019, the Mütter Museum, a part of the College of Physicians and Surgeons of Philadelphia, put together a comprehensive exhibit on the pandemic. Please go to their website using the link here: https://muttermuseum.org/exhibitions/spit-spreads-death. Please go to the 16-minute video showing a virtual tour of the exhibit (The 1918 Influenza Pandemic in Philadelphia Exhibit Tour). It should also be available through YouTube. Please take the virtual tour and answer the following questions:

   a. What was significant about the Liberty Loan Parade on September 28, 1918?

   b. How did flu enter the City of Philadelphia?

   c. What happened within 72 hours of the parade?

   d. What was one treatment for flu in 1918?

   e. Why were nurses valuable and why were there so few around during the 1918 pandemic?

   f. What was one mistaken assumption about African Americans and influenza?

   g. How did scientists reconstruct the 1918 flu strain in 2005?

   h. What was the most recent flu pandemic?

   i. Do you think that campaigns like "spit spreads death" worked in 1918? How about public messages on disease prevention used now over social media and other places?

5. Herd immunity is an important factor governing the spread of pathogens. Please go to the History of Vaccines website and follow the interactive on Herd Immunity. Please answer the questions on the website: www.historyofvaccines.org/content/herd-immunity-0

   At each step of the exercise, different numbers of individuals are vaccinated in the animation. If you press "play animation," you will see how many people get sick under different herd immunity situations. Record your observations of the three different herd immunity scenarios presented.

6. The author's grandmother was a little girl during the 1918 influenza pandemic, and now the author is living during the COVID-19 pandemic as she writes this book. Is going through a pandemic just a part of the human condition? Should we accept that pandemics will occur every so often on the earth, or should we work harder to prevent them?

References

Ackermann, H.-W., L. Berthiaume, and M. Tremblay. 1998. *Virus Life in Diagrams*. Boca Raton, FL: CRC press, Taylor & Francis Group.

Ahmed, R., M.B. Oldstone, and P. Palese. 2007. "Protective immunity and susceptibility to infectious diseases: Lessons from the 1918 influenza pandemic." *Nature Immunology* 8 (11):1188–93. doi: 10.1038/ni1530.

Alberts, B. 2012. "H5N1." *Science* 336 (6088):1521-. doi: 10.1126/science.336.6088.1521.

Ali, S.T., and B.J. Cowling. 2021. "Influenza virus: Tracking, predicting, and forecasting." *Annual Review of Public Health* 42 (1):43–57. doi: 10.1146/annurev-publhealth-010720-021049.

Apuzzo, M., M. Rich, and D. Yaffe-Bellany. 2020. "Failures on the Diamond Princess shadow another cruise ship outbreak." In *The New York Times*. New York, NY: The New York Times Company.

Baltimore, D. 1971. "Expression of animal virus genomes." *Bacteriological Reviews* 35 (3):235.

Barry, J.M. 2018. *The Great Influenza: The Epic Story of the Deadliest Plague in History*. New York, NY: Penguin Random House LLC.

Bernstein, M.F. 2008. "Why Princeton was spared." In *Princeton Alumni Weekly*. Princeton, NJ: Princeton University.

Bristow, N.K. 2021. "Pandemic then and now: Lessons from the 1918 influenza." *National WWI Museum and Memorial*. Accessed 24 July 2021. www.theworldwar.org/learn/wwi/influenza.

Britannica, E. 2021. "World War I: Killed, wounded and missing." *Encyclopaedia Britannica, Inc.* www.britannica.com/event/World-War-I/Killed-wounded-and-missing.

Brown, J. 2018. *Influenza: The Hundred Year Hunt to Cure the Deadliest Disease in History*. New York, NY: Touchstone.

Carney, J. 2020. "The Spanish Flu in Alaska: Why some villages were devastated and others unscathed." In *Anchorage Press*. Anchorage, AK: Wick Communications.

CDC, Centers for Disease Control and Prevention. 2021a. "FluSight: Flu forecasting." *Department of Health and Human Services*. Accessed 28 July 2021. www.cdc.gov/flu/weekly/flusight/index.html.

———. 2021b. "Highly pathogenic Asian avian influenza A (H5N1 in people)." *Department of Health and Human Services*. Accessed 29 July 2021. www.cdc.gov/flu/avianflu/h5n1-people.htm.

———. 2021c. "Types of influenza viruses." *Department of Health and Human Services*. Accessed 2 August 2021. www.cdc.gov/flu/about/viruses/types.htm.

———. 2021d. "U.S. influenza surveillance system: Purpose and methods." *U.S. Department of Health and Human Services*. Accessed 27 July 2021. www.cdc.gov/flu/weekly/overview.htm.

Clancy, S. 2008. "Genetics of the influenza virus." *Nature Education* 1 (1).

Couch, R.B. 1996. "Orthomyxoviruses." In *Medical Microbiology*, edited by S. Baron, 10. Galveston, TX: University of Texas Medical Branch at Galveston.

Crosby, A.W. 1989. *America's Forgotten Pandemic: The Influenza of 1918*. New York, NY: Cambridge University Press.

Dhakal, S., and S.L. Klein. 2019. "Host factors impact vaccine efficacy: Implications for seasonal and universal influenza vaccine programs." *Journal of Virology* 93 (21). doi: 10.1128/jvi.00797-19.

Eyler, J.M. 2009. "The fog of research: Influenza vaccine trials during the 1918–19 pandemic." *Journal of the History of Medicine and Allied Sciences* 64 (4):401–28. doi: 10.1093/jhmas/jrp013.

Falkow, S. 2012. "The lessons of Asilomar and the H5N1 'affair'." *mBio* 3 (5). doi: 10.1128/mBio.00354-12.

Fauci, A.S. 2012. "Research on highly pathogenic H5N1 influenza virus: The way forward." *mBio* 3 (5). doi: 10.1128/mBio.00359-12.

Fauci, A.S., and F.S. Collins. 2012. "Benefits and risks of influenza research: Lessons learned." *Science* 336 (6088):1522–3. doi: 10.1126/science.1224305.

Fouchier, R.A.M., A. García-Sastre, Y. Kawaoka, W.S. Barclay, N.M. Bouvier, I.H. Brown, I. Capua, et al. 2012. "Pause on avian flu transmission research." *Science* 335 (6067):400–1. doi: 10.1126/science.335.6067.400.

———. 2013. "Transmission studies resume for avian flu." *Science* 339 (6119):520–1. doi: 10.1126/science.1235140.

Gray, R. 2021. "The places that escaped the Spanish flu." *BBC*. Accessed 3 August 2021. www.bbc.com/future/article/20181023-the-places-that-escaped-the-spanish-flu.

Hatchett, R.J., C.E. Mecher, and M. Lipsitch. 2007. "Public health interventions and epidemic intensity during the 1918 influenza pandemic." *Proceedings of the National Academy of Sciences of the United States of America* 104 (18):7582–7. doi: 10.1073/pnas.0610941104.

Herfst, S., E.J.A. Schrauwen, M. Linster, S. Chutinimitkul, E. de Wit, V.J. Munster, E.M. Sorrell, et al. 2012. "Airborne transmission of influenza A/H5N1 virus between ferrets." *Science* 336 (6088):1534–41. doi: 10.1126/science.1213362.

Imai, M., T. Watanabe, M. Hatta, S.C. Das, M. Ozawa, K. Shinya, G. Zhong, et al. 2012. "Experimental adaptation of an influenza H5 HA confers respiratory droplet transmission to a reassortant H5 HA/H1N1 virus in ferrets." *Nature* 486 (7403):420–8. doi: 10.1038/nature10831.

Ison, M.G. 2017. "Antiviral treatments." *Clinics in Chest Medicine* 38 (1):139–53. doi: 10.1016/j.ccm.2016.11.008.

Kobasa, D., S.M. Jones, K. Shinya, J.C. Kash, J. Copps, H. Ebihara, Y. Hatta, et al. 2007. "Aberrant innate immune response in lethal infection of macaques with the 1918 influenza virus." *Nature* 445 (7125):319–23. doi: 10.1038/nature05495.

Kobasa, D., A. Takada, K. Shinya, M. Hatta, P. Halfmann, S. Theriault, H. Suzuki, et al. 2004. "Enhanced virulence of influenza A viruses with the haemagglutinin of the 1918 pandemic virus." *Nature* 431 (7009):703–7. doi: 10.1038/nature02951.

Kolata, G.B. 1999. *Flu: The Story of the Great Influenza Pandemic of 1918 and the Search for the Virus That Caused It*. New York, NY: Farrar, Straus and Giroux.

Krammer, F., G.J.D. Smith, R.A.M. Fouchier, M. Peiris, K. Kedzierska, P.C. Doherty, P. Palese, et al. 2018. "Influenza." *Nature Reviews Disease Primers* 4 (1):3. doi: 10.1038/s41572-018-0002-y.

Lazer, D., R. Kennedy, G. King, and A. Vespignani. 2014. "Big data. The parable of Google Flu: Traps in big data analysis." *Science* 343 (6176):1203–5. doi: 10.1126/science.1248506.

Lostroh, P. 2019. *Molecular and Cellular Biology of Viruses*. 1st ed. Boca Raton, FL: Taylor & Francis Group, LLC.

Machalaba, C.C., S.E. Elwood, S. Forcella, K.M. Smith, K. Hamilton, K.B. Jebara, D.E. Swayne, et al. 2015. "Global avian influenza surveillance in wild birds: A strategy to capture viral diversity." *Emerging Infectious Diseases* 21 (4):e1–7. doi: 10.3201/eid2104.141415.

Memorial, National WWI Museum and Memorial. 2021. "About WWI: Learn more about the conflict that changed the world." Accessed 24 July 2021. www.theworldwar.org/learn/wwi.

Minkoff, E.C., and P.J. Baker. 2004a. "Chapter 16: HIV and AIDS." In *Biology Today: An Issues Approach*, 573–609. New York, NY: Garland Science.

———. 2004b. "Chapter 17: New infectious threats." In *Biology Today: An Issues Approach*, 611–40. New York, NY: Garland Press.

Nelson, M.I., and M. Worobey. 2018. "Origins of the 1918 pandemic: Revisiting the swine 'mixing vessel' hypothesis." *American Journal of Epidemiology* 187 (12):2498–502. doi: 10.1093/aje/kwy150.

Office of Intramural Research, National Institutes of Health. 2021. "Dual-use research." *Department of Health and Human Services*. Accessed 4 August 2021. https://oir.nih.gov/sourcebook/ethical-conduct/special-research-considerations/dual-use-research.

Outka, E. 2020. *Viral Modernism: The Influenza Pandemic and Interwar Literature*. Edited by J. Berman and P. Saint-Amour, *Modernist Latitudes*. New York, NY: Columbia University Press.

Philadelphia, Mütter Museum of the College of Physicians of. 2020. "The 1918 influenza pandemic in Philadelphia exhibit tour." Accessed 28 July 2021. https://www.youtube.com/watch?v=pY2Jo4S15hU&t=901s.

Porter, K.A. 1967. *Pale Horse, Pale Rider: Three Short Novels*. New York, NY: Houghton Mifflin Harcourt Publishing Company.

Pritt, B.S., and M.C. Aubry. 2017. "Histopathology of viral infections of the lung." *Seminars in Diagnostic Pathology* 34 (6):510–7. doi: 10.1053/j.semdp.2017.06.005.

Reid, A.H., T.G. Fanning, J.V. Hultin, and J.K. Taubenberger. 1999. "Origin and evolution of the 1918 "Spanish" influenza virus hemagglutinin gene." *Proceedings of the National Academy of Sciences* 96 (4):1651–6. doi: 10.1073/pnas.96.4.1651.

Ross, M.H., and W. Pawlina. 2011. *Histology*. New York, NY: Lippincott Williams & Wilkins.

Russell, C.A., J.M. Fonville, A.E.X. Brown, D.F. Burke, D.L. Smith, S.L. James, S. Herfst, et al. 2012. "The potential for respiratory droplet—Transmissible A/H5N1 influenza virus to evolve in a mammalian host." *Science* 336 (6088):1541–7. doi: 10.1126/science.1222526.

Sheng, Z.M., D.S. Chertow, X. Ambroggio, S. McCall, R.M. Przygodzki, R.E. Cunningham, O.A. Maximova, J.C. Kash, D.M. Morens, and J.K. Taubenberger. 2011. "Autopsy series of 68 cases dying before and during the 1918 influenza pandemic peak." *Proceedings of the National Academy of Sciences of the United States of America* 108 (39):16416–21. doi: 10.1073/pnas.1111179108.

Short, K.R., K. Kedzierska, and C.E. van de Sandt. 2018. "Back to the future: Lessons learned from the 1918 influenza pandemic." *Frontiers in Cellular and Infection Microbiology* 8:343. doi: 10.3389/fcimb.2018.00343.

Spinney, L. 2017. *Pale Rider: The Spanish Flu of 1918 and How it Changed the World*. New York, NY: PublicAffairs, Hachette Book Group, Perseus Books LLC.

Taubenberger, J.K., J.V. Hultin, and D.M. Morens. 2007. "Discovery and characterization of the 1918 pandemic influenza virus in historical context." *Antiviral Therapy* 12 (4 Pt B):581–91.

Taubenberger, J.K., J.C. Kash, and D.M. Morens. 2019. "The 1918 influenza pandemic: 100 years of questions answered and unanswered." *Science Translational Medicine* 11 (502). doi: 10.1126/scitranslmed.aau5485.

Taubenberger, J.K., and D.M. Morens. 2006. "1918 influenza: The mother of all pandemics." *Emerging Infectious Diseases* 12 (1):15–22. doi: 10.3201/eid1201.050979.

———. 2020. "The 1918 influenza pandemic and its legacy." *Cold Spring Harbor Perspectives in Medicine* 10 (10). doi: 10.1101/cshperspect.a038695.

Taubenberger, J.K., A.H. Reid, A.E. Krafft, K.E. Bijwaard, and T.G. Fanning. 1997. "Initial genetic characterization of the 1918 "Spanish" influenza virus." *Science* 275 (5307):1793–6. doi: 10.1126/science.275.5307.1793.

Tumpey, T.M., C.F. Basler, P.V. Aguilar, H. Zeng, A. Solórzano, D.E. Swayne, N.J. Cox, et al. 2005. "Characterization of the reconstructed 1918 Spanish influenza pandemic virus." *Science* 310 (5745):77–80. doi: 10.1126/science.1119392.

Van Epps, H.L. 2006. "Influenza: Exposing the true killer." *Journal of Experimental Medicine* 203 (4):803. doi: 10.1084/jem.2034fta.

Varki, A. 2008. "Sialic acids in human health and disease." *Trends in Molecular Medicine* 14 (8):351–60. doi: 10.1016/j.molmed.2008.06.002.

Walker, M., and J. Healy. 2020. "A motorcycle rally in a pandemic? 'We kind of knew what was going to happen'." In *The New York Times*. New York, NY: The New York Times Company.

Webster, R.G., W.J. Bean, O.T. Gorman, T.M. Chambers, and Y. Kawaoka. 1992. "Evolution and ecology of influenza A viruses." *Microbiology Reviews* 56 (1):152–79. doi: 10.1128/mr.56.1.152-179.1992.

Wimmer, E., S. Mueller, T.M. Tumpey, and J.K. Taubenberger. 2009. "Synthetic viruses: A new opportunity to understand and prevent viral disease." *Nature Biotechnology* 27 (12):1163–72. doi: 10.1038/nbt.1593.

Wright, L. 2021. *The Plague Year: America in the Time of Covid*. New York, NY: Alfred A. Knopf.

Yu, X., T. Tsibane, P.A. McGraw, F.S. House, C.J. Keefer, M.D. Hicar, T.M. Tumpey, et al. 2008. "Neutralizing antibodies derived from the B cells of 1918 influenza pandemic survivors." *Nature* 455 (7212):532–6. doi: 10.1038/nature07231.

Zimmer, C. 2011. *A Planet of Viruses*. 2nd ed. Chicago, IL: University of Chicago Press.

4

Poliovirus

Learning Outcomes:

4.1 Describe the Details of the Poliovirus Life Cycle and the Disease It Causes, Poliomyelitis (Polio)

4.2 Describe How the Poliovirus Affects Its Victims in the Short Term and Long Term

4.3 Discuss Possible Treatments for Polio before Vaccine

4.4 Interpret the Historical Factors That Contributed to the Spread of the Poliovirus Starting in the Late 19th Century and Peaking in 1940s and 1950s

4.5 Understand How Scientists Raced to Understand Polio through Experimentation, Created a Polio Vaccine, and Eventually Attempted to Eradicate It from the Planet: 1908–1950; 1951–1955 (The Polio Vaccine Race, Salk-IPV); 1956–2000 (Sabin-OPV; Polio Eradication Program)

4.6 Examine the March of Dimes and Mass Vaccination Campaigns

4.7 Describe Worldwide Race to Eradicate Polio and Recent Barriers

4.8 Determine the Lessons Learned from Poliovirus and How Polio Is Still Affecting Society Today, Including Post-Polio Syndrome

4.9 Understand How Other Enteroviruses Are Impacting People Today, as Well as How Genetically Modified Poliovirus May Actually Be Used to Help Cancer Patients

4.1 Describe the Details of the Poliovirus Life Cycle and the Disease It Causes, Poliomyelitis (Polio)

4.1.1 General Background

As an enterovirus, poliovirus enters the body through the digestive system (the mouth) and then multiplies in the pharynx region or lymphatic tissue in the walls of the gastrointestinal tract, before being excreted in waste to potentially be spread to others. When someone is infected with poliovirus, they may present with a headache, sore throat, and/or nausea, or be asymptomatic. Roughly 1% (or a little less) of the time, the virus will enter the central nervous system (CNS; brain and spinal cord) by way of the bloodstream, leading to muscle pain and spasms and potentially causing paralysis, often of the legs. The disease caused by the poliovirus is known as infantile paralysis or poliomyelitis, which became shortened to polio (Oshinsky 2005; Jacobs 2015; Wilson 2005; Paul 1971; Yin-Murphy and Almond 1996). A person with poliovirus can shed virus in their feces for several weeks (CDC 2021b; Yin-Murphy

DOI: 10.1201/9781003172260-4

and Almond 1996). Unlike some other pathogens, poliovirus is not killed by stomach acid or bile, so it can pass through the entire digestive tract (Yin-Murphy and Almond 1996). Polio has now been eradicated from the United States, but hundreds of thousands of people contracted polio in the early to mid-20th century, peaking in the 1940s and 1950s.

Some survivors recalled having a headache and a stiff neck in the evening, and then waking up the next day to partial paralysis. A few former polio patients indicated that they were initially misdiagnosed as having another illness as well (Gould 1995). Scientists know that poliovirus can induce an interferon response initially, which explains the febrile-like illness noted by these polio survivors (Yin-Murphy and Almond 1996). A spinal tap (to obtain cerebrospinal fluid) became the standard for correctly diagnosing polio in the early to mid-20th century (Wilson 2005). Currently, poliovirus can be detected from throat, feces, or cerebrospinal fluid samples that are then used to culture the virus *in vitro* in the laboratory or used in a polymerase chain reaction (PCR) test to detect the poliovirus genome. Sequencing can be used to determine the type of polio, and even the typical geographical location for that strain of the virus (CDC 2021a). People infected with poliovirus also make antibodies against the virus that can be detected in bodily secretions (Yin-Murphy and Almond 1996).

When a child suspected of having polio arrived at the hospital, they were typically placed in isolation, away from their family. The child may have experienced gradual paralysis occurring in the limbs, or difficulty with certain functions like breathing or swallowing during the acute phase of the disease. After moving onto the recovery phase, months of physical therapy, surgeries, and other rehabilitation would take place to see what motor neuron function could be recovered. The children in rehabilitation in the mid-20th century in the United States often formed their own communities in these wards (Wilson 2005).

Specifically, a cell type known as the motor neuron is affected in polio (Oshinsky 2005; Gould 1995; Jacobs 2015). The path that the virus uses to enter the body, multiply, and then move to the CNS took researchers many years to work out. Scientists did not even have the tools needed to do the experiments initially. The details of this scientific research will be described in one of the upcoming sections of the chapter.

Before the polio vaccine, little could be done to prevent outbreaks since the poliovirus was poorly understood. Typical public health guidance included things like avoiding crowds, washing your hands, and not using pools or swimming holes (Oshinsky 2005; Wilson 2005). As Oshinsky remarks in his book, *Polio: An American Story* (p. 5): "No disease drew as much attention, or struck the same terror, as polio. And for good reason. Polio hit without warning. There was no way of telling who would get it and who would be spared."

4.1.2 Virus Classification

Poliovirus is in a family of viruses called picornaviruses within the *Enterovirus* genus. The Coxsackievirus virus is also in the *Enterovirus* genus. Another well-known genus of picornaviruses includes the rhinoviruses causing the common cold (Paul 1971; Yin-Murphy and Almond 1996). Picornaviruses are Baltimore Class IV viruses that contain positive-strand, single-stranded RNA viruses, meaning that their genome is equivalent to an mRNA strand and is read as such by the cellular machinery. Picornaviruses are naked viruses in that they do not have an envelope around them. The viral particle is a 20-sided three-dimensional shape known as an icosahedron that can bind to its receptor on the host cell, and then proteins at or near the surface of the capsid help create a pore so the virus can directly transfer its genome through the cell membrane into the host cell cytoplasm. This relatively simple virus also has a small genome, and the entire genome is translated

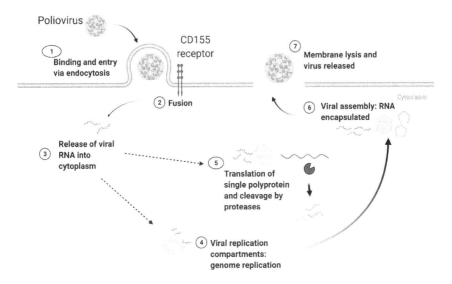

FIGURE 4.1

Life cycle of poliovirus.

Shown here are the steps of the poliovirus life cycle. First, the virus binds to the CD155 receptor and enters the cell. The viral RNA is then released into the cytoplasm where it can be used as a template for translation of a single polyprotein that is then cut into smaller proteins by a protease. Then the genome is replicated in viral replication compartments associated with internal membranes in the cell. The viral proteins and RNA are then encapsulated into the icosahedral shell, and the viral particles burst out of the cell membrane to infect other cells.

Created using Biorender.com.

as one large polyprotein that is then cut by proteases into smaller proteins to do the work of viral replication and particle assembly. When the virus makes a copy of itself, it does so within a viral replication complex that forms to help the virus avoid detection by the immune system (Lostroh 2019; Yin-Murphy and Almond 1996; Racaniello 2006; Baltimore 1971). Then, when the virus leaves the cell, it lyses the cell, bursting open the cell membrane with the help of proteins known as viroporins (Lostroh 2019; Nieva, Madan, and Carrasco 2012). Even though poliovirus is not membrane-bound, cellular membranes are critical for its life cycle, and recent structural biology studies have explored the poliovirus viral replication complexes in detail, which are believed to come from the Golgi intracellular membrane (Belov et al. 2012). The cellular receptor for poliovirus has been identified as a protein known as CD155, which is expressed in a wide variety of tissue types like the brain, spinal cord, skeletal muscle, and kidneys as well as tonsils, small intestine, and large intestine (Mueller, Wimmer, and Cello 2005; Racaniello 2006) (Figure 4.1).

4.2 Describe How the Poliovirus Affects Its Victims in the Short Term and Long Term

In 1916, Dr. Robert Lovett became well known for first publishing the details of the stages of poliomyelitis (acute, convalescent, and chronic). The acute stage occurs within the first few days of poliovirus infection, and it is not yet clear the extent of the damage done by the virus. In the convalescent or recovery phase, it is possible for some or most bodily capabilities to return. Finally, when the patient stabilizes, any remaining muscle weakness or paralysis would likely persist for the person's lifetime as a part of a chronic condition (Gould 1995; Oshinsky 2005; Paul 1971). Modern guidelines for physicians break down the acute stage of polio into two phases: minor illness in which the patient might have a fever and a few other symptoms not involving the nervous system or major illness where involvement of the brain and/or spinal cord can happen. If paralysis occurs, it will peak at about two to four days after it starts to occur, with recovery lasting up to six months later when progress begins to level off and the predicted outcome for the patient becomes clearer. Also, since poliovirus can attack the brain stem and/or the anterior horn section of the spinal cord, paralysis can be classified as spinal, bulbar (brain stem-based) or spino-bulbar (both) (Routh, Oberste, and Patel 2014). Poliovirus can also affect the cerebral cortex, in addition to the brain stem and spinal cord (Yin-Murphy and Almond 1996).

Dr. W.H. Frost and his colleagues at the Public Health Service publicized several critical details about the spread of polio at about the same time after the 1916 epidemic in the United States. First, poliovirus primarily was spread from person to person, not through an animal vector. Second, there were many people acting as carriers, who may not have known that they were sick. These individuals may have had no symptoms, or the symptoms would be mild. Those cases resulting in paralysis are in the minority (Gould 1995). A recognizable case of poliomyelitis that does not result in paralysis is also known as non-paralytic or abortive poliomyelitis. A case that causes paralysis is called paralytic or true poliomyelitis (Oshinsky 2005; Paul 1971).

The most recent statistics from the Centers for Disease Control and Prevention (CDC) indicate that approximately 72% of people with poliovirus show no symptoms at all. Approximately 25% of individuals with poliovirus show the flu-like symptoms mentioned previously such as fever and sore throat. A very small number of those with poliovirus show neurological symptoms including features like life-threatening paralysis. Some form of paralysis affects approximately one out of every 200 people with poliovirus (CDC 2021b). Some scientists studying how the poliovirus causes disease even consider the entry of the poliovirus, an enterovirus, into the nervous system as a type of accident (Racaniello 2006; Mueller, Wimmer, and Cello 2005).

The CDC also clarifies that indicating someone has the disease, polio, means that they are actually displaying some form of paralysis (CDC 2021b). One should note that nervous tissue is typically not capable of regenerating, so dead nerve cells cannot be replaced, unlike tissues in the body capable of replacing themselves (Paul 1971). The human nervous system can be divided into two parts: the central nervous system (CNS) and the peripheral nervous system (PNS). The CNS includes the brain and spinal cord, and the PNS includes all the nerves either sending information to the CNS or sending information out from the CNS, as well as the sense organs. The main cell types of the nervous system include the neuron, also called a nerve cell, and the support cells known as glial cells. As mentioned earlier, poliovirus attacks the motor neurons, which are responsible for sending signals to muscles and glands, including both involuntary and voluntary movements. Motor neurons have a particular orientation related to their ability to convey information: the cellular projections called dendrites receive information into the cell, the information is processed in the cell body, and then the signal goes out to another neuron or directly to muscle via an axon. The orientation of motor neurons is important for understanding the significance of different parts of the spinal cord. The spinal cord is in the vertebral column. If one were to take a cross section of the spinal cord, one would see that there is gray matter on the inside, around a

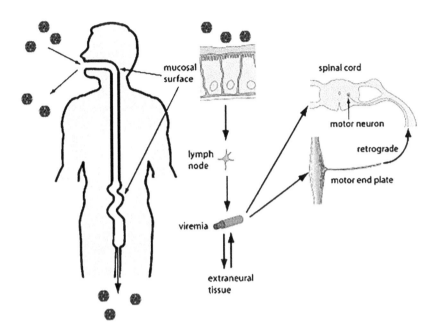

FIGURE 4.2
How poliovirus enters the body, reproduces, and causes disease.

When poliovirus enters the body, it makes copies of itself at mucosal surfaces including those in the pharynx and gastrointestinal tract. The virus then goes into lymph nodes and from there can get into the bloodstream. Poliovirus can attack the central nervous system either right from the blood or by getting into motor neuron axons at neuromuscular junctions. The virus can also multiply in soft tissue outside of nerves (extraneural tissue).

Source: Racaniello, V.R. 2006. "One hundred years of poliovirus pathogenesis." *Virology* 344 (1):9–16. doi: 10.1016/j. virol.2005.09.015. PMID: 16364730. (Permission obtained through RightsLink.)

central canal, with white matter around the gray matter core. The cell bodies and dendrites are in the gray matter, and the axons are in the white matter. The ventral horn or anterior part of the spinal cord has the axons of the motor neurons to send signals for movement away from the spinal cord. The sensory neurons bringing signals in are on the opposite side (Ross and Pawlina 2011). A French doctor named Charcot studied spinal cord samples taken from children who died of polio in the late 19th century and determined that there was damage to the anterior part of the gray matter of the spinal cord, what he already knew as the location important for motor neuron function. No bacteria were present, so Charcot's findings also suggested that polio was a viral disease (Jacobs 2015; Paul 1971) (Figure 4.2).

4.3 Discuss Possible Treatments for Polio before Vaccine

In the acute stage of polio, a physician might need to put the patient in an iron lung to assist with breathing if weakness of the diaphragm muscles occurs. Some doctors like Lovett emphasized the need for bed rest during this stage. During convalescence or

A.

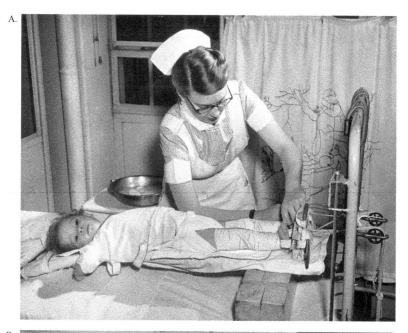

B.

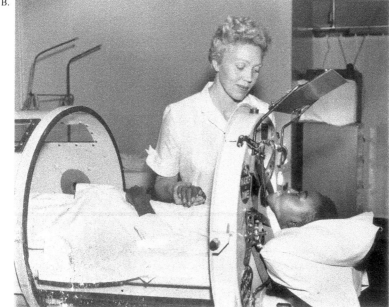

FIGURE 4.3
Young polio patients in the United States in the mid-20th century.

Shown in (A) is an image of a child with polio being treated with leg splints in 1948.

Photo credit: George D. McDowell Collection, Philadelphia Evening Tribune, SCRC170, Organizations-Community Chest-1948-1949, "Adventures of a ten-dollar bill-what happens to your red feather contribution/ P386047M." Special Collections Research Center, Temple University Libraries, Philadelphia, PA. Used with permission.

Shown in (B) is an image of a child with polio in an iron lung. "Boy in an Iron Lung is attended by a nurse, Herman Kiefer Hospital, Detroit, Michigan," (NCP 4147-1). OHA 250 New Contributed Photographs. Otis Historical Archives, National Museum of Health and Medicine. Used with permission. No photograph date available.

recovery, muscle manipulation and mineral baths/hydrotherapy were used. The United States president Franklin Delano Roosevelt (FDR), a polio survivor, helped to make hydrotherapy popular (Gould 1995; Oshinsky 2005). Some healthcare providers decided to splint the affected limbs or place them in casts at this stage of the disease, which potentially could affect recovery if kept on for too long (Oshinsky 2005; Paul 1971). A nurse/physical therapist from Australia named Sister Elizabeth Kenny advocated for getting the child's muscles moving as soon as possible with light exercise and applying hot packs to the muscles. Her methods were controversial but popular among the public in the 1930s and 1940s (Gould 1995; Oshinsky 2005; Wilson 2005; Paul 1971). If a patient entered the chronic stage of the illness without being able to breathe on his or her own, the patient might need to be in the iron lung for life. Crutches or a wheelchair might be needed if partial paralysis remained in the limbs (Oshinsky 2005) (Figure 4.3).

4.4 Interpret the Historical Factors That Contributed to the Spread of the Poliovirus Starting in the Late 19th Century and Peaking in 1940s and 1950s

Poliovirus was known to strike in the summer, just like when it struck FDR in the summer of 1921. The virus was known to spread when someone failed to wash their hands after using the bathroom, contaminating the food or water used by others. Surprisingly, many attributed the development of better standards for delivering clean water and removing human wastes from urban areas with the emergence of poliovirus epidemics. Despite the benefits of modern sanitation, the improved cleanliness meant that young children did not encounter the virus at a very young age when they were still protected by their mother's antibodies against poliovirus (Colt 2009; Oshinsky 2005; Jacobs 2015; Wilson 2005; Paul 1971). Medical historians noted that depictions or accounts of paralysis of the limbs in early literature and art may have been polio, with these accounts going all the way back to the time of the ancient Egyptians (Oshinsky 2005; Jacobs 2015). In his book, A *History of Poliomyelitis*, Paul notes that both changes in human protection against poliovirus and in the way that poliovirus can spread in a population led to "bringing a disease to the surface which had been in existence long before, although more or less hidden" (p. 10).

Polio was first documented in modern history in Scandinavia in the late 19th century (Gould 1995; Paul 1971), although others indicated that sporadic case clusters may have been occurring since the mid-1800s in Western Europe and the United States.

The first major U.S. epidemic occurred in Vermont in 1894. A respected Vermont doctor at the time, Dr. Charles Caverly, indicated that most cases occurred in males, displaying symptoms mentioned earlier such as tiredness, headache, fever, and a stiff neck. He also had identified the presence of mild so called "abortive" cases of poliomyelitis (Oshinsky 2005; Jacobs 2015; Paul 1971). New York had its first epidemic in 1916 (Gould 1995; Oshinsky 2005; Jacobs 2015; Paul 1971). During the epidemic, the city focused on improving general hygiene practices because public health officials did not know how to prevent the spread of the poliovirus in a targeted way. In the meantime, immigrants were blamed for spreading the disease. Rich people sent their children away for the summer to live outside New York City (Oshinsky 2005; Gould 1995). However, after the epidemic, the Public Health Service was able to summarize their findings during the epidemic and report that there was no animal or insect host for the virus, poliovirus infection was more common than first realized because of all the asymptomatic cases, and that most of the transmission came from these asymptomatic cases (Paul 1971).

In the summer of 1921, FDR became ill with polio most likely while visiting a Boy Scout camp. After his recovery, he became committed to helping other polio survivors in their recovery by setting up a retreat in Warm Springs, Georgia, for hydrotherapy (Gould 1995; Oshinsky 2005; Jacobs 2015). FDR helped change attitudes towards polio survivors by increasing the public awareness and funding for rehabilitation (Wilson 2005; Paul 1971). He established a nonprofit organization with his law partner Basil O'Connor called the Georgia Warm Springs Foundation that hosted a number of "Birthday Balls" on FDR's birthday to raise money annually for the foundation for several years. In 1938, FDR decided to change his fundraising strategy in the fight against polio, starting the National Foundation for Infantile Paralysis (NFIP) or National Foundation, with the fundraising arm better known as the March of Dimes. This organization's goals extended those of the Birthday Balls, including raising money for curing polio and polio treatment (Jacobs 2015; Oshinsky 2005). The National Foundation turned polio into "America's greatest medical crusade" (Oshinsky 2005). There was no infrastructure in place to deal with the thousands of polio survivors in the United States when the National Foundation was founded, and this private organization helped fund millions of dollars' worth of research and facilities for patient rehabilitation, as well as even paying patient medical bills (Oshinsky 2005).

Close friends and family of FDR debated if the illness made any difference in FDR's personality since polio struck him when he was 39 years old, well into adulthood (Gould 1995). Although potentially devastating for any individual, having a prominent figure like FDR get paralytic polio ended up being a hugely important event in moving the United States towards polio awareness, treatment, and then eventually a vaccine trial, privately funded by NFIP.

4.5 Understand How Scientists Raced to Understand Polio through Experimentation, Created a Polio Vaccine, and Eventually Attempted to Eradicate It from the Planet: 1908–1950; 1951–1955 (The Polio Vaccine Race, Salk-IPV); 1956–2000 (Sabin-OPV; Polio Eradication Program)

4.5.1 1908–1950

The scientists Landsteiner and Popper found the infectious agent for poliomyelitis in 1908. Like other virus research at the time, it had to be conducted without being able to see the virus, but instead by identifying an infectious entity that could pass through a fine pore filter, unlike bacteria. The researchers took a sample from the spinal cord of a polio victim, filtered it, and then injected it into two monkeys' brains. They both became ill (Oshinsky 2005; Gould 1995; Jacobs 2015; Paul 1971).

Flexner of the Rockefeller Institute became famous for repeating Landsteiner's experiments and conducting additional groundbreaking polio research. The work was challenging because it involved direct introduction of the poliovirus into monkeys, since they were not a natural host for the virus (Oshinsky 2005). There was not much progress in polio research for quite a while. Monkeys seemed to be the only useful model system, and they were expensive (Gould 1995). Flexner became sidetracked by his observations of poliomyelitis as it spread in an artificial experimental situation in monkeys in the laboratory rather than in natural human cases. For example, Flexner never wavered from his belief that poliovirus was entering the brain through the olfactory nerves in the nose, which was not supported by the research results of other scientists (Paul 1971).

The year 1935 was not a good one for polio research. That year, the researchers Park and Brodie tested a vaccine candidate made of killed virus on monkeys and then moved onto humans, including themselves and a group of children in their vaccine trial (Oshinsky 2005; Jacobs 2015; Paul 1971; Gould 1995). Brodie described an account of the initial vaccine testing of a formalin-treated poliovirus on monkeys and then children in the *American Journal of Public Health and the Nation's Health* (Brodie 1935). However, when Park and Brodie attempted to scale up the trials, they were so poorly organized that the results were hard to interpret, and some children may have even gotten polio from the vaccination. A competitor of Park and Brodie, John Kolmer, tested a live virus vaccine on himself, his family, and other children around the same time, with similar results (Oshinsky 2005; Jacobs 2015; Paul 1971). This was a major setback in the quest for a polio vaccine, and it would take almost 20 years before the success of the Salk vaccine (Oshinsky 2005). However, Salk would revisit the idea of a polio vaccine created using an inactivated virus, as first studied by Park and Brodie, when he developed his own vaccine in the 1950s (Paul 1971).

At this point, the National Foundation, under a new director, Thomas Rivers, shifted its focus to basic research projects (Oshinsky 2005). In the next few years, NFIP focused on three major areas of research to bring the world closer to a polio vaccine. These areas of basic research include determining the types of polioviruses, finding the route taken through the body to cause disease in the CNS, and discovering how to maintain the virus in tissue culture cells. Jonas Salk's first big project with the NFIP involved doing strain typing (Gould 1995; Oshinsky 2005; Paul 1971). Knowing the types of polioviruses is critical to designing a vaccine and testing for immunity in patients, since the different types are all recognized slightly differently by our immune systems (Paul 1971).

This narrowing of the focus of the NFIP on basic research reminds us that even though the public was pushing for a disease cure, the groundwork for understanding a disease is laid through basic research, to better understand the virus and develop necessary tools to manipulate it. Developing an *in vitro* culture method was critical to being able to create a vaccine. Up to this point, monkeys were the primary system used for poliovirus research. Using monkeys was a costly process, involving transfer of animal nervous tissue. Monkeys would continue to be used even after culturing methods were developed, like in testing vaccine safety, for example. However, tissue-culturing methods had been tested since the 1930s. Sabin and Olitsky published their findings of growing poliovirus in cultured nervous tissue (Oshinsky 2005; Sabin and Olitsky 1936; Paul 1971). Many scientists thought that poliovirus could only be grown in nervous tissue, until Enders, Weller, and Robbins were able to culture the virus in skin, muscle, and tissue (Oshinsky 2005). Their discovery earned them the Nobel Prize in Physiology or Medicine in 1954 (Nobel Prize Outreach AB, 2021).

Finding the path of poliovirus into the body and through the body was also critical in stopping polio. Researchers needed to figure out how poliovirus gets to the central nervous system. When scientists tried to block the nose or develop a prophylactic spray, the experiments failed (Gould 1995). Many scientists, like Flexner, relied strictly on the monkey studies to point to olfactory tissue and the upper respiratory tract as the point of entry for poliovirus. In contrast, Sabin and Ward conducted autopsy studies of human polio victims in 1941 and determined that the alimentary canal was actually the point of entry (Oshinsky 2005). The details from seven autopsy cases in which 20 different kinds of tissue were carefully dissected in each autopsy were reported. Strikingly, the predominance of poliovirus in the walls of the gastrointestinal tract, and not in the upper respiratory tract, indicated that poliovirus was getting in through the digestive system and not the respiratory system (Sabin and Ward 1941). Dorothy Horstmann performed experiments on chimpanzees in which she introduced the virus to monkeys through the mouth, and then found the virus in their blood within several days (Horstmann 1952; Oshinsky 2005). The work of Horstmann, along with Bodian, Howe, and Morgan at Johns Hopkins University, solidified the theory that poliovirus entered the CNS via the bloodstream (Oshinsky 2005; Jacobs 2015; Paul 1971). Isabel Morgan, daughter of the famous geneticist Thomas Hunt Morgan, developed a vaccine using killed poliovirus that effectively immunized monkeys against the disease (Oshinsky 2005; Gould 1995; Jacobs 2015; Paul 1971). However, in 1949, Morgan made the decision to leave Hopkins to resettle in New York and raise a family, and no one immediately picked up with her research the lab, bringing the work to a halt (Oshinsky 2005). Hilary Koprowski, working at Lederle Labs, was testing a live attenuated poliovirus vaccine that he eventually gave to a small group of institutionalized children in 1950 in a controversial vaccine trial. In the post–World War II era, other polio researchers raised concern over consent for such studies, but none of the children became ill and the world moved ever closer to a vaccine for the masses (Oshinsky 2005; Jacobs 2015).

4.5.2 1951–1955 The Polio Vaccine Race

Three main research teams were competing to be the first to produce a polio vaccine for the United States: Albert Sabin of the University of Cincinnati, who was developing a live vaccine, Jonas Salk of the University of Pittsburgh, who was developing an inactivated or killed vaccine, and Hilary Koprowski of Lederle Labs, who was also developing a live vaccine (Oshinsky 2005). Eventually, Salk won the race, and his national vaccine trials in 1954 involved over a million schoolchildren (Oshinsky 2005).

In 1951, as Salk wrapped up his work with the typing project for NFIP, he received additional funding to accelerate his work on developing a vaccine. Salk expanded his lab, adding key personnel like Bazeley, Ward, and Youngner, among others, so that they could use the Enders method of growing poliovirus in non-nerve cells in tissue culture. They developed a method to culture monkey kidney cells that seemed to work well for growing the virus (Oshinsky 2005; Jacobs 2015). Since poliovirus has three possible circulating types, I, II, and III, all three would need to be represented in the vaccine. Salk carefully selected the strains to use to represent each type, choosing the controversial Mahoney strain to represent Type I. This strain was a highly virulent strain that Salk thought would be great to induce immune protection, but other researchers feared that it was a higher risk choice for manipulation to make a part of a vaccine. Salk and his team figured out how much formaldehyde, at what temperature, and for how long was needed to inactivate the virus. The vaccine was then injected into monkeys, and if no monkeys became ill, they were sacrificed one month later, and their tissues examined for evidence of the virus. The results of these experiments were presented at the first NFIP Immunization Committee meeting in 1951. Some of the other scientists on the committee questioned Salk's method, encouraging the use of a live attenuated virus in the vaccine over Salk's method of using inactivated virus. One of his strongest critics was Albert Sabin, an advocate for a live virus vaccine as the only way to go (Oshinsky 2005). The NFIP decided to continue Salk's project anyway, without seeking endorsement of the other scientists for the project. Basil O'Connor and other key leaders in the NFIP supported Salk and would push the project on to get their vaccine (Oshinsky 2005).

Salk tested his vaccine on two different homes for disabled children in 1952. Sensitive to the issue of patient consent, Salk is said to have personally met with the children's parents or guardians when he could. In addition, the children at one of the homes were polio survivors, so their vaccines were chosen based on what strain of the poliovirus they had already had, an attempt to raise their antibody levels against the virus rather than induce them anew. This approach was considered lower risk than giving the vaccine to non-polio survivors. The pilot trials work (Oshinsky 2005; Jacobs 2015).

Public pressure mounted even more for a vaccination campaign, given that there were 57,000 cases of polio reported in the United States in 1952, and the average age of the person getting polio was going up as well for unknown reasons (Wilson 2005; Oshinsky 2005). For example, in the 1916 epidemic, most cases were in children under the age of four, but in the 1940s and 50s, there were many cases in the range of five to nine years of age and in children greater than ten years old (Wilson 2005; Paul 1971). Salk presented the results of his pilot trial in 1953 to the NFIP Immunization Committee. Again, many of the other scientists seemed to be stuck in their own belief that a dead virus could not give a sufficient sustainable immune response. Some scientists encouraged Salk to proceed cautiously and not risk his career for the wishes of the NFIP. On some level, this was good advice, but Salk was confident in his method and results, only wanting a little more time to prepare for field trials. He eventually participated in interviews with the press to start to get the word out about the vaccine he was testing. Basil O'Connor of the NFIP formed a new vaccine advisory committee to prepare for large-scale vaccine trials, working around the other NFIP-funded scientists who questioned Salk's approach (Oshinsky 2005; Jacobs 2015).

Planning for the 1954 vaccine field trials got underway. With the permission of their parents, almost 1.5 million first, second, and third graders from 211 counties around the United States participated in the field trials. Some children received the actual vaccine and others acted as controls, in a trial design representing a compromise between what government officials and what Salk and the NFIP wanted for a study design. Children in these grades were selected because they were in the age group with the highest incidence of polio in the seasonal outbreaks. The use of both observed controls, children who were monitored to see if they got polio but were given no injections, and placebo controls, where half the children were not given the vaccine but instead a control injection, was an unusual study design. The placebo-controlled studies were double blind, in that neither the doctors nor the children knew who got the vaccine and who got the placebo until the end of the study. In the observed controls, the second graders got the vaccine, and the children in the first and third grades acted as observed controls. Because of the risk of contracting polio, public buy-in for the placebo type control was harder to find, even though this is the typical model for a rigorous medical trial. Nevertheless, through the participation of thousands of volunteers like doctors, school officials, and local public officials, the data from both approaches were successfully collected in an organized way that could be evaluated (Meldrum 1998; Oshinsky 2005; Jacobs 2015).

Before giving the vaccine to the children, each batch of vaccine was triple-checked for safety, with the vaccines being made by two companies: Eli Lilly and Parke-Davis. Salk initially tested the vaccine in the Pittsburgh area with 5,000 children, and then the large-scale trial started. The participating schoolchildren became known as "Polio Pioneers" and were given a special card and button for their participation (Jacobs 2015).

Thomas Francis of the University of Michigan was responsible for analyzing the results of the vaccine trial. The results were announced at the University of Michigan on April 12, 1955, the ten-year anniversary of FDR's death (Oshinsky 2005; Jacobs 2015; Paul 1971). The vaccine worked (Francis et al. 1955)! Church bells rang out across the country (Oshinsky 2005; Gould 1995; Jacobs 2015). Now a mass vaccination campaign across the United States could begin. Salk did not pursue a patent for his vaccine either, indicating that the vaccine really belonged to the people, a decision unheard of in today's pharmaceutical industry (Oshinsky 2005; Jacobs 2015). Salk received a presidential citation from Eisenhower in 1955 (Jacobs 2015). The impact of the vaccination campaign was quickly seen in the United States, with the cases of paralytic polio in the country dropping off precipitously after the 1950s (CDC 2021b) (Figure 4.4).

However, one cannot mention the 1955 mass vaccination campaign using the Salk vaccine without bringing up the tragic incident in which 11 people died from polio due to an issue with several batches of the vaccine created by Cutter Laboratories in California (Gould 1995; Oshinsky 2005; Paul 1971). When the polio vaccine was first approved for mass distribution, the federal government left the plans up to private companies, including Cutter Labs. Then, some children who had recently received a polio vaccine came down with polio, and their vaccines were specifically tracked back to Cutter labs. At this point, the United States government did step in and temporarily halt vaccine distribution. The Public Health Service created a Polio Surveillance Unit to review what happened at Cutter Labs once they were identified as the source of bad vaccine. Unlike the triple checking of the polio vaccine used in Salk's 1954 field trial, vaccines now made by companies were reviewed in a much shorter process. No single specific reason was ever found for the defective vaccine, but changes in either the storage of or protocol for inactivating the virus with formaldehyde most likely resulted in the error (Oshinsky 2005; Bodian et al. 1955).

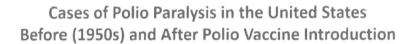

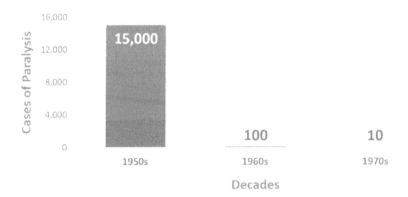

FIGURE 4.4

Cases of paralytic polio in the United States before and after vaccine introduction.

Shown in this image are the cases of paralytic polio seen in the United States in the 1950s, 1960s, and 1970s. Note that the development of the polio vaccine in 1955, followed by a mass vaccination campaign, led to a dramatic reduction in the cases of paralytic polio in the 1960s and 1970s.

From www.cdc.gov/polio/what-is-polio/polio-us.html

Credit: Centers for Disease Control and Prevention (CDC), material in the public domain (www.cdc.gov/media/subtopic/questions.htm).

Sabin used the Cutter incident as an opportunity to renew his objections to the use of the virulent Mahoney strain in Salk's vaccine. Even though no other "Cutter" incidents occurred and the Salk vaccine was otherwise safe, the fears and insecurities raised by the incident created an opening for others to offer an alternative (Oshinsky 2005).

4.5.3 1956–2000 Sabin-OPV and the Global Polio Eradication Program

Although the rivalry between Salk and Sabin was more or less intense, depending on your source of information, there was actually room for both of their approaches in saving the world from polio. Sabin was working on a live attenuated vaccine taken orally, following the same path of entry as the natural poliovirus as an enterovirus through the gastrointestinal tract. Since it was a live vaccine, which still underwent viral replication, it could also confer passive immunity to those around the child in the days after vaccination. Sabin was also planning a vaccine to be taken as a single dose, unlike the three shots required by the Salk vaccine (Oshinsky 2005). It is important to note that the development of a cheaper vaccine, Sabin's vaccine, readily accessible to the rest of the world, was also critical to controlling poliomyelitis (Paul 1971). Unable to get approval for a mass vaccination program in the United States, Sabin eventually went to Russia and formed a working relationship with Mikail Chumakov, the head of the Polio Research Institute in Moscow. In 1959, 10 million Russian children were vaccinated using the Sabin vaccine, either as a single dose or in three separate doses for each type. Dorothy Horstmann, a well-respected American polio researcher, gave a preliminary evaluation of the vaccine trials for the World Health Organization (WHO) and reported that the vaccine had appeared to reduce the number of cases of paralytic polio in the Soviet Union (Oshinsky 2005; Horstmann 1991; Jacobs 2015).

Back in the U.S. in 1959, polio became "a disease of the unvaccinated" where new cases arose in children who had not been vaccinated, mainly in poor urban areas. A couple of live virus vaccines were being tested in trials around the world, such as by Koprowski, but Sabin and Cox got permission to do trials on a live virus vaccine in the U.S. in 1960, which was then approved to start the process of being licensed for distribution. In 1961, the American Medical Association then made the decision to support their Council on Drugs' recommendation to replace the Salk vaccine with the Sabin vaccine (Oshinsky 2005; Jacobs 2015) (Figure 4.5).

The use of the oral polio vaccine (OPV) was in place in the United States until the year 2000 when the recommendation was changed back to exclusively the inactivated polio vaccine (IPV). From 1961 to 2000, there were reports of a very small number of cases of paralytic polio, mostly in adults, caused by exposure to someone who had recently taken the OPV or by OPV itself. These cases did not change the recommendation for the vaccine strategy for many years (Blume and Geesink 2000; Alexander et al. 2004). Researchers estimated that between 1961 and 1989, there were nine cases per year in the United States (out of the millions of polio vaccine doses administered) of polio acquired directly or indirectly from the vaccine, also known as vaccine-associated paralytic poliomyelitis (VAPP). An epidemiological study found that no cases of VAPP have occurred in the United States since the switch to IPV in the year 2000 (Alexander et al. 2004).

Other countries, like the Netherlands, kept using IPV and even worked to improve it so it could be combined with other vaccines for patient delivery (Blume and Geesink 2000). Salk himself had a hand in working on a better version of the IPV vaccine called enhanced potency IPV or eIPV (Jacobs 2015). The cheaper, more effective OPV developed by Sabin is still used in many parts of the world as a part of the WHO's campaign to eradicate polio. Although the WHO missed their original deadline of the year 2000 to eradicate the

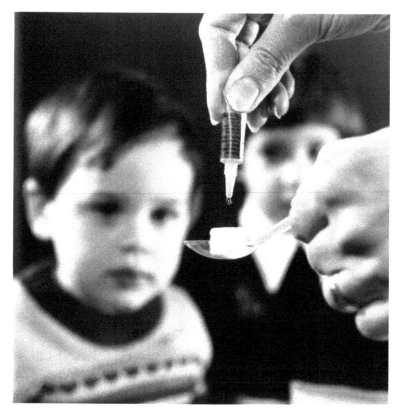

FIGURE 4.5
Oral polio vaccine (OPV) to be given to a child.

Shown here is the oral polio vaccine being dropped on a sugar cube so it can be administered to the child in the background.

Photo credit: "Wellcome polio vaccine," CC BY4.0 (https://wellcomecollection.org/works/qps38n3k).

poliovirus, they are still actively working to immunize people in the remaining countries where polio is endemic (Blume and Geesink 2000).

In Asia and Africa, there have been outbreaks of vaccine-derived polio, leading some scientists to call for a new oral polio vaccine, in particular against serotype 2, which has been the primary source of the vaccine-derived poliovirus circulating in those places. The new vaccine would be made in such a way to reduce the chance of reversion to a paralytic polio-causing strain (Donlan and Petri 2020; Macklin et al. 2020). Another strategy is to reintroduce IPV and begin to phase out OPV containing type 2, in favor of a bivalent OPV—only against type 1 and type 3 (Kew and Pallansch 2018). Other scientists have cautioned that resistant strains may arise from type 1 and type 3 as well, favoring immunization with IPV followed by a trivalent OPV using all three polio strain types (Chumakov et al. 2021). As one can see, completing eradication of polio from the planet is a complicated issue, and it may still take years to see what the best approach is for eliminating the OPV-derived cases.

In the end, both Salk and Sabin made huge contributions to the reduction of death and suffering caused by polio, although neither scientist won the Nobel Prize. One might ask if their rivalry was an example of healthy competition driving scientific research forward or unhealthy posturing holding scientific research back. Either way, their rivalry, like other scientific rivalries, did reveal to us the real human factor always present in scientific research. In certain accounts, it has been mentioned that Sabin protested Salk's vaccine trial strategy from the beginning (Oshinsky 2005). However, others have pointed out that Sabin emphasized his main concern was the use of the Mahoney strain in the inactivated vaccine, as well as his belief that a live polio vaccine was needed to eradicate polio. Sabin claimed not to have had a grudge against Salk personally, and that Sabin was working on many other infectious diseases as well over the years, not being in a singular battle with Salk over polio (Jimenez 2014). The rivalry may have also been built up by the press (Jacobs 2015). Others will argue that Sabin was the real innovator who had the courage to push for a type of vaccination strategy that could be administered to the whole world (Matysiak 2005; Institute 2021). After his work with the polio vaccine, Salk went on to form an institute in La Jolla, California, known as the Salk Institute, where he hoped to bring together those studying the sciences and the humanities to collaborate. He also continued research, even participating in the development of a candidate AIDS vaccine in the 1980s (Jacobs 2015).

4.6 Examine the March of Dimes and Mass Vaccination Campaigns

The fundraising arm of the National Foundation for Infantile Paralysis, the March of Dimes, was able to successfully complete their mission of protecting America's children from polio. During the Great Depression and even World War II, the foundation adapted and kept raising money to fight polio through an amazing marketing campaign. Impressively, the NFIP privately funded Salk's vaccination trials, something that would be done today through significant collaboration with either national or international governmental partners. Certain aspects of disease fundraising, such as using "Poster Children," was first used by the March of Dimes as well (Oshinsky 2005). The March of Dimes also affected the public's awareness of and attention to one particular disease, polio, among many other diseases that can affect children. Their successful mission illustrated that public perception of a disease is critical to raising the political will and capital to tackle an expensive task like eliminating a disease. One modern fundraising comparison might be to the "Ice Bucket Challenge" campaign for amyotrophic lateral sclerosis (ALS), which swept the United States in 2014, raising $115 million dollars for ALS research (The ALS Association 2019). Now, imagine a sustained fundraising challenge happening from 1938 to 1955! After the Salk vaccine came out, the National Foundation for Infantile Paralysis changed its name to National Foundation and shifted its focus to birth defects and arthritis, continuing its mission to help America's children. It is known today exclusively as the March of Dimes (Jacobs 2015; Rose 2010) (Figure 4.6).

The testing of a new vaccine on children also raises ethical issues in the conducting of scientific research. A new biomedical product would likely not be first tested on children today. We will discuss the ethics of medical research and other issues of public health in Chapter 8.

A.

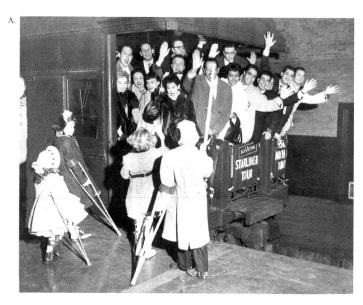

B.

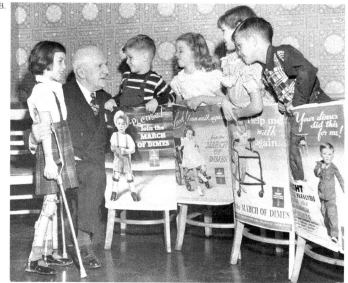

FIGURE 4.6
March of Dimes campaign photographs.

Shown here are two March of Dimes campaign photographs used in the *Philadelphia Evening Tribune* in the 1950s. In A, one sees children who survived polio (on crutches) greeting celebrities on a train pulling out of 30th Street Station. The celebrities were a part of the 1956 RCA Victor Starliner Tour. In B, children who survived polio hold up posters at an event, along with Joseph F. Gallagher, the Philadelphia chairperson for the March of Dimes in 1950.

Photo credits: (A) George D. McDowell Collection, Philadelphia Evening Tribune, SCRC170, Polio victims greet entertainers on tour for infantile paralysis/P401106B, Special Collections Research Center, Temple University Libraries, Philadelphia, PA. Used with permission.

(B) George D. McDowell Collection, Philadelphia Evening Tribune, SCRC170, Children with polio hold posters to support the March of Dimes/P401107B, Special Collections Research Center, Temple University Libraries, Philadelphia, PA. Used with permission.

4.7 Describe Worldwide Race to Eradicate Polio and Recent Barriers

Some may ask: why do we need to eradicate any disease? Well, if eradication were declared, then countries would no longer need to spend the time and money vaccinating their people. The world has all the scientific tools needed to eradicate polio, including knowledge of the virus itself and a vaccine.

When one examines the biology of a virus to see if it lends itself to eradication, polio is a good candidate. For example, it has no natural animal reservoir outside of humans, so if eradicated from humans it would be eradicated from the planet. In addition, when someone is infected with poliovirus, they eventually clear the infection; it is not maintained in the body in a latent state like with some viruses such as herpesviruses (Kew and Pallansch 2018). The next step has been the part that has been difficult to complete: having the political will and the organizational infrastructure necessary to distribute the vaccine to all the children of the world (Closser 2010; Kew and Pallansch 2018). It is important to note that people must be protected from all three types of polioviruses for eradication to work. The existing IPV protects against all three types, but there are different variations of the OPV, each one protecting against one, two, or three types of wild poliovirus. In addition to eradication through vaccination, what is known as "containment," making sure that stocks of the poliovirus are not around in labs or other research centers, is a part of the eradication plan as well (Poliovirus 2020).

The Global Polio Eradication Initiative (GPEI) is a "public-private partnership led by national governments with six partners—the World Health Organization (WHO), Rotary International, the U.S. Centers for Disease Control and Prevention (CDC), the United Nations Children's Fund (UNICEF), Bill & Melinda Gates Foundation, and Gavi, the vaccine alliance" (WHO 2021b). According to their website, GPEI has vaccinated 2.5 billion children (WHO 2021b). The GPEI was formed in 1988 after the success of regional polio vaccination campaigns and the completed eradication of another virus, smallpox, in 1977 (Kew and Pallansch 2018). In 1994, the WHO region of the Americas was declared free of wild poliovirus. India reported their last polio case in 2011, and the WHO region of South-East Asia was declared polio-free in 2014 (2021c). Another major step forward in the GPEI came in 2020 when wild polio was eradicated from Africa. On August 25, 2020, the WHO Africa region was declared free of wild polio since no new cases of wild polio had been reported in four years. With this declaration, 90% of the people of the world were now considered free from wild polio. The only two countries left in the world with circulating wild polio are Pakistan and Afghanistan (WHO 2021a). However, the world will still need to address the issue of vaccine-derived poliovirus (Donlan and Petri 2020; Macklin et al. 2020) (Figure 4.7).

Many people who are a part of the GPEI have been working earnestly to eliminate polio in Pakistan. In one author's account of her work in Pakistan in 2006 and 2007, the failure to eliminate polio from the country is tied to significant "management issues" on the ground, rather than cultural issues or a lack of knowledge of the problem. She also adds that the same global inequality issues that promote the transmission of diseases in poorer countries can also inhibit the eradication of a disease. In addition, there can be issues when outside organizations like the WHO dictate the structure and plan for a vaccine initiative inside a country (Closser 2010). Another issue mentioned in Closser's account includes the need for many more vaccinations per individual where poliovirus is endemic. Most vaccination is done seasonally, with teams of vaccinators fanning out across areas where polio cases have been reported. Some children are vaccinated every time, up to ten or more

A.

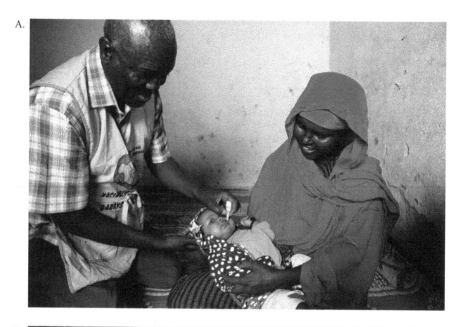

B.

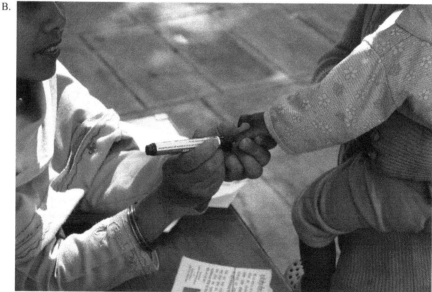

FIGURE 4.7
Children being vaccinated through the Global Polio Eradication Initiative (GPEI).

Shown in these photos are children being vaccinated with oral polio vaccine as a part of the United Nations' Global Polio Eradication Initiative. In (A) one sees a two-month-old child who is a part of a nomadic community in Somalia being vaccinated in 2019. In (B) one sees a child's finger being marked after receiving vaccine in Nepal in 2011.

Photo credits: (A) © World Health Organization/Ilyas Ahmed, 2019. Used with permission.

(B) © World Health Organization/Homero Hernandez, 2011. Used with permission.

vaccinations over time. However, certain children like nomads, refugees, and the poor may be left out when vaccinations are distributed. Unlike smallpox where a "ring vaccination" strategy can be used, many cases of polio are asymptomatic, so it is more difficult to vaccinate everyone in a particular area who may have been exposed to a polio case. The children of Pakistan face risks from many other childhood diseases too, and because of the low number of cases overall, polio has been held to an endemic level disease at this point, rather than one causing epidemics (Closser 2010). Hopefully, Pakistan and Afghanistan can finally move to elimination status in the coming years, despite these challenges.

4.8 Determine the Lessons Learned from Poliovirus and How Polio Is Still Affecting Society Today, Including Post-Polio Syndrome

The recovery and chronic phases of the illness for a polio survivor varied tremendously depending on the individual and the kind of treatment accessible to them. Personal accounts by survivors sometimes mention the discrimination that they faced because of their new disability, while others did not have the same experience. In many instances, survivors of paralytic polio were able to go back to their lives and finish school, get a job, and start a family (Wilson 2005). As Wilson states in his book *Living with Polio* (p. 169), "Here, one of the biggest hurdles was to learn to deal with the stigma of being a cripple." Polio survivors, especially children, just wanted to "fit in" with their old neighborhood and community, and typically did not have contact with other polio survivors after leaving the hospital. At the same time, there were estimated to be over a million polio survivors in the United States in the late 20th century (Wilson 2005).

For some polio survivors, their battle with the disease recurred later in life. Some survivors experienced new symptoms such as pain, tiredness, and changes in muscle strength different from what happened when they first contracted polio, sometimes 20–30 years earlier. This was known as post-polio syndrome (Wilson 2005; International 2021).

4.9 Understand How Other Enteroviruses Are Impacting People Today, as Well as How Genetically Modified Poliovirus May Actually Be Used to Help Cancer Patients

Although poliovirus has been eliminated for 90% of the world's population, it is important to note that there are other enteroviruses that are an emerging threat. The enterovirus D68, also known as EV-D68, was first discovered in California in 1962. It is a member of the picornavirus family like poliovirus and displays characteristics of both enteroviruses and rhinoviruses in some respects, since it is primarily a mild respiratory illness that can cause neurological symptoms like acute flaccid myelitis (AFM) involving muscle weakness and paralysis. However, AFM itself is poorly understood. Although research is ongoing, scientists believe that EV-D68 is responsible for most cases of AFM (Cassidy et al. 2018; CDC 2021c; Baggen et al. 2018). The CDC indicates that many cases of AFM began to be reported in the United States in 2014 (CDC 2021c). It is not known why cases of AFM are on the rise.

Future studies of the picornavirus family of viruses need to focus not only on polio, but also on the non-poliovirus enteroviruses and how to control infection and/or develop a vaccine against these viruses.

Since the development of genetic engineering, scientists have been able to manipulate viruses to study them. We will discuss more details of genetic engineering in Chapter 7. In 1981, scientists cloned the entire poliovirus genome and expressed it in tissue culture cells creating infectious poliovirus particles. In addition, the same group sequenced the poliovirus genome (Racaniello and Baltimore 1981a, 1981b; Mueller, Wimmer, and Cello 2005). To attempt to get around the need for using monkeys as an animal model, scientists have created CD155 transgenic mice expressing the poliovirus receptor to create an alternative animal model for laboratory research. These mice have been used to better understand poliovirus replication and how it gets to the nervous system (Racaniello 2006).

Scientists have also started manipulating poliovirus to develop a type of oncolytic virus that can kill cancerous cells. Some scientists are developing attenuated poliovirus strains that can actually kill tumors like neuroblastoma in mouse models (Toyoda et al. 2007). Other scientists have found that many solid tumors express the CD155 receptor, the receptor for poliovirus, and are trying to use attenuated poliovirus as a type of cancer immunotherapy, stimulating the immune system to go after CD155-expressing cells (Gromeier and Nair 2018). Hopefully, a virus like poliovirus, which has caused so much human suffering, can now be used, through genetic engineering, to help cure diseases like cancer.

4.10 Summary

Poliomyelitis is caused by the poliovirus that enters the body through the GI tract, causing no symptoms in most people it infects. In a small number of people who contract the poliovirus, paralysis can occur. Research on poliovirus began in earnest in the early 20th century following small outbreaks in the United States and Europe, and then a major epidemic in the United States in 1916. Seasonal cases of polio increased until the mid-1950s. Public health officials had few answers in stopping the spread of the virus, and people lived in fear every summer up until the mid-20th century when Jonas Salk and his team developed a polio vaccine through the support of the National Foundation for Infantile Paralysis. Over a million U.S. schoolchildren participated in a large vaccine trial in 1954 using an inactivated or killed polio vaccine (IPV) developed by Salk and his team that successfully prevented polio. Implementation of this vaccine caused a rapid decline in the cases of polio in the United States. IPV was replaced with an oral polio vaccine (OPV) developed by Albert Sabin in the 1960s and was used in the United States until the year 2000 when the medical community once again recommended the use of IPV. Around the world, the OPV helped reduce the incidence of polio and is still used in the campaign to eradicate polio from the planet. Roughly 90% of the world's people are now free from fear of polio.

Discussion Questions:

1. Based on what you read about the history of polio, why was basic research needed before a polio vaccine could be invented?

2. Polio research involved *in vitro* studies using cells grown in petri dishes and *in vivo* studies using monkeys. What are the advantages and disadvantages of these two approaches?

3. Do you think Dr. Jonas Salk is an American hero? Why or why not?

4. Was the competition between Salk and Sabin good for or detrimental to scientific innovation?

5. How has the public perception of people with disabilities, such as paralysis, changed since the 1950s?

6. How is the social climate present during the polio epidemics of the 20th century similar to and different from the COVID-19 pandemic social climate?

7. How do social determinants of health impact your chances of getting polio? In 1950? In 2021?

References

AB, Nobel Prize Outreach. 2021. "The Nobel prize in physiology or medicine 1954." Accessed 3 September 2021. www.nobelprize.org/prizes/medicine/1954/summary/.

Alexander, L.N., J.F. Seward, T.A. Santibanez, M.A. Pallansch, O.M. Kew, D.R. Prevots, P.M. Strebel, et al. 2004. "Vaccine policy changes and epidemiology of poliomyelitis in the United States." *JAMA* 292 (14):1696–701. doi: 10.1001/jama.292.14.1696.

Association, The ALS. 2019. "Ice Bucket Challenge dramatically accelerated the fight against ALS." Accessed 12 September 2021. www.als.org/stories-news/ice-bucket-challenge-dramatically-accelerated-fight-against-als.

Baggen, J., H.J. Thibaut, J. Strating, and F.J.M. van Kuppeveld. 2018. "The life cycle of non-polio enteroviruses and how to target it." *Nature Reviews Microbiology* 16 (6):368–81. doi: 10.1038/s41579-018-0005-4.

Baltimore, D. 1971. "Expression of animal virus genomes." *Bacteriological Reviews* 35 (3):235.

Belov, G.A., V. Nair, B.T. Hansen, F.H. Hoyt, E.R. Fischer, and E. Ehrenfeld. 2012. "Complex dynamic development of poliovirus membranous replication complexes." *Journal of Virology* 86 (1):302–12. doi: 10.1128/jvi.05937-11.

Blume, S., and I. Geesink. 2000. "A brief history of polio vaccines." *Science* 288 (5471):1593–4.

Bodian, D., T. Francis, Jr., C. Larson, J.E. Salk, R.E. Shope, J.E. Smadel, and J.A. Shannon. 1955. "Interim report, public health service technical committee on poliomyelitis vaccine." *JAMA* 159 (15):1444–7. doi: 10.1001/jama.1955.02960320020007.

Brodie, M. 1935. "Active immunization against poliomyelitis." *American Journal of Public Health and the Nation's Health* 25 (1):54–67.

Cassidy, H., R. Poelman, M. Knoester, C.C. Van Leer-Buter, and H.G.M. Niesters. 2018. "Enterovirus D68—The new polio?" *Frontiers in Microbiology* 9:2677. doi: 10.3389/fmicb.2018.02677.

CDC, Centers for Disease Control and Prevention. 2021a. "Diagnostic methods." Accessed 19 September 2021. www.cdc.gov/polio/what-is-polio/lab-testing/diagnostic.html.

———. 2021b. "What is polio?" Accessed 19 September 2021. www.cdc.gov/polio/what-is-polio/.

———. 2021c. "Acute flaccid myelitis (AFM)." Accessed 21 September 2021. www.cdc.gov/acute-flaccid-myelitis/what-cdc-is-learning.html.

Chumakov, K., E. Ehrenfeld, V.I. Agol, and E. Wimmer. 2021. "Polio eradication at the crossroads." *The Lancet Global Health* 9 (8):e1172-e5. doi: 10.1016/s2214-109x(21)00205-9.

Closser, S. 2010. *Chasing Polio in Pakistan: Why the World's Largest Public Health Initiative May Fail.* xiii, 232 pages: Illustrations vols. Nashville, TN: Vanderbilt University Press.

Colt, S. 2009. "American experience. The polio crusade." In, 1 videodisc of (DVD) (54 min.): Sound, color with black and white sequences; 4 3/4 in. master 1 videocassette of 1 (Betacam SP) (min.): Sound, color with black and white sequences; 1/2 in. duplication copy 1 videocassette of 1 (VHS) (min.): Sound, color with black and white sequences; 1/2 in. viewing copy. [Boston, MA; Alexandria, VA]: WGBH Educational Foundation; Distributed by PBS Home Video.

Donlan, A.N., and W.A. Petri. 2020. "Mucosal immunity and the eradication of polio." *Science* 368 (6489):362–3. doi: 10.1126/science.abb8588.

Francis, T., Jr., R.F. Korns, R.B. Voight, M. Boisen, F.M. Hemphill, J.A. Napier, and E. Tolchinsky. 1955. "An evaluation of the 1954 poliomyelitis vaccine trials." *American Journal of Public Health and the Nation's Health* 45 (5 Pt 2):1–63.

Gould, T. 1995. *A Summer Plague: Polio and its Survivors.* New Haven, CT: Yale University Press.

Gromeier, M., and S.K. Nair. 2018. "Recombinant poliovirus for cancer immunotherapy." *Annual Review of Medicine* 69:289–99. doi: 10.1146/annurev-med-050715-104655.

Horstmann, D.M. 1952. "Poliomyelitis virus in blood of orally infected monkeys and chimpanzees." *Proceedings of the Society for Experimental Biology and Medicine* 79 (3):417–9.

———. 1991. "The Sabin live poliovirus vaccination trials in the USSR, 1959." *Yale Journal of Biology and Medicine* 64 (5):499–512.

Institute, Sabin Vaccine. 2021. "The legacy of Albert B Sabin." Accessed 12 September 2021. www.sabin.org/legacy-albert-b-sabin.

International, Post-Polio Health. 2021. "What is post-polio syndrome?" Accessed 12 September 2021. https://post-polio.org/education/what-is-post-polio-syndrome/.

Jacobs, C.D. 2015. *Jonas Salk: A Life.* Cary, NC: Oxford University Press, Incorporated.

Jimenez, M.R. 2014. "Biographical memoirs: Albert B. Sabin 1906–1993." Washington, DC: The National Academies Press.

Kew, O., and M. Pallansch. 2018. "Breaking the last chains of poliovirus transmission: Progress and challenges in global polio eradication." *The Annual Review of Virology* 5 (1):427–51. doi: 10.1146/annurev-virology-101416-041749.

Lostroh, P. 2019. *Molecular and Cellular Biology of Viruses.* 1st ed. Boca Raton, FL: Taylor & Francis Group, LLC.

Macklin, G.R., K.M. O'Reilly, N.C. Grassly, W.J. Edmunds, O. Mach, R. Santhana Gopala Krishnan, A. Voorman, et al. 2020. "Evolving epidemiology of poliovirus serotype 2 following withdrawal of the serotype 2 oral poliovirus vaccine." *Science* 368 (6489):401–5. doi: 10.1126/science.aba1238.

Matysiak, A. 2005. "The myth of Jonas Salk." *MIT Technology Review.* Accessed 12 September 2021. www.technologyreview.com/2005/07/01/230689/the-myth-of-jonas-salk/.

Meldrum, M. 1998. "'A calculated risk': The Salk polio vaccine field trials of 1954." *BMJ* 317 (7167):1233–6.

Mueller, S., E. Wimmer, and J. Cello. 2005. "Poliovirus and poliomyelitis: A tale of guts, brains, and an accidental event." *Virus Research* 111 (2):175–93. doi: 10.1016/j.virusres.2005.04.008.

Nieva, J.L., V. Madan, and L. Carrasco. 2012. "Viroporins: Structure and biological functions." *Nature Reviews Microbiology* 10 (8):563–74. doi: 10.1038/nrmicro2820.

Oshinsky, D.M. 2005. *Polio: An American Story.* New York, NY: Oxford University Press USA—OSO.

Paul, J.R. 1971. *A History of Poliomyelitis, Yale Studies in the History of Science and Medicine; 6.* New Haven: Yale University Press.

Poliovirus, U.S. National Authority for Containment of. 2020. "Polio disease and poliovirus." *CDC Centers for Disease Control and Prevention.* Accessed 19 September 2021. www.cdc.gov/cpr/polioviruscontainment/diseaseandvirus.htm.

Racaniello, V.R. 2006. "One hundred years of poliovirus pathogenesis." *Virology* 344 (1):9–16. doi: 10.1016/j.virol.2005.09.015.

Racaniello, V.R., and D. Baltimore. 1981a. "Cloned poliovirus complementary DNA is infectious in mammalian cells." *Science* 214 (4523):916–9. doi: 10.1126/science.6272391.

———. 1981b. "Molecular cloning of poliovirus cDNA and determination of the complete nucleotide sequence of the viral genome." *Proceedings of the National Academy of Sciences of the United States of America* 78 (8):4887–91. doi: 10.1073/pnas.78.8.4887.

Rose, D. 2010. "A history of the march of dimes." *March of Dimes*. Accessed 12 September 2021. www.marchofdimes.org/mission/a-history-of-the-march-of-dimes.aspx.

Ross, M.H., and W. Pawlina. 2011. *Histology*. New York, NY: Lippincott Williams & Wilkins.

Routh, J.A., M.S. Oberste, and M. Patel. 2014. "Chapter 12: Poliomyelitis." *Centers for Disease Control and Prevention CDC*. Accessed 19 September 2021. www.cdc.gov/vaccines/pubs/surv-manual/index.html.

Sabin, A.B., and P.K. Olitsky. 1936. "Cultivation of poliomyelitis virus in vitro in human embryonic nervous tissue." *Proceedings of the Society for Experimental Biology and Medicine* 34 (3):357–9.

Sabin, A.B., and R. Ward. 1941. "The natural history of human poliomyelitis: I. Distribution of virus in nervous and non-nervous tissues." *The Journal of Experimental Medicine* 73 (6):771.

Toyoda, H., J. Yin, S. Mueller, E. Wimmer, and J. Cello. 2007. "Oncolytic treatment and cure of neuroblastoma by a novel attenuated poliovirus in a novel poliovirus-susceptible animal model." *Cancer Research* 67 (6):2857–64. doi: 10.1158/0008-5472.can-06-3713.

WHO, World Health Organization. 2021a. "Global polio eradication initiative applauds WHO Africa region for wild polio-free certification." Accessed 14 September 2021. www.who.int/news/item/25-08-2020-global-polio-eradication-initiative-applauds-who-african-region-for-wild-polio-free-certification.

———. 2021b. "Global polio eradication initiative." Accessed 14 September 2021. https://polioeradication.org/.

———. 2021c. "History of polio." Accessed 14 September 2021. https://polioeradication.org/polio-today/history-of-polio/.

Wilson, D.J. 2005. *Living with Polio: The Epidemic and Its Survivors*. Chicago, IL: University of Chicago Press.

Yin-Murphy, M., and J.M. Almond. 1996. "Picornaviruses." In *Medical Microbiology*, edited by S. Baron. Galveston, TX: University of Texas Medical Branch at Galveston.

5

HIV/AIDS

Learning Outcomes:

5.1 Describe the Details of the Human Immunodeficiency Virus Compared to Other Viruses

5.2 Discuss How HIV Is Transmitted

5.3 Explore How HIV Impacts the Immune System and Leads to AIDS

5.4 Interpret Historical Factors Related to the Emergence of HIV in the United States and Its Global Spread

5.5 Follow the Scientists' Race to Discover What Causes AIDS

5.6 Determine How You Would Trace the Origins of HIV

5.7 Examine Ongoing Efforts to Control HIV/AIDS—Antiviral Drugs and Prevention of Infection

5.8 Will We Ever Have an HIV Vaccine?

5.9 Understand the Impact of HIV/AIDS on Society in the United States and around the World

When you bring up the term "pandemic" in 2022, most people think about the novel coronavirus, SARS-CoV-2. However, there is another virus in the world that has killed approximately 36 million people since it was first discovered in 1981 in the United States, and that is the human immunodeficiency virus (HIV) (WHO 2021b; Zimmer 2011). The World Health Organization (WHO) officially calls HIV a "global epidemic" (WHO 2021a). However, scientists throughout the world routinely refer to HIV/AIDS as a pandemic in scientific articles and textbooks. Nevertheless, although large numbers of cases of HIV have not been seen in an extremely short period of time, such as with a sudden seasonal flu pandemic, the continued steady presence of new HIV infections throughout the world indicates that it is one of the major ongoing threats to global health.

There is no cure for HIV, but current treatments have in effect turned an HIV-positive status into a "manageable chronic condition," one that never progresses to acquired immunodeficiency syndrome (AIDS) if antiretroviral therapy (ART) is taken, albeit for life (WHO 2021b). In this chapter, we will look at the characteristics of the HIV retrovirus, how it is transmitted, how it can damage the immune system to cause AIDS, and how it can be treated. Of the 37 million people in the world living with HIV, 73% are keeping HIV at bay with ART (WHO 2021b). We will explore how HIV was discovered as the cause of AIDS and the scientific progress made on treating and finding a cure for HIV infection. Like no other virus, HIV has been referenced in the products of popular culture in the late 20th and early 21st centuries such as books, television, and movies. We will explore the public perception of HIV and AIDS, and how that changed over time when an HIV-positive status no longer became a death sentence.

5.1 Describe the Details of the Human Immunodeficiency Virus Compared to Other Viruses

The human immunodeficiency virus first manifested itself in humans in the form of acquired immunodeficiency syndrome. The "acquired" part of the name indicates that the disease is not congenital, meaning not genetically inherited at birth. "Immunodeficiency" indicates that the major hallmark of the disease is a loss of function of the immune system, and finally "syndrome" is used to indicate a collection of symptoms that result from the immunodeficiency. HIV actually attacks a specific kind of cell in the immune system, known as T-helper or CD4 cells (Minkoff and Baker 2004; Zimmer 2011; Walker 2008a). In addition to the T-helper cells, macrophages and dendritic cells can also be affected (Cruse and Lewis 2009).

As mentioned in Chapter 2, T cells are a part of the acquired or adaptive immune response, participating in cell-mediated immunity (Coico and Sunshine 2015). All animals in general have some type of innate immunity, but vertebrates, beginning with the jawless fishes, evolved the capability of an acquired immune response (Buchmann 2014). In this branch of the immune system, antigen-presenting cells, including macrophages and dendritic cells, can take antigens and break them into pieces, and then display them outwardly for T-helper (CD4+) cells to respond. The T-helper cell uses the CD4 molecule as a receptor to interact with the presented antigen fragment and then mobilize the cytotoxic T (CD8) cells to kill the infected host cell in several ways (Biointeractive 2021; Cruse and Lewis 2009; Walker 2008a). One can imagine if those T-helper cells are gone as in the case of AIDS, then the immune system communication network breaks down and the body cannot sufficiently respond to recognize and destroy infected cells.

HIV is a retrovirus. Humans are born with what are known as "endogenous retroviruses" in their genome, in addition to possibly acquiring "exogenous retroviruses" like human T-cell leukemia virus (HTLV) and HIV during their lifetimes. Endogenous retroviruses include fragments or whole retroviruses that embedded in our DNA during human evolution and rarely cause disease (Cloyd 1996). HIV is in the *Lentivirus* genus, a type of enveloped retrovirus that uses reverse transcriptase to make a DNA copy of its genome that then inserts into the host cell genome (Zimmer 2011; Lostroh 2019; Cloyd 1996). Lentiviruses are known for causing chronic infections with a long incubation period, primarily attacking the immune system or the nervous system (Tang, Kuhen, and Wong-Staal 1999; Cruse and Lewis 2009). Lentiviruses are of the Baltimore classification Class VI, which is a single-stranded RNA virus that uses a DNA intermediate for replication (Baltimore 1971). Lentiviruses possess the three critical genes found in any retrovirus: *gag*, *pol*, and *env*, which are necessary for making the structural proteins and enzymes required by the virus (Tang, Kuhen, and Wong-Staal 1999).

HIV has an envelope displaying spike proteins and contains two copies of its positive sense single-stranded RNA genome (Lostroh 2019; Cloyd 1996). To enter cells, HIV binds to the CD4 receptor on the surface of the T-helper cells as well as a chemokine co-receptor, such as CCR5, and then uses a fusion peptide to make an opening to enter the cell. Once the virus enters the cells, reverse transcription occurs, and the viral genome can move to the nucleus and integrate into the host cell genome using an enzyme known as an integrase. Other viral proteins are made using the host cell's translational machinery, and then the viral protein chains are cleaved by a protease when the virus matures. Once the viral particle is assembled, it buds out of the host cell and moves onto another cell (Lostroh

2019; Minkoff and Baker 2004; Cloyd 1996; Walker 2008a) (Ackermann, Berthiaume, and Tremblay1998) (Figure 5.1).

Reverse transcriptase was mentioned in Chapter 1 of this book as an enzyme first discovered by cancer biologists studying RNA tumor viruses. These researchers also confirmed the existence of the proviral form of the virus, where its genome is stably integrated into the genome of the host cell (Weinberg 2014; Nobel Media AB 2021). Reverse transcriptase is known for lacking "proofreading" capability, meaning that errors in the transferring of the code from RNA to DNA are not corrected (Walker 2008a; Ojikutu 2008a). These errors become a source of variation in the genetic code of the HIV virus. Overall, the HIV life cycle will become important later because antiretroviral drugs have been developed that block many steps of the pathway, including preventing spike proteins from binding to cells, blocking reverse transcriptase activity, and disabling the protease needed to mature HIV proteins (Lostroh 2019).

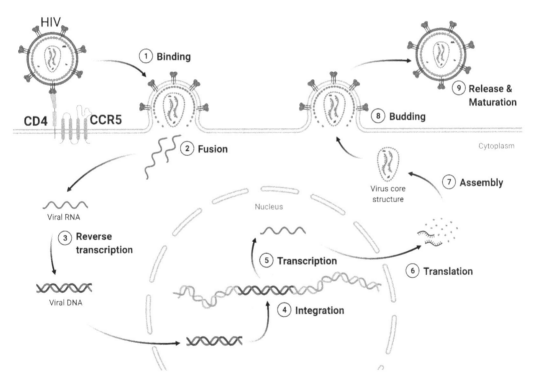

FIGURE 5.1
HIV life cycle.

Shown is the life cycle of a retrovirus like HIV. First, the virus binds to the T-helper cell using the CD4 receptor and a co-receptor like CCR5. Then the virus enters the cell, and reverse transcriptase makes a DNA copy of the viral genome, which enters the nucleus and integrates into the host cell's genome. The viral genes are transcribed, and the mRNA is exported to the nucleus. The viral proteins are translated and then assembled into the virus core structure. The virus buds from the cell membrane so it can then infect the next cell.

Created using Biorender.com.

5.2 Discuss How HIV Is Transmitted

HIV is transmitted through select bodily fluids such as blood or semen passed from person to person during sex without a condom. It can also be transmitted by sharing needles in intravenous drug use or an unsafe medical procedure such as one involving transfer of blood or tissue. HIV can also be transmitted from mother to child *in utero*. However, sharing food or water, getting bitten by a mosquito, and kissing and hugging are *not* considered at-risk behaviors for acquiring HIV (WHO 2021b; Zimmer 2011; Minkoff and Baker 2004; Cloyd 1996; CDC 2021d). If a healthcare worker is accidentally stuck with a needle or if anyone thinks they may have been exposed to HIV, they can take antiviral drugs for a brief period as a preventative measure against HIV infection (Lostroh 2019; CDC 2021c). Research has also been conducted on what is known as "discordant couples," where one person is HIV positive and the other is HIV negative. From this research, scientists have found that certain types of contact from which HIV can be acquired are higher risk than others and that there is a relationship between the amount of HIV in the blood and the risk of transmission. These findings on the viral concentration-dependent nature of risk led to studies indicating that treatment of the HIV-positive partner with antiretroviral therapy can stop the spread of HIV to the HIV-negative partner. ART, in combination with avoiding the highest risk behaviors, can help reduce the number of infected individuals in the overall population (Kumi Smith et al. 2018; Lostroh 2019). Screening donated blood, providing education on safe sexual practices, and preventing intravenous drug users from sharing needles can also reduce infection rates (Cloyd 1996).

To determine if someone has acquired HIV, several different tests are available. For many years, antibody-based tests such as an ELISA and western blot analysis have been used to detect antibodies against HIV in a person's blood (Minkoff and Baker 2004). Antibody tests have been available since 1985 (Alexander 2016; UNAIDS 2021a). A PCR test is also available (Cloyd 1996). PCR is a type of nucleic acid–based test. In general, antibody-based tests, nucleic acid–based tests, and tests detecting both HIV antigen and antibodies against HIV can now be done. Rapid tests are available for detecting antibodies as well as antigens and antibodies (CDC 2021c). If someone does test positive for HIV, the current recommended course of treatment is to begin antiretroviral therapy (WHO 2021b).

5.3 Explore How HIV Impacts the Immune System and Leads to AIDS

There are three stages to HIV/AIDS. The acute stage, the chronic or asymptomatic stage, and the AIDS stage (CDC 2021a) (Figure 5.2). In the weeks immediately following infection with HIV (acute stage), no symptoms or general flu-like symptoms might arise. Fever, coughing, and diarrhea may occur. However, lymph node swelling, called lymphadenopathy, may indicate something is happening with the immune system. When the immune system is severely weakened, it can allow susceptibility to other diseases such as tuberculosis or even cancers like lymphoma or Kaposi's sarcoma (KS), called opportunistic infections (WHO 2021b; Zimmer 2011). Before HIV was discovered, swollen lymph nodes and other symptoms were mysteriously seen in people who were otherwise healthy (Shilts 1987).

HIV is said to cause "both chronic lytic and latent infections" in the sense that it is never cleared from the body once a person is infected, with some cell types where HIV

Stage	1	2	3
Description	**Acute phase**	**Chronic phase**	**AIDS**
	Increase in HIV in blood	Asymptomatic	Increase in HIV in blood
	May have symptoms like the flu	Decrease in HIV in blood, but still reproducing	CD4+ cells drop
		ART can prevent progression to Stage Three	Highly susceptible to opportunistic infections
CD4+/T-Helper Cell Count (cells/µl) If ≥ 6 years old	≥500	200–499	<200

FIGURE 5.2
Stages of HIV/AIDS.

The three stages of HIV/AIDS are shown, along with a description of each stage. Physicians can monitor the T-helper cells in the patient's blood to identify progression to the next phase.

Stage details can be found at the CDC HIV Basics website. Cell counts from Centers for Disease Control and Prevention (CDC). Revised surveillance case definition for HIV infection—United States, 2014. Morbidity and Mortality Weekly Report 2014 Apr 11;63 (RR-03):1–10. PMID: 24717910 (www.cdc.gov/mmwr/preview/mmwrhtml/rr6303a1.htm).

continually replicates and some cell types where HIV can be latent (Lostroh 2019). However, it may take years before untreated HIV infection progresses to AIDS. Some estimates indicate that the incubation period could be as long as eight to ten years after acquiring HIV before some people would develop AIDS without ART (Walker 2008a; Ojikutu 2008a).

Initially, the amount of HIV viral particles detected in the blood typically peaks a few weeks after infection, and then begins to drop off as the virus is controlled by the immune system at least temporarily, known as the early phase of infection. During the chronic stage of the infection, the amount of virus in the blood stabilizes at some level, known as the viral set point. This set point is an important indicator of the patient's prospects (Simon and Ho 2003). Tracking the amount of virus in the blood could give some indication of whether the person would begin to move into an AIDS progression period (Walker 2008a). Blood tests indicating less than 200 T-helper cells per microliter of blood would mean that a person's immune system is in serious trouble and may be entering Stage 3 AIDS (Cruse and Lewis 2009).

If a person with AIDS gets a secondary disease caused by a microbe at that point, the weakened immune system could not fight it off like a person with a normal immune system (Minkoff and Baker 2004). Examples of opportunistic infections would include fungal infections caused by *Candida* (yeast infections) or parasitic infections caused by *Toxoplasma gondii*, severe cytomegalovirus infection (CMV), or even tuberculosis, one of the main causes of death worldwide in people with AIDS (Minkoff and Baker 2004; Shilts 1987). In the early days of AIDS in the United States before treatment became available, many people died excruciating deaths from severe opportunistic infections taking over their bodies leading to panic, fear, and confusion in cities where the first case clusters occurred (Shilts 1987; France 2016).

Because of the development of antiretroviral therapy, a person in the chronic stage of infection may never progress to AIDS if ART is taken as directed by a physician for life. If ART is not used, months or years later the levels of HIV can begin to rise in the blood and then the T-helper cells die off, leaving the person vulnerable to opportunistic infections that can ultimately cause their death as the final phase of AIDS progression (Lostroh 2019; Minkoff and Baker 2004; Cruse and Lewis 2009; Walker 2008a).

Over time, some people have emerged, sometimes known as outliers, who did not acquire HIV despite engaging in high-risk behaviors for acquiring HIV (Lostroh 2019). One such person was Stephen Crohn, who did not acquire HIV even though he may have been exposed to it many times. Scientists studied Crohn and found he possessed the rare delta 32 mutation in the HIV co-receptor CCR5 (Walker 2008a; Ojikutu 2008a). Unfortunately, Crohn took his own life in 2013 (Schwartz 2013). This mutation is very rare, and a person needs to have two copies of the delta 32 mutation to see the effect. Although the mutation is thought to have come from the Vikings in northern Europe originally, the mutation has been found in people with geographic origins in other parts of Europe as well as western Asia (Novembre, Galvani, and Slatkin 2005; Huang et al. 1996; Martinson et al. 1997). These human outliers can be important for understanding HIV/AIDS infection and trying to find new ways to stop the virus.

5.4 Interpret Historical Factors Related to the Emergence of HIV in the United States and Its Global Spread

In June 1981, doctors in Los Angeles submitted a report for publication with the CDC's *Morbidity and Mortality Weekly Report* describing a cluster of cases of a rare kind of *Pneumocystis* pneumonia (PCP) in what were once healthy young homosexual men. These men also had in common cytomegalovirus (CMV) infection and some type of *Candida* infection. Then, in July 1981, physicians mainly in New York but also in California reported a case cluster of 26 homosexual men with an unusual cancer known as Kaposi's sarcoma, normally only seen in older men of Mediterranean geographic origin. Infections like CMV and PCP were occurring in these men as well (Gottlieb et al. 1981; Zimmer 2011; Ojikutu 2008a; Friedman-Kien et al. 1981; Minkoff and Baker 2004; Shilts 1987).

Some patients from the growing case clusters in both New York and Los Angeles had decreased T-helper cell blood counts. At this point, physicians, scientists, and public health officials scrambled to figure out what was in common among all these patients. Some people searched for a common chemical exposure or drug in their environment, a change in the course of an illness caused by a pathogen that the patient already had, or something about how they lived their lives that would lead to this disease (Minkoff and Baker 2004; Shilts 1987; Ojikutu 2008a).

Over time, more and more people displayed the symptoms of infection by this mysterious virus even in other parts of the country. Some people had a fever and swollen lymph nodes for months or years. More and more physicians then began to realize that their patients did not have the flu or another well-known viral infection. A common symptom that brought people to the physician's office or hospital was shortness of breath, and it was determined that they had PCP like the first cases in Los Angeles in 1981. The CDC tracked the use of certain medications, like a powerful drug called pentamidine, which was rarely prescribed. It was used primarily for cancer patients with very weakened immune systems who came down with PCP. Now, the CDC saw a spike in requests for pentamidine around the United States, with no or little explanation for how the person may have acquired PCP. Other patients had different opportunistic infections taking over their bodies, or the rare cancer Kaposi's sarcoma characterized by purple bumps on the skin, as reported in the case cluster in New York. Contact tracing in New York and Los Angeles led public health officials to a Canadian flight attendant with AIDS, who had had over 250 sexual partners a year for several years. These officials realized that he, among others, could have potentially passed on a pathogen to many people. Air travel between Los Angeles, New York, and San Francisco meant that a pathogen could spread to many parts of North America, and the delay in showing signs of AIDS meant that a person could pass the infection to others for quite a while before knowing they were ill (Ojikutu 2008a; Shilts 1987).

Later genomics analysis of over 2,000 viral RNA samples from the United States in the 1970s indicated that because of the genomic diversity in the HIV-1 group M (main) sequences identified, most likely HIV came to the United States from an epidemic already happening in the Caribbean. Also, the intense focus on the Canadian flight attendant as a possible "patient zero" seemed to be unfounded, and he was not considered to be the primary case first seen in North America (Worobey et al. 2016). Much of the focus on the flight attendant is linked back to the account of the early days of AIDS in a popular book by Randy Shilts (Shilts 1987).

Contact tracers narrowed in on certain groups in the United States that may have been affected, including men who had sex with men, Haitians, and intravenous drug users (Shilts 1987; Ojikutu 2008b). However, this group-centered approach, rather than an approach centered on high-risk behaviors, led U.S. officials down an erroneous path that ended up labeling certain groups of people as being more susceptible to the virus than others. AIDS was even called GRID (gay-related immune defficiency) briefly in the early days, which unsettled some people at the CDC (Shilts 1987; Minkoff and Baker 2004). These misconceptions of those who can be infected with HIV persist today among some people, although, from the start, any human could acquire HIV in a high-risk situation. Ignoring this fact put many people at risk of acquiring HIV and still puts people at risk today.

As the virus spread, hemophiliacs, blood transfusion recipients, and children born of mothers with HIV/AIDS began to show up in hospitals with AIDS themselves. Early on, they may not have been recognized as having AIDS since they were not labeled as being a part of a high-risk group. Attention began to shift to protecting the blood supply for the general population. Randy Shilts's book, *The Band Played On*, ended its account of events in the fall of 1985 around the time of the revelation that the famous actor Rock Hudson died of AIDS (Shilts 1987). By mid-1985, there had been over 12,000 cases of AIDS reported in the United States, and over 6,000 of those people had already died (Shilts 1987). This realization brought AIDS to the American public's attention yet again, but many still were in denial of the gravity of the situation and the need for more funding for research and treatment. A U.S. representative from California, Henry Waxman, was quoted in 1982 indicating that the government would have had a different response if the disease had not been seen as mainly affecting gay males. It seemed like little had changed (Shilts 1987). People with AIDS (PWA) began to travel to Mexico to seek out experimental drugs to treat their disease (Shilts 1987). A fictionalized account of the quest of one real person with AIDS, Ron Woodroof, to find an experimental cure for AIDS, as well as help organize others to get treatment, was made into a film called *Dallas Buyers Club* (Vallee 2013).

People began to have hope when certain FDA-approved treatments that seemed to prolong the life of PWA started to become available in the late 1980s. The drug azidothymidine (AZT) can act as an analog for one of the building blocks of DNA, thymidine, disrupting the synthesis of the new DNA chain. It was first developed as an anti-cancer drug but was shelved because it was ineffective as a form of chemotherapy. Then, researchers began trying AZT to inhibit HIV reverse transcriptase activity and found that it worked. AZT began being used to treat patients in 1987 (Ojikutu 2008b; Lostroh 2019; UNAIDS 2021a). AZT and other drugs that followed (protease inhibitors) helped make being HIV positive a manageable condition (Ojikutu 2008b; France 2016). However, it has been noted that AZT became the costliest drug on the market when it was released (Vallee 2013; France 2016). We will now talk about how scientists first figured out the link between HIV and AIDS so that the lifesaving treatments could be developed.

5.5 Follow the Scientists' Race to Discover What Causes AIDS

At the time HIV emerged, Robert Gallo ran a laboratory at the National Cancer Institute in the United States and had already discovered a type of retrovirus called human T-cell leukemia I (HTLV-I) that caused excess cell proliferation of T cells, leading to a type of cancer. Although many people were still trying to figure out something about a person's lifestyle that could lead to AIDS, scientists like Gallo became focused on finding a viral cause for AIDS after hemophiliacs began getting AIDS. This suggested that there was something in human blood, a virus, that was causing AIDS (Minkoff and Baker 2004; Shilts 1987).

In the meantime, a group working in France was able to find and characterize the virus and determined that it was different from HTLV-I and other similar tumor viruses. The French researchers settled on the name lymphadenopathy-associated virus (LAV) (Shilts 1987). Gallo's group was in fierce competition with the French researchers, but Gallo thought the virus would turn out to be another leukemia virus, calling it HTLV-III (Shilts 1987). Gallo himself admits that he went down the wrong path with HIV initially because he assumed that he would not be dealing with another kind of human retrovirus, right after his discovery of the human T-cell leukemia virus (NIH 2021a). The French group lead by Luc Montagnier had successfully detected reverse transcriptase enzymatic activity in white blood cells cultured in the lab from the lymph nodes of people in the early stages of AIDS, a signature of a retrovirus. The same retroviral activity was seen in the blood of patients at more advanced stages of AIDS. They isolated the virus and introduced it to white blood cells where it was able to kill the T-helper cells, unlike how a tumor virus would behave. The research group observed the virus using electron microscopy and, based on all of the virus's characteristics, were the first to determine it was a lentivirus. They also found that the isolated virus elicited a positive response for binding to antibodies taken from PWA. It is important to note that this research group went on to isolate HIV from all different kinds of people: those who acquired HIV through sexual transmission, hemophiliacs who acquired HIV through contaminated blood products, children who obtained the virus from their mothers *in utero*, as well as blood transfusion patients who acquired the virus from contaminated donated blood (Nobel Media AB 2021). The development of antibody testing meant that blood could be tested to see how prevalent HIV was in each geographic area, and blood samples could now be screened for HIV (Shilts 1987).

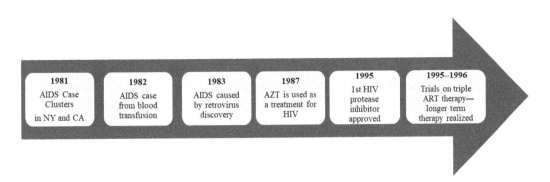

FIGURE 5.3
Timeline of HIV/AIDS key events.

Six major events in the early history of HIV/AIDS are shown. Additional timeline information can be found at www.niaid.nih.gov/

The Gallo and Montagnier research groups published their initial findings back to back in *Science* in 1983 (Gallo et al. 1983; Barré-Sinoussi et al. 1983; HHS 2021).

Robert Gallo is credited with the co-discovery of HIV in many circles and was responsible for creating a blood test for HIV that helped screen blood critical for the treatment of many people, such as hemophiliacs. He received the Lasker Award (often considered a prize that can lead up to a Nobel Prize) for his discovery of HTLV-I, as well as for the discovery of HIV-1 (NIH 2021b). Some will note how the exchange of ideas and discussion of data at the early HIV/AIDS conferences helped drive the field forward and that others were involved in the HIV discovery as well, including Jay Levy of the University of California at San Francisco (NIH 2021a). Jonas Salk himself became involved in helping Robert Gallo and Luc Montagnier come to an agreement on the sharing of credit for the discovery of HIV, as well as the royalties. President Ronald Reagan of the United States and Prime Minister Jacques Chirac of France announced the co-discovery agreement together, although it was an uneasy truce (Shilts 1987; Jacobs 2015; France 2016). Still, Gallo and Montagnier have written review articles together on HIV/AIDS (Gallo and Montagnier 1988; Gallo and Montagnier 2003). Gallo and Montagnier highlighted how their laboratories did build on each other's work, like how both groups contributed to the knowledge of the T cell *in vitro* growth conditions needed to study HIV in the lab (Gallo and Montagnier 2003). The Nobel Committee ended up having what might be the final say though by giving the Nobel Prize in Physiology or Medicine to just Montagnier and Barré-Sinoussi, not Gallo, for the discovery of HIV (AB 2008). A timeline with the major events in the early days of HIV/AIDS can be found in Figure 5.3.

5.5.1 Review Koch's Postulates

Whenever a new viral pathogen is proposed, Koch's postulates are used as the scientific standard to establish a direct link between the viral pathogen and the disease. In summary, if one follows Koch's postulates, the pathogen must be associated with all or almost all of the cases of the disease, and then the pathogen itself is isolated and used to recreate the disease in another organism (Minkoff and Baker 2004). In this case, scientists had to determine if HIV was really causing AIDS. It is important to note that the start of the process is detecting the virus in all or almost all of people who have AIDS, and then not finding the virus in people without AIDS. Once antibody tests were developed, HIV or antibody against HIV could be detected in almost everyone with AIDS or any stage leading up to AIDS. In addition, people who died of an AIDS-related dementia were found to have HIV in their brains during an autopsy (Minkoff and Baker 2004). HIV has been cultured in the lab in T-helper cells, causing the death of that cell population as expected and permitting necessary *in vitro* studies of HIV, but finding a good animal model organism to mimic the human system to study HIV has been problematic.

Several immune system characteristics are needed if you want to recapitulate AIDS in an animal model. The animal would have to have key cellular components like receptors that allow for HIV infection of the cells and then support the HIV life cycle with their cellular machinery. Also, it has been found that some animals naturally have some "restriction factors" that prevent HIV infection, while those factors have been overridden by HIV in humans. For example, mice, rats, and rabbits do not become infected with HIV naturally (Hatziioannou and Evans 2012).

Researchers have tried two main approaches to finding an animal model for studying HIV/AIDS. First, scientists have made rodents (more commonly mice than rats) with a "humanized" immune system, in a challenging and time-sensitive process in which the mouse's immune system is destroyed before maturing and replaced with cells and tissues of the human immune system, which can fully develop in the animal. Mice are a popular choice when a mammalian model is needed for biomedical research given that they are small, easy to maintain in a research facility, and have large litter sizes (Hatziioannou and Evans 2012; Agarwal et al. 2020; Dash et al. 2021). Although other animals, like cats, are known to be susceptible to a similar virus known as feline immunodeficiency virus (FIV), there are major limitations to this model, including the types of cells infected by FIV versus HIV as well as the course of the illness potentially being longer with FIV versus HIV (Hatziioannou and Evans 2012). In the second approach, nonhuman primates are studied using simian immunodeficiency virus (SIV) or a modified version of SIV that looks like HIV called SHIV. Four different species of Asian macaques are used commonly (Hatziioannou and Evans 2012). However, some researchers have noted that vaccine trials first tested in nonhuman primates and then brought to human clinical trials have failed, indicating that a better animal model approach is needed. Advances in the sophistication of the humanized mouse models may become the go-to animal model in the future (Agarwal et al. 2020).

5.6 Determine How You Would Trace the Origins of HIV

One of the first clues in trying to find the animal origins of HIV came when researchers observed AIDS-type symptoms in nonhuman primates housed at a research center. It turns out that they had a primate lentivirus related to HIV called simian immunodeficiency virus (Zimmer 2011; Hatziioannou and Evans 2012; Peeters, Jung, and Ayouba 2013). It is generally accepted that HIV came from chimpanzees (Simon and Ho 2003; Hatziioannou and Evans 2012). Researchers determined that the transfer of SIV from chimpanzees to humans in southeastern Cameroon was the origin of the major group of HIV-1 (Sharp and Hahn 2010; Sharp and Hahn 2011). There are many similarities between SIV and HIV, including the structure of their genomes, relatedness in the tree of life from a gene sequence point of view, route of transmission of the virus itself, and the initial geographic location of cases (Gao et al. 1999).

HIV may have arisen from the transmission of a virus from other primates to humans more than once, since the versions of HIV seen in the human population are not all derived from one HIV strain. There are two major types of HIV. HIV-1 is found throughout the world including the United States, Europe, and central Africa, and HIV-2 is primarily found in West Africa (Cruse and Lewis 2009; Zimmer 2011; Cloyd 1996; Hatziioannou and Evans 2012). HIV-1 is most like SIV isolated from chimpanzees and gorillas, whereas HIV-2 is most like SIV isolated from a primate known as a sooty mangabey (Peeters, Jung, and Ayouba 2013; Sharp and Hahn 2010).

The spillover of a virus from an animal reservoir to a human host usually happens in a few steps before the virus switches over to being perpetuated in the human host. For example, the virus may be introduced to humans, but then not initially transmitted to other people. In the next step, the virus may be introduced to humans, and then cause a small local outbreak where the virus moves from person to person only in that small area. However, there is potential for an epidemic with the third step, where the virus is introduced to humans and then transmitted from person to person for a longer period and over a greater geographic distance (Parrish et al. 2008).

Humans may have become infected with the simian version of the virus by eating or handling infected meat (Sharp and Hahn 2010; Zimmer 2011). There is also an indication of transfer among primates such as from chimpanzees to gorillas (Zimmer 2011). It seems like the virus moved from other primates to humans at least four times (Lostroh 2019). HIV-1 can be divided into four major groups known as M (main group), N, O, and P (Zimmer 2011; Parrish et al. 2008; Peeters, Jung, and Ayouba 2013; Sharp and Hahn 2010).

Having access to a viral genome isolated from a patient, as well as sequence data from earlier patient isolates and even related viral sequences, allows a scientist to conduct something known as "molecular clock" analysis. This analysis is based on the idea that mutations (changes in the DNA or RNA sequence) in any genome occur at relatively the same rate over time across species. The more time that passes, the more mutations. Eventually, a neutral mutation (not conferring an advantage or disadvantage to the organism) becomes "fixed in the population," and the rate of these changes is known as the substitution rate (Ho 2008). Therefore, one can look at a gene sequence from one species and then from a related species and determine the time when they last had a common ancestor in the tree of life. If you see fewer sequence differences between two genomes, then they are more closely related than sequences where you see many differences (Ho 2008; Zimmer 2011). Many scientists conduct their analysis using a "relaxed clock model" where even if the mutations are not occurring at a regular rate in every organism, a correction can be made, such as through using an average substitution rate (Ho 2008).

The time when SIV first contacted humans is still debated, but some molecular clock studies indicate that group M for HIV-1 could have been around since the 1920s to 1930s, probably first being seen around Kinshasa (then known as Leopoldville), which is now the capital of the Democratic Republic of Congo. However, the HIV outbreak did not start expanding rapidly to a wider geographic area until the 1960s–1970s (Parrish et al. 2008; Faria et al. 2014; Sharp and Hahn 2010; Korber et al. 2000; Sharp and Hahn 2011). A broader time range of 1884–1924 was reported in other molecular clock analyses (Worobey et al. 2008). Finally, an even earlier range of 1881–1918 has been proposed by other groups (Gryseels et al. 2020). Researchers also noted the importance of Kinshasa as an economic and transportation center for the Belgian Congo, which could have also contributed to the spread of the pathogen (Faria et al. 2014). From its origins as an epidemic in Africa, HIV/

AIDS became a pandemic that was uncontrolled in the early 1980s, and researchers worldwide were in search of a way to control the virus using antiretroviral therapy.

5.7 Examine Ongoing Efforts to Control HIV/AIDS—Antiviral Drugs and Prevention of Infection

As mentioned earlier, initially there was no way of stopping the progression of HIV infection to AIDS and being HIV positive was typically a death sentence. However, the development of antiretroviral drugs gave hope that the virus could be controlled, and eventually the development of protease inhibitors and the use of combination therapy helped lead to the closing of AIDS wards in hospitals around the United States (France 2016). In the United States, HIV diagnoses notably declined between 1993 and 1998, and deaths steeply declined from 1995 to 1998 (Torian et al. 2011) (Figure 5.4).

In this section, I will describe the different classes of antiretroviral drugs used to treat HIV/AIDS, as well as some new preventative and treatment strategies that have been used

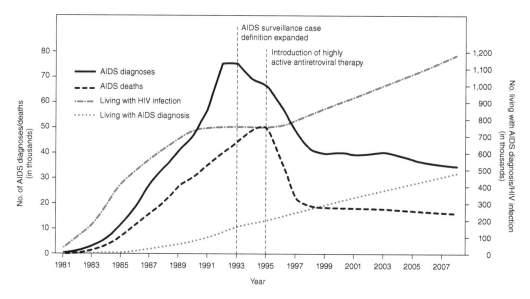

FIGURE 5.4

The number of AIDS diagnoses and deaths, and those living with either HIV infection or an AIDS diagnosis, 1981–2008.

Beginning in 1981, the CDC started tracking the number of AIDS diagnoses (solid line) and deaths (dashed line) in the United States, which both rose through the mid-1990s. Then, diagnoses began to decline in 1993, followed by the decline of deaths in 1995. After 1995, when the first protease inhibitors were developed, the number of people living with HIV infection began to increase (alternating dashed and dotted line) after leveling off around 1989. The number of people living with an AIDS diagnosis has gradually increased from 1985 onward (dotted line).

Credit: Torian, L., M. Chen, P. Rhodes, and H.I. Hall. 2011. "HIV surveillance—United States, 1981–2008." *Morbidity and Mortality Weekly Report* 60 (21):689–93 (www.cdc.gov/mmwr/preview/mmwrhtml/mm6021a2. htm).

MMWR graphics are in the public domain, www.cdc.gov/mmwr/about.html

to reduce HIV infection rates in high-risk populations or make being HIV positive a manageable condition. The general goals of antiretroviral therapy include limiting the replication of HIV so that T-helper cells do not die off and the immune system is still functional. If this happens, then the HIV-positive person can effectively live like someone who is HIV negative (Gulick and Flexner 2019). The development of a vaccine is still the ultimate goal of many scientists, but there are other ways in which the AIDS pandemic has been managed to a certain degree. However, this approach requires money to pay for the ART for the rest of their lives, as well as the individual's commitment to the regular treatment schedule.

In addition to drug cost challenges and patient "adherence" issues, HIV is capable of mutating even while in a person, allowing it to become resistant to ART (Lostroh 2019). Another way of saying this is that because of its high mutation rate, the HIV genome varies from person to person ("inter-individual") and even within a person ("intra-individual") (Simon and Ho 2003). For these reasons, new drug therapies are continuing to be developed to replace older generations of drugs.

5.7.1 Classes of Drugs

Nucleoside/nucleotide analogs are drugs that are competitive inhibitors of the reverse transcriptase that is needed to copy the HIV genome. One of the most famous drugs in this category is AZT (Ojikutu 2008b; Lostroh 2019). AZT can be used to reduce the chance of mother-to-child transmission of HIV, which can occur *in utero*, during birth, or just after birth (Ojikutu 2008b). Other categories of drugs include non-nucleoside inhibitors of reverse transcriptase, drugs that block fusion of the virus with the cell, and drugs that block the integration of the genome into the host's cellular genome, among others. One can look at every stage of the HIV life cycle as a possible point of attack for an antiretroviral drug (Lostroh 2019; Gulick and Flexner 2019). Another important class of anti-HIV drugs are the protease inhibitors that block the viral enzyme called a protease that is needed for the maturing of the virus. Protease inhibitors were developed through "rational drug design," meaning that the crystal structure of the protease was resolved, and then a drug was designed to block it, rather than testing an existing compound for its effectiveness against the virus (Lostroh 2019).

5.7.2 Combination Therapy

The combination therapy called highly active antiretroviral therapy (HAART), combination antiretroviral therapy (cART), or retroviral therapy (ART) was considered a major breakthrough in treatment, and then also actual prevention of HIV infection (Lostroh 2019; Simon and Ho 2003). In this approach, more than one antiretroviral drug, typically three, are given at the same time in a drug cocktail (Gulick and Flexner 2019). Using more than one drug at a time helps slow down the onset of HIV resistance to the ART drugs, as well as reduces the speed with which the virus can make copies of itself, which can put off AIDS onset. However, this is where the patient adherence issue comes in, because sticking to the strict daily medication regimen required for this treatment can be quite challenging (Ojikutu 2008b; Gulick and Flexner 2019).

5.7.3 New Treatments and Approaches

The development of pre-exposure prophylaxis, also known as PrEP, has been another game changer in HIV prevention strategy. PrEP was approved in 2013, after a clinical trial in 2010 with men who have sex with men indicated that there was a 44% reduction in HIV-negative individuals acquiring HIV from an HIV-positive partner if the PrEP regimen was used (UNAIDS 2021a; Lostroh 2019; Grant et al. 2010). PrEP typically involves two antiretroviral drugs (Gulick and Flexner 2019). This research also informed recommendations released in 2012 for what are known as "serodiscordant" or "discordant" couples, where one partner is HIV positive and the other is HIV negative (UNAIDS 2021a).

Like with other antiretroviral drug therapies, long-acting therapies are being tested now too to see if side effects are manageable, if they interact with other drugs, if they can be taken during pregnancy, and how quickly drug resistance develops (Gulick and Flexner 2019). In 2018, an intravaginal ring that can supply a long-acting version of antiretroviral therapy to females was developed (UNAIDS 2021a). A long-acting injectable antiretroviral therapy was approved by the Food and Drug Administration (FDA) in 2021. The injectable therapy, known as CABENUVA, is a combination of cabotegravir, an integrase inhibitor, and rilpivirine, a non-nucleoside reverse transcriptase inhibitor (FDA 2021; Healthcare 2021). Clinical trials yielded promising results for patients who started oral ART and then were switched to the long-acting therapy in the first long-acting injectable regimen (FLAIR) trial, as well as for patients on an oral therapy who switched to the long-acting drug to maintain their suppression of HIV in the antiretroviral therapy as long-acting suppression (ATLAS) trial for either four or eight weeks (Orkin et al. 2020; Swindells et al. 2020; Rizzardini et al. 2020; Gulick and Flexner 2019; Overton et al. 2021; Rial-Crestelo, Pinto-Martínez, and Pulido 2020).

Another treatment approach, which has also been used to treat COVID-19, is the use of broadly neutralizing antibodies (bNABs). These are antibodies purified from individuals who had the disease, in this case HIV-positive individuals. The isolated antibodies bind to HIV proteins, like HIV membrane proteins, and neutralize them. These kinds of antibodies can be made in the body as a part of the passive immune response to a vaccine, but scientists are trying to deliver the antibodies themselves in lieu of a vaccine as a treatment for HIV (Gulick and Flexner 2019; Simon and Ho 2003; Burton 2019). Some scientists are also making "multi-specific antibodies" that go after more than one HIV-1 target protein at the same time, as well as engineering existing antibodies to bind better to their target antigen (Padte et al. 2018). Clinical trials using broadly neutralizing antibodies found that this treatment did not protect the majority of at-risk individuals from acquiring HIV. However, the researchers did determine that the antibody therapy worked against about 30% of the HIV-1 strains known to be present in the population in the clinical trial geographic area. These results indicate that the breadth of coverage against HIV strains needs to be expanded, perhaps through combinations of antibodies (Corey et al. 2021). However, researchers believe that if antibodies with long-lived protection can be developed at a lower cost, this could be a viable therapy or even preventative tool against HIV (Karuna and Corey 2020). Humanized mice are also being used to try to find better antibodies for this type of therapy (Dash et al. 2021; Gawron et al. 2019).

Even if one has access to treatment, ART is not capable of fully eliminating HIV from the body. During ART, HIV is said to hide in reservoirs in the body such as resting T-helper cells or in certain areas of the body like the brain that the antiretroviral drugs cannot access (Simon and Ho 2003; Lostroh 2019). If ART is stopped, within two weeks, the amount of virus "rebounds" in the blood, presumably from the cells and tissues where the drug could not act on the virus (Chun, Moir, and Fauci 2015).

It is important to note that there is at least one example of a patient who was cured of HIV, and the most famous example is known as the "Berlin Patient." This individual, named Timothy Ray Brown, went through chemotherapy as a treatment for leukemia. He then had a bone marrow transplant to replace his hematopoietic (blood) stem cells. The bone marrow donor happened to carry two copies of the CCR5-delta 32 mutation, making the donated cells resistant to HIV infection. After the patient's recovery, no HIV was detected in his body (Chun, Moir, and Fauci 2015; Gallagher 2021). Unfortunately, Brown died in 2020 when the leukemia returned. There are reports of another patient being cured in a similar manner, but the circumstances of the cure are considered too expensive and risky for the patient to be used routinely (Gallagher 2021). Given the extreme rarity of a cure using ART, an HIV vaccine is still desperately needed by the world.

5.8 Will We Ever Have an HIV Vaccine?

The search for an HIV/AIDS vaccine has gone on since 1981. Jonas Salk even wanted to participate in finding a vaccine against HIV, taking the approach of vaccinating people who were HIV positive so that they do not develop AIDS, called an "immunotherapeutic" approach. The vaccine unfortunately failed (Jacobs 2015). An anti-HIV vaccine tested in clinical trials in Thailand (RV144) used the strategy of inducing an immune response against several HIV proteins, and it seemed to be somewhat effective in preventing infection. The results were published in 2009, indicating a rate of infection that was 31% lower than the rate seen in those who took the placebo vaccine. However, this level of protection was below the typical 50% protection threshold used for most commercially available vaccines. The vaccine induced antibody production but also tried to boost the cytotoxic T cell–mediated immune response of the body (Lostroh 2019; Karasavvas et al. 2012; Rerks-Ngarm et al. 2009). Another 2007 vaccine trial that also used an approach focused on provoking the cytotoxic T cell response actually had to be stopped because the vaccine ended up increasing the risk of acquiring HIV (Walker 2008b; Lostroh 2019; Sekaly 2008).

Considering the many failed attempts at creating an effective HIV vaccine, public health officials have begun to shift to other strategies to end the AIDS pandemic. Back in 2015, UNAIDS was emphasizing the "90–90–90" goal to end the AIDS pandemic by the year 2030. In this initiative, the aim was to make sure that 90% of people who had acquired HIV knew that they had it, 90% of those people (HIV-positive individuals) would be on antiretroviral therapy, and that 90% of those people (HIV-positive individuals on ART) were successfully using antiretroviral therapy to keep their viral load below a detectable level as evaluated by testing (Fauci and Marston 2015; UNAIDS 2021b). Scientists have also talked about increasing prevention, diagnosis, and treatment initiatives among high-risk populations, targeting initiatives to any case clusters that are present, and readily using tools that are now available such as PrEP (Fauci and Marston 2015; Eisinger and Fauci 2018; Eisinger, Dieffenbach, and Fauci 2019). Others have pointed out that if a person brings their viral load to an undetectable point by successfully adhering to their ART regimen, then they are very unlikely to transmit HIV to their partner. The slogan "undetectable = untransmittable" has been used to help spread awareness of this important point (Eisinger, Dieffenbach, and Fauci 2019). Also, the knowledge that a person who keeps HIV at an undetectable amount is most likely not going to transmit it to a sexual partner is said to improve the self-esteem of someone who is HIV positive, as well as help decrease the stigma associated with being HIV positive (Eisinger, Dieffenbach, and Fauci 2019). All these ideas, including continuing the search for an HIV vaccine, most likely will be needed to end the HIV/AIDS pandemic, but it can be done. So why is it taking so long? An update on the latest world initiatives to end the HIV/AIDS pandemic are described at the end of the chapter.

5.9 Understand the Impact of HIV/AIDS on Society in the United States and around the World

Now that it has been 40 years since the first reports of AIDS, what has been done and what more needs to be done to end HIV/AIDS? Importantly, antiretroviral therapy has turned being HIV positive into a chronic condition for millions of people. However, there is still a huge "treatment gap" in terms of how many people know they are HIV positive and how many of them are receiving treatment. In addition, new HIV cases are still occurring regularly, more frequently in "black and brown communities" and "marginalized communities" in the U.S., indicating that health disparities and access to healthcare are playing a role in the emergence of new cases (Brangham, Coles, and Mufson 2021). Also, mistrust of the medical community among marginalized people is still a big issue when it comes to many kinds of disease treatment. For example, almost all HIV-positive African Americans enrolled in a clinical trial on adherence to HIV ART who were surveyed about COVID-19 indicated mistrust in medical information related to the topic, and many were also hesitant to get the COVID-19 vaccine (Bogart et al. 2021).

As of 2020, there were still 1.5 million new HIV infections every year on the planet (WHO 2021b). The WHO indicates that their global priorities include providing treatment equitably and finding ways to finance treatment, since ART must be taken for life. The WHO also funds initiatives looking at HIV and tuberculosis co-infection and working to prevent mother-to-child transmission of the virus through UNICEF (WHO 2021b). Of the over 35 million people in the world who are HIV positive, most of them are living in Africa (Ojikutu 2008a; Lostroh 2019). A recent estimate indicates that 25 million out of the 37 million people living with HIV are in Africa (WHO 2021b). There are at least 1.7 million children who have HIV in the world. A July 2021 report indicates that 46% were not on any antiretroviral therapy, and many HIV-positive mothers did not even have their children tested (UNAIDS 2021d).

According to the CDC, over a million people in the United States have HIV as of 2019 and the number of cases is still steadily increasing every year. For example, in New York State alone, there were 2,330 new cases in 2019. People 13 to 24 years of age account for 21% of the newly diagnosed HIV-positive individuals in the United States. Among those with HIV, 42% are Black/African American, 29% Latino, 25% White, and just under 5% of another or multiracial background (CDC 2021a).

Unlike the other viral diseases discussed in this book, people with AIDS did not garner sympathy universally from the public at the time AIDS and then HIV were first discovered in the early 1980s, and many still face HIV stigma and discrimination today. First, as a sexually transmitted disease, cultural perceptions of the appropriate time, place, and kind of sexual contact between human beings affected some people's perceptions of those who came down with AIDS. For example, PWA may have been "blamed" for getting HIV because of engaging in sexual activity. In addition, because the initial case clusters arising in the United States occurred in men who had sex with men and those who used intravenous drugs, AIDS became erroneously labeled as a "gay" disease or a disease found in drug addicts, leading some people to mistakenly believe that they were not susceptible to such a disease. However, as mentioned previously, as HIV spread, it became clear that anyone could get HIV under the right transmission conditions.

The social implications of these misconceptions ended up being huge and devastating for PWA, something our society should never forget, leading to housing, employment, insurance, and other kinds of discrimination directed at people with HIV, at a time when they were most vulnerable. Depictions of that discrimination can be seen in films such as *Philadelphia* and *Dallas Buyers Club* and in books such as *And the Band Played On* and *How to Survive a Plague* (Demme 1993; Vallee 2013; France 2016; Shilts 1987). One way to fight discrimination is to actively work against HIV stigma, including carefully choosing the words you use to describe a person living with HIV. The CDC even provides a language guide link from their "HIV Stigma and Discrimination" website (CDC 2021b).

The HIV/AIDS pandemic changed many people's attitudes towards health information privacy too, given the risk of discrimination based on one's HIV status. How is one's right to keep their health status private balanced with public health needs? How should partner notification programs work if a person finds out that they are HIV positive? The preferred approach might be different depending on if a person is a public health official, a friend, or a healthcare professional. Also, should exposing someone to potentially acquiring HIV be illegal? The United States and the world still need to address these issues. Also, what is one's overall "right to health," including access to preventative care, treatment, and support services within a society (Gostin 2005)? These are all complex issues with no easy answers.

The early years of the AIDS crisis in the U.S., from 1980 to 1985, were documented in the book by Randy Shilts called *And the Band Played On*. In his account, Shilts follows the lives of men primarily in Los Angeles and New York as their friends begin dying around them from a mysterious illness (AIDS), along with the scientists and physicians seeking to learn the cause of AIDS in these patients. At that time, no drugs were on the market to treat AIDS, making AIDS a fatal disease. To push for research on the cause of AIDS as well as treatment, PWA, as well as their friends and loved ones, had to form their own advocacy groups such as Gay Men's Health Crisis in New York (GMHC). GMHC was organized by Larry Kramer and others, and their first president was Paul Popham. These groups had to constantly push government officials for more money into funding scientists and physicians working on AIDS and AIDS-related diseases, while raising their own funds as well. In addition, PWA faced discrimination in hospitals where some people refused to treat AIDS patients or neglected them even near the end of their lives. Members of the community had to step in to care for individuals who had no family willing to help them in their final hours (Shilts 1987). An additional account of the early days of AIDS, as well as the fight to make effective medication available to everyone who needed it in the late 1980s and 1990s, can be found in David France's book *How to Survive a Plague* (France 2016).

In his book, David France documents the work of the AIDS Coalition to Unleash Power (ACT UP) in advocating for PWA. ACT UP formed its own "Treatment +Data Committee," later becoming the independent Treatment Action Group, to research promising drugs and go directly to pharmaceutical companies to demand release of those drugs to PWA. In addition, some people sought any means possible to bring drugs to the people who needed it, even if it meant finding ways to supply or make their own. France describes the release of the first AIDS drug, AZT, and how ACT UP protested the huge cost of the drug, limiting access for those who needed it. Their efforts continued until the development of protease inhibitors and ultimately the drug cocktails that allowed HIV-positive individuals to survive for long periods with their disease never progressing to AIDS. However, the high cost of ART has continued to be an issue (France 2016).

The friends and family of those who had died of AIDS, and other advocates who wanted to advance biomedical research on HIV/AIDS, started other grassroots movements to remember these individuals, including two of the most famous remembrances, the AIDS Quilt and World AIDS Day. The idea for the AIDS quilt came from Cleve Jones (mentioned in *And the Band Played On*) after seeing a display of the names of people who died of AIDS at an event. Jones made the first panel of the quilt in honor of his friend Marvin Feldman in 1985. The quilt became a powerful symbol of each person lost, with each panel said to be the approximate size of a human's grave, as well as a symbol of the enormity of the loss, when all the panels were displayed together. By the time the AIDS quilt was first displayed on the National Mall in Washington, D.C., in 1987, there were over 1,900 panels, and then at the last display of the full quilt in the same location in 1996 there were 40,000 panels. Since that time, the quilt has been displayed in sections around the world and is cared for by the National AIDS Memorial. An interactive AIDS quilt is available for viewing through their website (Memorial 2021) (Figure 5.5). World AIDS Day has been celebrated

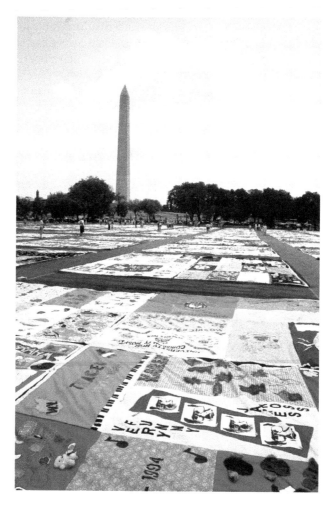

FIGURE 5.5

Commemorating the lives of those lost to HIV/AIDS—AIDS Memorial Quilt.

Shown above is a display of AIDS Memorial Quilt panels in Washington, D.C., on June 27, 2004.

Photo credit: DBKing (licensed under CC BY 2.0; https://creativecommons.org/licenses/by/2.0/legalcode).

Original image can be found at https://wordpress.org/openverse/photos/be7a1324-9284-4e6f-9aca-0e7fdd9eab 3f?referrer=creativecommons.org and www.flickr.com/photos/65193799@N00/14419883

every December 1 since 1988 as a day to remember those who died of AIDS and show support for those who are HIV positive and PWA. It was the first day designated internationally centered on one global health issue. Participants often wear a red ribbon on that day. Activities around the world include educating people about HIV/AIDS and volunteering at and attending events about HIV/AIDS research advances (UNAIDS 2021e).

One can also find many references to HIV/AIDS routinely in popular culture. Larry Kramer, an AIDS activist, wrote a play called *The Normal Heart* that was made into a film (France 2016; Shilts 1987; Murphy 2014). Other famous works using HIV/AIDS as a theme include the stage musical *Rent* written by Jonathan Larson adapted into a film of the same name and the play *Angels in America* written by Tony Kushner turned into television miniseries (Columbus 2005; Nichols 2003). We must never forget the people who suffered in the early years of the HIV/AIDS pandemic and the millions of productive and creative years of life that were lost because treatment was not available sooner.

Because of all the treatment options available, many wonder when we will be able to end the AIDS pandemic altogether. How will the United States and other countries address the issue of access to treatment? Why is being HIV positive more common among the poor and people of color, and how can we change that? The group UNAIDS released a report in 2021 entitled "Global AIDS Strategy 2021–2026—End Inequalities. End AIDS." In this report, the group's goals for the next five years are described, all centered around eliminating AIDS, at least as a major public health threat, by 2030. Priorities include providing equal access for all to HIV/AIDS preventative care, testing, and treatment. In addition, UNAIDS will work towards continuing to reduce HIV stigma and discrimination against people who are HIV positive, in the hope of getting more people tested and treated for HIV. Finally, reducing gender inequality and gender-based violence and promoting better overall health and social services around the world will help reduce inequalities that put some people more at risk than others are for acquiring HIV (UNAIDS 2021c).

5.10 Conclusion

As scientists celebrated the eradication of smallpox in 1980, little did they know that they were about to discover another scourge known as HIV/AIDS in 1981. Scientists have remarked on this timing as an indication that we will always face emerging virus threats (Fine and Heymann 2020). Although the discovery of AIDS and then HIV led to a harrowing race to detect the virus and then treat HIV infection, scientists are now closing in on this killer and working hard to halt it through ART, rigorous testing, and education on preventative measures. Improving healthcare around the world and focusing on healthcare as a human right will help defeat HIV/AIDS.

5.11 Summary

Human immunodeficiency virus (HIV) is a type of retrovirus known as a lentivirus that causes acquired immunodeficiency syndrome (AIDS). HIV attacks T-helper cells that are a part of the immune system, preventing the body from fighting other pathogens.

AIDS was first discovered in the United States in two clusters of patients exhibiting out-of-control infections from opportunistic pathogens characteristic of people with compromised immune systems. Soon, HIV was seen in patients such as hemophiliacs who were most likely acquiring HIV from a contaminated blood supply. Isolates from these patients helped lead to the discovery of HIV, the implementation of HIV testing to detect the virus or antibodies against the virus, and then the development of the first antiretroviral drugs to fight the virus. Initial treatment approaches were not successful long term due to mutation of the virus causing resistance to treatment, but the development of protease inhibitors and combination drug therapies in the mid-1990s led to a steep decline in AIDS deaths in those who had access to treatment. Many people suffered in the early days of the HIV/AIDS pandemic, and they are remembered in works of literature and art, such as the AIDS quilt, and through remembrances like World AIDS Day. Future research is geared towards finding an HIV vaccine, making antiretroviral therapy (ART) available to all who need it, and preventing new HIV infection through education and addressing healthcare disparities around the world.

Discussion Questions:

1. Do you think the goal of eradicating HIV from the earth is attainable? Explain why or why not.
2. What are the major roadblocks and challenges that have prevented the development of an HIV vaccine?
3. How do we fight discrimination based on one's HIV status?
4. Compare and contrast the HIV/AIDS pandemic to the COVID-19 pandemic.
5. Go to the interactive AIDS Memorial Quilt website at https://www.aidsmemorial.org/interactive-aids-quilt where you can search by name, or click on one of the featured 40 stories for 40 years of the AIDS pandemic https://www.aidsmemorial.org/40-40a
   a. Take some time to learn about this individual.
   b. What did they enjoy about life based on the graphics and photos used in the quilt panel or story?
   c. How do their friends and family remember them in the quilt or story?

References

AB, Nobel Media. 2021. "The Nobel prize in physiology or medicine 1975." Accessed 4 February 2021. www.nobelprize.org/prizes/medicine/1975/press-release/.

AB, Nobel Prize Outreach. 2008. "Nobel prize in physiology or medicine 2008 press release." Accessed 15 October 2021. www.nobelprize.org/prizes/medicine/2008/press-release/.

Ackermann, H.-W., L. Berthiaume, and M. Tremblay. 1998. *Virus Life in Diagrams*. Boca Raton, FL: CRC press, Taylor & Francis Group.

Agarwal, Y., C. Beatty, S. Biradar, I. Castronova, S. Ho, K. Melody, and M.T. Bility. 2020. "Moving beyond the mousetrap: Current and emerging humanized mouse and rat models for investigating prevention and cure strategies against HIV infection and associated pathologies." *Retrovirology* 17 (1):8. doi: 10.1186/s12977-020-00515-3.

Alexander, T.S. 2016. "Human immunodeficiency virus diagnostic testing: 30 years of evolution." *Clinical and Vaccine Immunology* 23 (4):249–53. doi: 10.1128/cvi.00053-16.

Baltimore, D. 1971. "Expression of animal virus genomes." *Bacteriological Reviews* 35 (3):235.

Barré-Sinoussi, F., J.C. Chermann, F. Rey, M.T. Nugeyre, S. Chamaret, J. Gruest, C. Dauguet, et al. 1983. "Isolation of a T-lymphotropic retrovirus from a patient at risk for acquired immune deficiency syndrome (AIDS)." *Science* 220 (4599):868–71. doi: 10.1126/science.6189183.

Biointeractive, H. 2021. "The immune system." *Howard Hughes Medical Institute*. Accessed 11 October 2021. www.biointeractive.org/classroom-resources/immune-system.

Bogart, L.M., B.O. Ojikutu, K. Tyagi, D.J. Klein, M.G. Mutchler, L. Dong, S.J. Lawrence, D.R. Thomas, and S. Kellman. 2021. "COVID-19 related medical mistrust, health impacts, and potential vaccine hesitancy among black Americans living with HIV." *Journal of Acquired Immune Deficiency Syndromes* 86 (2):200–7. doi: 10.1097/qai.0000000000002570.

Brangham, W., D. Coles, and C. Mufson. 2021. "After 40 years of AIDS, progress has been made but major problems remain." In *PBS NewsHour*, 11 min 21 sec. Arlington, VA: NewsHour Productions LLC.

Buchmann, K. 2014. "Evolution of innate immunity: Clues from invertebrates via fish to mammals." *Frontiers in Immunology* 5:459.

Burton, D.R. 2019. "Advancing an HIV vaccine; advancing vaccinology." *Nature Reviews Immunology* 19 (2):77–8.

CDC, Centers for Disease Control and Prevention. 2021a. "HIV basics." *Department of Health and Human Services*. Accessed 11 October 2021. www.cdc.gov/hiv/basics/statistics.html#:~:text=About%20 37.9%20million%20people%20were,the%20start%20of%20the%20epidemic.

———. 2021b. "HIV stigma and discrimination." *Health and Human Services*. Accessed 19 October 2021. www.cdc.gov/hiv/basics/hiv-stigma/index.html.

———. 2021c. "HIV testing." *Department of Health and Human Services*. Accessed 11 October 2021. www.cdc.gov/hiv/basics/transmission.html.

———. 2021d. "HIV transmission." *Department of Health and Human Services*. Accessed 11 October 2021. www.cdc.gov/hiv/basics/transmission.html.

Chun, T.W., S. Moir, and A.S. Fauci. 2015. "HIV reservoirs as obstacles and opportunities for an HIV cure." *Nature Immunology* 16 (6):584–9. doi: 10.1038/ni.3152.

Cloyd, M.W. 1996. "Human retroviruses." In *Medical Microbiology*, edited by S. Baron. Galveston, TX: University of Texas Medical Branch at Galveston.

Coico, R., and G. Sunshine. 2015. *Immunology: A Short Course*. 7th ed. Hoboken, NJ: John Wiley & Sons, Incorporated.

Columbus, C. (director). Rosenthal, J., DeNiro, R., Columbus, C., Radcliffe, M, and Barnathan, M. (producers). 2005. "*Rent.*" [Film].135 min. Culver City, CA: Sony Pictures Releasing.

Corey, L., P.B. Gilbert, M. Juraska, D.C. Montefiori, L. Morris, S.T. Karuna, S. Edupuganti, et al. 2021. "Two randomized trials of neutralizing antibodies to prevent HIV-1 acquisition." *The New England Journal of Medicine* 384 (11):1003–14. doi: 10.1056/NEJMoa2031738.

Cruse, J.M., and R.E. Lewis. 2009. *Illustrated Dictionary of Immunology*. Boca Raton, FL: CRC Press, Taylor & Francis Group.

Dash, P.K., S. Gorantla, L. Poluektova, M. Hasan, E. Waight, C. Zhang, M. Markovic, et al. 2021. "Humanized mice for infectious and neurodegenerative disorders." *Retrovirology* 18 (1):13. doi: 10.1186/s12977-021-00557-1.

Demme, J. (director). Demme, J. and E. Saxon (producers). 1993. "*Philadelphia.*" [Film] 126 min. Culver City, CA: TriStar Pictures.

Eisinger, R.W., C.W. Dieffenbach, and A.S. Fauci. 2019. "HIV viral load and transmissibility of HIV infection: Undetectable equals untransmittable." *JAMA* 321 (5):451–2. doi: 10.1001/jama.2018.21167.

Eisinger, R.W., and A.S. Fauci. 2018. "Ending the HIV/AIDS pandemic." *Emerging Infectious Diseases* 24 (3):413.

Faria, N.R., A. Rambaut, A. Suchard Marc, G. Baele, T. Bedford, J. Ward Melissa, J. Tatem Andrew, et al. 2014. "The early spread and epidemic ignition of HIV-1 in human populations." *Science* 346 (6205):56–61. doi: 10.1126/science.1256739.

Fauci, A.S., and H.D. Marston. 2015. "Focusing to achieve a world without AIDS." *JAMA* 313 (4):357–8.

FDA, Food and Drug Administration. 2021. "FDA approves first extended-release, injectable drug regimen for adults living with HIV." *Department of Health and Human Services.* Accessed 9 November 2021. www.fda.gov/news-events/press-announcements/fda-approves-first-extended-release-injectable-drug-regimen-adults-living-hiv.

Fine, P., and D. Heymann. 2020. "Smallpox: Lessons from eradication." In *Jenner Conversations,* edited by G. Williams. Berkeley, England: Jenner Museum.

France, D. 2016. *How to Survive a Plague: The Inside Story of How Citizens and Science Tamed AIDS.* New York, NY: Vintage Books, a division of Penguin Random House LLC.

Friedman-Kien, A., L. Laubenstein, M. Marmor, K. Hymes, J. Green, A. Ragaz, . . ., and J. Goedert. 1981. "Kaposi's sarcoma and pneumocystis pneumonia among homosexual men—New York City and California." *Morbidity and Mortality Weekly Report* 30 (25):305–8.

Gallagher, J. 2021. "Berlin patient: First person cured of HIV, Timothy Ray Brown, dies." *BBC.* Accessed 27 October 2021. www.bbc.com/news/health-54355673.

Gallo, R.C., and L. Montagnier. 1988. "AIDS in 1988." *Scientific American* 259 (4):40–51.

———. 2003. "The discovery of HIV as the cause of AIDS." *New England Journal of Medicine* 349 (24):2283–5. doi: 10.1056/NEJMp038194.

Gallo, R.C., P.S. Sarin, E.P. Gelmann, M. Robert-Guroff, E. Richardson, V.S. Kalyanaraman, D. Mann, et al. 1983. "Isolation of human T-cell leukemia virus in acquired immune deficiency syndrome (AIDS)." *Science* 220 (4599):865–7. doi: 10.1126/science.6601823.

Gao, F., E. Bailes, D.L. Robertson, Y. Chen, C.M. Rodenburg, S.F. Michael, L.B. Cummins, et al. 1999. "Origin of HIV-1 in the chimpanzee Pan troglodytes troglodytes." *Nature* 397 (6718):436–41. doi: 10.1038/17130.

Gawron, M.A., M. Duval, C. Carbone, S. Jaiswal, A. Wallace, J.C. Martin, 3rd, A. Dauphin, et al. 2019. "Human anti-HIV-1 gp120 monoclonal antibodies with neutralizing activity cloned from humanized mice infected with HIV-1." *Journal of Immunology* 202 (3):799–804. doi: 10.4049/jimmunol.1801085.

Gostin, L.O. 2005. *The AIDS Pandemic: Complacency, Injustice, and Unfulfilled Expectations.* Chapel Hill, NC: Univ of North Carolina Press.

Gottlieb, M.S., H.M. Schanker, P.T. Fan, A. Saxon, J.D. Weisman, and I. Pozalski. 1981. "*Pneumocystis* pneumonia—Los Angeles." *Morbidity and Mortality Weekly Report* 30 (21):1–3.

Grant, R.M., J.R. Lama, P.L. Anderson, V. McMahan, A.Y. Liu, L. Vargas, P. Goicochea, M. Casapía, J.V. Guanira-Carranza, and M.E. Ramirez-Cardich. 2010. "Preexposure chemoprophylaxis for HIV prevention in men who have sex with men." *New England Journal of Medicine* 363 (27):2587–99.

Gryseels, S., T.D. Watts, J.M. Kabongo Mpolesha, B.B. Larsen, P. Lemey, J.J. Muyembe-Tamfum, D.E. Teuwen, and M. Worobey. 2020. "A near full-length HIV-1 genome from 1966 recovered from formalin-fixed paraffin-embedded tissue." *Proceedings of the National Academy of Sciences of the United States of America* 117 (22):12222–9. doi: 10.1073/pnas.1913682117.

Gulick, R.M., and C. Flexner. 2019. "Long-Acting HIV drugs for treatment and prevention." *Annual Review of Medicine* 70:137–50. doi: 10.1146/annurev-med-041217-013717.

Hatziioannou, T., and D.T. Evans. 2012. "Animal models for HIV/AIDS research." *Nature Reviews Microbiology* 10 (12):852–67. doi: 10.1038/nrmicro2911.

Healthcare, V. 2021. "Clinical trials for CABENUVA." Accessed 9 November 2021. https://cabenuvahcp.com/clinical-trials/.

HHS, D.o.H.a.H.S. 2021. "A timeline of HIV and AIDS." Accessed 26 September 2021. www.hiv.gov/hiv-basics/overview/history/hiv-and-aids-timeline.

Ho, S. 2008. "The molecular clock and estimating species divergence." *Nature Education* 1 (1):168.

Huang, Y., W.A. Paxton, S.M. Wolinsky, A.U. Neumann, L. Zhang, T. He, S. Kang, et al. 1996. "The role of a mutant CCR5 allele in HIV-1 transmission and disease progression." *Nature Medicine* 2 (11):1240–3. doi: 10.1038/nm1196-1240.

Jacobs, C.D. 2015. *Jonas Salk: A Life.* Cary, NC: Oxford University Press, Incorporated.

Karasavvas, N., E. Billings, M. Rao, C. Williams, S. Zolla-Pazner, R.T. Bailer, R.A. Koup, S. Madnote, D. Arworn, and X. Shen. 2012. "The Thai phase III HIV type 1 vaccine trial (RV144) regimen induces antibodies that target conserved regions within the V2 loop of gp120." *AIDS Research and Human Retroviruses* 28 (11):1444–57.

Karuna, S.T., and L. Corey. 2020. "Broadly neutralizing antibodies for HIV prevention." *Annual Review of Medicine* 71:329–46.

Korber, B., M. Muldoon, J. Theiler, F. Gao, R. Gupta, A. Lapedes, B.H. Hahn, S. Wolinsky, and T. Bhattacharya. 2000. "Timing the ancestor of the HIV-1 pandemic strains." *Science* 288 (5472):1789–96. doi: 10.1126/science.288.5472.1789.

Kumi Smith, M., B.L. Jewell, T.B. Hallett, and M.S. Cohen. 2018. "Treatment of HIV for the prevention of transmission in discordant couples and at the population level." *Advances in Experimental Medicine and Biology* 1075:125–62. doi: 10.1007/978-981-13-0484-2_6.

Lostroh, P. 2019. *Molecular and Cellular Biology of Viruses*. 1st ed. Boca Raton, FL: Taylor & Francis Group, LLC.

Martinson, J.J., N.H. Chapman, D.C. Rees, Y.T. Liu, and J.B. Clegg. 1997. "Global distribution of the CCR5 gene 32-basepair deletion." *Nature Genetics* 16 (1):100–3. doi: 10.1038/ng0597-100.

Memorial, N.A. 2021. "The history of the quilt." Accessed 11 October 2021. www.aidsmemorial.org/quilt-history.

Minkoff, E.C., and P.J. Baker. 2004. "Chapter 16: HIV and AIDS." In *Biology Today: An Issues Approach*, 573–609. New York, NY: Garland Science.

Murphy, R. (director). Ferguson, S. (producer). 2014. *"The normal heart."* [Film]. 2 hr 13 min. New York, NY: Home Box Office (HBO). https://www.hbo.com/movies/the-normal-heart.

Nichols, M. (director). Costas, C.D. (producer). 2003. *"Angels in America."* [Film]. 352 min. New York, NY: Home Box Office (HBO). https://www.hbo.com/angels-in-america.

NIH, National Institutes of Health. 2021a. "Discovery of HIV." *Office of NIH History and Stetten Museum*. Accessed 20 October 2021. https://history.nih.gov/display/history/Discovery+of+HIV.

———. 2021b. "NIH eminent scientist profiles: Robert C. Gallo (1937–)." *Office of NIH History and Stetten Museum*. Accessed 20 October 2021. https://history.nih.gov/pages/viewpage.action?pageId=11600169.

Novembre, J., A.P. Galvani, and M. Slatkin. 2005. "The geographic spread of the CCR5 delta32 HIV-resistance allele." *PLoS Biology* 3 (11):e339. doi: 10.1371/journal.pbio.0030339.

Ojikutu, B.O. 2008a. "Lecture 1: From outbreak to epidemic." *Howard Hughes Medical Institute*. Accessed 11 October 2021. www.biointeractive.org/professional-learning/science-talks/aids-evolution-epidemic.

———. 2008b. "Lecture 3: Drugs and HIV evolution." *Howard Hughes Medical Institute*. Accessed 11 October 2021. www.biointeractive.org/professional-learning/science-talks/aids-evolution-epidemic.

Orkin, C., K. Arasteh, M. Górgolas Hernández-Mora, V. Pokrovsky, E.T. Overton, P.M. Girard, S. Oka, et al. 2020. "Long-acting cabotegravir and rilpivirine after oral induction for HIV-1 infection." *New England Journal of Medicine* 382 (12):1124–35. doi: 10.1056/NEJMoa1909512.

Overton, E.T., G. Richmond, G. Rizzardini, H. Jaeger, C. Orrell, F. Nagimova, F. Bredeek, et al. 2021. "Long-acting cabotegravir and rilpivirine dosed every 2 months in adults with HIV-1 infection (ATLAS-2M), 48-week results: A randomised, multicentre, open-label, phase 3b, non-inferiority study." *Lancet* 396 (10267):1994–2005. doi: 10.1016/s0140-6736(20)32666-0.

Padte, N.N., J. Yu, Y. Huang, and D.D. Ho. 2018. "Engineering multi-specific antibodies against HIV-1." *Retrovirology* 15 (1):60. doi: 10.1186/s12977-018-0439-9.

Parrish, C.R., E.C. Holmes, D.M. Morens, E.C. Park, D.S. Burke, C.H. Calisher, C.A. Laughlin, L.J. Saif, and P. Daszak. 2008. "Cross-species virus transmission and the emergence of new epidemic diseases." *Microbiology and Molecular Biology Reviews* 72 (3):457–70. doi: 10.1128/mmbr.00004-08.

Peeters, M., M. Jung, and A. Ayouba. 2013. "The origin and molecular epidemiology of HIV." *Expert Review of Anti-infective Therapy* 11 (9):885–96. doi: 10.1586/14787210.2013.825443.

Rerks-Ngarm, S., P. Pitisuttithum, S. Nitayaphan, J. Kaewkungwal, J. Chiu, R. Paris, N. Premsri, et al. 2009. "Vaccination with ALVAC and AIDSVAX to prevent HIV-1 infection in Thailand." *New England Journal of Medicine* 361 (23):2209–20. doi: 10.1056/NEJMoa0908492.

Rial-Crestelo, D., A. Pinto-Martínez, and F. Pulido. 2020. "Cabotegravir and rilpivirine for the treatment of HIV." *Expert Review of Anti-infective Therapy* 18 (5):393–404.

Rizzardini, G., E.T. Overton, C. Orkin, S. Swindells, K. Arasteh, M. Górgolas Hernández-Mora, V. Pokrovsky, et al. 2020. "Long-acting injectable cabotegravir + rilpivirine for HIV maintenance therapy: Week 48 pooled analysis of phase 3 ATLAS and FLAIR trials." *Journal of Acquired Immune Deficiency Syndromes* 85 (4):498–506. doi: 10.1097/qai.0000000000002466.

Schwartz, J. 2013. "Stephen Crohn, who furthered AIDS study, dies at 66." In *The New York Times*. New York, NY: The New York Times Company.

Sekaly, R.-P. 2008. "The failed HIV Merck vaccine study: A step back or a launching point for future vaccine development?" *The Journal of Experimental Medicine* 205 (1):7–12. doi: 10.1084/jem.20072681.

Sharp, P.M., and B.H. Hahn. 2010. "The evolution of HIV-1 and the origin of AIDS." *Philosophical Transactions of the Royal Society B* 365 (1552):2487–94. doi: 10.1098/rstb.2010.0031.

———. 2011. "Origins of HIV and the AIDS pandemic." *Cold Spring Harbor Perspectives in Medicine* 1 (1):a006841-a. doi: 10.1101/cshperspect.a006841.

Shilts, R. 1987. *And The Band Played On: Politics, People, and the AIDS Epidemic*. New York, NY: St. Martin's Griffin.

Simon, V., and D.D. Ho. 2003. "HIV-1 dynamics in vivo: Implications for therapy." *Nature Reviews Microbiology* 1 (3):181–90. doi: 10.1038/nrmicro772.

Swindells, S., J.F. Andrade-Villanueva, G.J. Richmond, G. Rizzardini, A. Baumgarten, M. Masiá, G. Latiff, et al. 2020. "Long-acting cabotegravir and rilpivirine for maintenance of HIV-1 suppression." *New England Journal of Medicine* 382 (12):1112–23. doi: 10.1056/NEJMoa1904398.

Tang, H., K.L. Kuhen, and F. Wong-Staal. 1999. "Lentivirus replication and regulation." *Annual Review of Genetics* 33 (1):133–70. doi: 10.1146/annurev.genet.33.1.133.

Torian, L., M. Chen, P. Rhodes, and H.I. Hall. 2011. "HIV surveillance—United States, 1981–2008." *Morbidity and Mortality Weekly Report* 60 (21):689–93.

UNAIDS. 2021a. "40 years of the AIDS response." *UNAIDS*. Accessed 26 October 2021. www.unaids.org/en/resources/infographics/40-years-of-the-AIDS-response.

———. 2021b. "90–90–90: Treatment for all." *UNAIDS*. Accessed 14 November 2021. www.unaids.org/en/resources/909090.

———. 2021c. "Global AIDS strategy 2021–2026—End inequalities. End AIDS." *The Joint United Nations Programme on HIV/AIDS*. Accessed 19 October 2021. www.unaids.org/en/resources/documents/2021/2021-2026-global-AIDS-strategy.

———. 2021d. "New report reveals stark inequalities in access to HIV prevention and treatment services for children-partners call for urgent action." *UNAIDS*. Accessed 19 October 2021. www.unaids.org/en/resources/presscentre/pressreleaseandstatementarchive/2021/july/20210721_start-free-stay-free-aids-free.

———. 2021e. "World AIDS day." Accessed 19 October 2021. www.unaids.org/en/World_AIDS_Day.

Vallee, J.-M. (director). Brenner, B. and Winter, R. (producers). 2013. *"Dallas Buyers Club"* [Film]. 117 min. Universal City, CA: Focus Features. https://www.focusfeatures.com/dallasbuyersclub.

Walker, B.D. 2008a. "Lecture 2: AIDS and the HIV life cycle." *Howard Hughes Medical Institute*. Accessed 11 October 2021. www.biointeractive.org/professional-learning/science-talks/aids-evolution-epidemic.

———. 2008b. "Lecture 4: Vaccines and HIV evolution." *Howard Hughes Medical Institute*. Accessed 11 October 2021. www.biointeractive.org/professional-learning/science-talks/aids-evolution-epidemic.

Weinberg, R.A. 2014. *Biology of Cancer*. 2nd ed. New York, NY: Garland Science, Taylor & Francis Group.

WHO, World Health Organization. 2021a. "HIV data and statistics." Accessed 26 September 2021. www.who.int/teams/global-hiv-hepatitis-and-stis-programmes/hiv/strategic-information/hiv-data-and-statistics.

———. 2021b. "HIV/AIDS." Accessed 26 September 2021. www.who.int/news-room/fact-sheets/detail/hiv-aids.

Worobey, M., M. Gemmel, D.E. Teuwen, T. Haselkorn, K. Kunstman, M. Bunce, J.J. Muyembe, et al. 2008. "Direct evidence of extensive diversity of HIV-1 in Kinshasa by 1960." *Nature* 455 (7213):661–4. doi: 10.1038/nature07390.

Worobey, M., T.D. Watts, R.A. McKay, M.A. Suchard, T. Granade, D.E. Teuwen, B.A. Koblin, W. Heneine, P. Lemey, and H.W. Jaffe. 2016. "1970s and 'Patient 0' HIV-1 genomes illuminate early HIV/AIDS history in North America." *Nature* 539 (7627):98–101. doi: 10.1038/nature19827.

Zimmer, C. 2011. *A Planet of Viruses*. 2nd ed. Chicago, IL: University of Chicago Press.

6

SARS-CoV-2 and COVID-19

Learning Outcomes:

6.1 Describe the Details of Novel Coronavirus (SARS-CoV-2) Compared to Other Viruses

6.2 Understand How SARS-CoV-2 Is Transmitted among Humans, Discover How SARS-CoV-2 Affects the Body, and Understand What Tests and Treatments Are Available

6.3 Examine the Historical Factors Leading to the Development and Continuation of the COVID-19 Pandemic

6.4 Follow the Race to Develop a COVID-19 Vaccine

6.5 Differentiate the Course of the Pandemic before and after Mass Vaccination Campaigns Begin in the United States

6.6 Discuss Whether the COVID-19 Pandemic Could Have Been Prevented and What the World Learned from the COVID-19 Pandemic

6.7 Recognize the Impact of the COVID-19 Pandemic on the United States and the World, and What Our Societies Will Look Like Post-Pandemic

In this book, we have discussed epidemics and pandemics, many of which took place before humans even knew what viruses were. Now, in the 21st century, we have more research tools and techniques, medicines, and types of health interventions than ever, yet the COVID-19 pandemic still made life difficult for almost every human being on the planet, even those who did not acquire the virus. What is SARS-CoV-2, and how did it create the COVID-19 pandemic unchecked? What are the current treatments for COVID-19 and how did researchers develop a vaccine so fast? How has our society forever changed during the COVID-19 pandemic? We will explore these questions and other details in this chapter.

6.1 Describe the Details of Novel Coronavirus (SARS-CoV-2) Compared to Other Viruses

Coronaviruses are a family of large single-stranded RNA viruses (Class IV Baltimore classification) with a lipid envelope covering studded with spike proteins, thus giving the virus the "crown-like" appearance behind its name (corona means crown in several languages going back to Latin and Greek) (Figure 6.1). These spike proteins help the virus attach to our cells, in particular cells that display the ACE2 receptor (Christakis 2020; Baltimore 1971; Rabadan 2021; Wright 2021; Callaway 2020; Cyranoski 2020). Cells in the

DOI: 10.1201/9781003172260-6

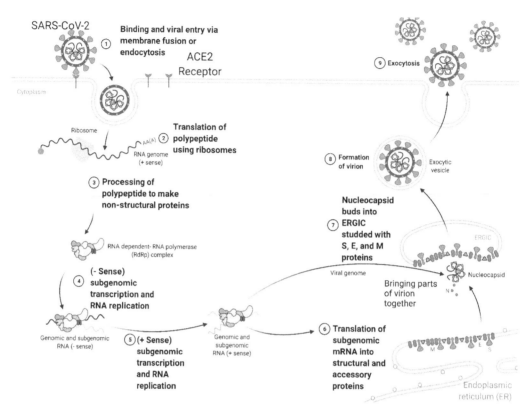

FIGURE 6.1

Life cycle of SARS-CoV-2.

Shown here is the life cycle of the coronavirus, SARS-CoV-2. First, the virus binds to the cell using the ACE2 receptor and enters the cell. Then, a polypeptide is translated and processed so that nonstructural proteins like the RNA-dependent RNA polymerase can copy the genome. A – sense copy of viral genes is transcribed, and the RNA replicated, followed by a + sense copy. The transcription and replication are occurring at membrane structures that form in response to the virus (not shown). + sense RNA is used as a template for translation of SARS-CoV-2 structural and accessory proteins at the ER. Then, the spike (S), envelope (E), and membrane (M) proteins begin to assemble at the membrane in a structure known as an ER-Golgi intermediate compartment (ERGIC). The whole virion takes shape and is then released by exocytosis.

Created using Biorender.com using a template based on Hartenian, E., D. Nandakumar, A. Lari, M. Ly, J.M. Tucker, and B.A. Glaunsinger. 2020. "The molecular virology of coronaviruses." *Journal of Biological Chemistry* 295 (37):12910–12934. doi: 10.1074/jbc.REV120.013930. Epub 2020 Jul 13. PMID: 32661197; PMCID: PMC7489918.

lungs, digestive tract, and brain all have ACE2 receptors, in addition to endothelial cells, the cells that line blood vessels (Wright 2021; Cyranoski 2020). The viral particle itself is about 100–125 nanometers in diameter (Rabadan 2021; Cyranoski 2020; Bar-On et al. 2020). Once the coronavirus attaches to cells, it enters through our own cellular trafficking network and is processed in a specialized structure known as an endosome. Then the viral genome (RNA-based) is released so the viral proteins can be translated using the host's own machinery. A viral enzyme also makes a negative strand (template) copy of the RNA genome, so that the coronavirus subgenome can be transcribed and translated to make the proteins needed for the new virion particles. Once the subgenome is copied and new viral proteins are made, the virus assembled in the cytoplasm buds out as a membrane-bound virion using the ER and Golgi, and then makes it way to the plasma membrane to be released from the cell (LabXchange 2021a; Cyranoski 2020; Callaway 2020; Ackermann, Berthiaume, and Tremblay 1998). When compared to other viral pathogens, SARS-CoV-2 is said to have a lower mutation rate than influenza A, and it can proofread its RNA genome to fix errors. However, it has a fast rate of replication once in a host cell (Abdelrahman, Li, and Wang 2020).

SARS-CoV-2 is very similar to two other coronaviruses that have affected humans in the past 20 years, including the original SARS, SARS-CoV, which became an epidemic mostly in Asia in 2002–2003, and MERS-CoV which has been found in regional outbreaks in the Middle East (Wardeh, Baylis, and Blagrove 2021; Christakis 2020; Wright 2021). All three, SARS-CoV, SARS-CoV-2, and MERS-CoV, cause respiratory illness with varying degrees of severity. There are also four more coronaviruses, HKU1, NL63, OC43, and 229E, that can infect humans but only cause mild illness such as seen with the common cold (Wardeh, Baylis, and Blagrove 2021; Christakis 2020; Rabadan 2021; Cyranoski 2020; Krammer 2020; Abdelrahman, Li, and Wang 2020).

SARS-CoV was first discovered among humans in November 2002 in southeastern China (about 600 miles from Wuhan). This pathogen was spread mainly through travel. There was an infamous incident in which a doctor who had treated SARS patients took a trip to the Metropole Hotel in Hong Kong in February 2003, bringing SARS-CoV with him, and eventually spread the virus to several hotel guests via airborne transmission. The hotel guests then spread the virus to other countries when they traveled home by plane. It is said that about 50% of all SARS cases can be traced back to this hotel incident. Ultimately, just over 8,000 people contracted SARS-CoV, and 774 people died. The virus was deemed under control by July 2003 (Rabadan 2021; Christakis 2020; Enserink 2013; Normile 2013b, 2013a; Abdelrahman, Li, and Wang 2020).

When SARS-CoV is compared to SARS-CoV-2 as a pathogen, it appears that SARS-CoV causes a higher case fatality rate than SARS-CoV-2, and that people with SARS-CoV generally had symptoms while those with SARS-CoV-2 may not, at least 50% of the time. These two differences may be some of the reasons that SARS did not turn into a pandemic (Christakis 2020). However, one can see that there are major similarities between the two pathogens, including their probable animal origin in bats (Zhou et al. 2020; Normile 2013b; Abdelrahman, Li, and Wang 2020). The movie *Contagion* is loosely based on the SARS epidemic (Soderbergh 2011).

Middle Eastern respiratory syndrome (MERS) was first described in humans in 2012. This virus also came from bats, with camels being an intermediate vector. So far, cases have been largely confined to the Middle East (mainly Saudi Arabia) or people who traveled there. The symptoms of MERS are very similar to SARS and COVID-19, but it has a higher case fatality rate (Christakis 2020; Abdelrahman, Li, and Wang 2020). As of the beginning of 2020, there were 2,519 cases of MERS resulting in 866 fatalities (Abdelrahman, Li, and Wang 2020).

As we saw with most other viruses (poliovirus and smallpox are notable exceptions), animals often act as a reservoir or vector for coronaviruses without necessarily affecting the animal (Figure 6.2). When a virus makes a leap from one species to another, it is known as zoonosis. Zoonosis is encouraged by increased human activity in areas where potential animal vectors are found (LabXchange 2021b). Sequence analysis of SARS-CoV-2 indicated that it is most closely related to a virus isolated from horseshoe bats (Zhou et al. 2020; Rabadan 2021; Mallapaty 2021; Andersen et al. 2020). Similar sequences have been found in pangolins and civets, however, which may be intermediate animal vectors (Lam et al. 2020; Cyranoski 2020; Zhou et al. 2020; Zhang, Wu, and Zhang 2020; Andersen et al. 2020).

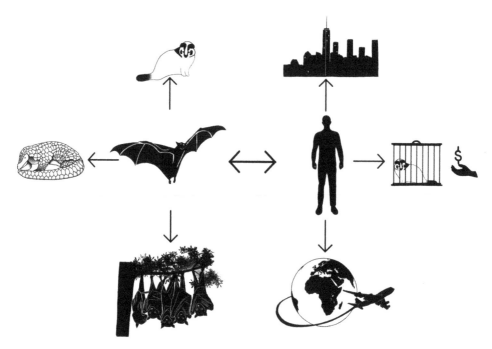

FIGURE 6.2
Contributing factors to the spread of SARS-CoV-2.

Shown here are factors that may contribute to the spread of SARS-CoV-2 among humans. Bats are a known vector for coronaviruses, and they may interact with pangolins (far left) and civets (top left) that could act as intermediate vectors for the transfer of the virus to humans, such as in an animal market (far right). Bats also live in colonies of thousands or millions, leading to transfer of viruses among them (lower left). If a human is exposed to a coronavirus through interaction with a bat or other animal, and the virus is capable of human-to-human transmission, that person could spread the virus to other people in crowded spaces found in cities or through travel to other places.

Source: Created by Jasneet Punia, used with permission.

Civets, a cat-like mammal, are a known intermediary for SARS-CoV (Huang et al. 2020; Cyranoski 2020; Normile 2013b).

A coronavirus can recombine its genome with genomic sequences from another coronavirus in the same cell in either people or an animal, in theory (Cyranoski 2020). Studies making predictions about other potential animal hosts for SARS-CoV-2 find that mink, pigs, rabbits, and cats, among other animals, might also be potential reservoirs (Wardeh, Baylis, and Blagrove 2021; Phillips 2021). (During April 2020, five tigers and three lions tested positive for COVID-19 at the Bronx Zoo in New York City. They displayed coughing symptoms. It was thought that they acquired the virus from a staff person at the zoo [News 2020; Wright 2021].) However, one risk of SARS-CoV-2 establishing infection in other animals, like mink, is that the virus can mutate in this animal and then turn around and infect people again, perhaps in a more virulent form (Mallapaty 2021; Phillips 2021).

Aside from other possible animal vectors, bats are infamous for carrying many viruses, including coronaviruses. Scientists speculate that the lifestyle of the bat, being a flying mammal that lives in close contact with other bats, having a potentially long life, and being able to limit the capacity of the virus to copy itself in the bat's cells, all contribute to the bat being a good vector for viruses that could make a leap to another mammal, like us (LabXchange 2021b; Streicker and Gilbert 2020; Irving et al. 2021). In addition, there are increasingly more opportunities for humans to come into contact with bats because of climate change, the expansion of cities into more rural areas, and the selling of bats at market (Streicker and Gilbert 2020). Bats have caused outbreaks of not only SARS-CoV-2, SARS, and MERS, but also Ebola, Marburg, Nipah, and Hendra viruses, indicating that this mammal is a major reservoir for potentially dangerous viruses that need to be monitored worldwide (Irving et al. 2021).

6.2 Understand How SARS-CoV-2 Is Transmitted among Humans, Discover How SARS-CoV-2 Affects the Body, and Understand What Tests and Treatments Are Available

SARS-CoV-2, like other respiratory viruses, is airborne and can be spread through respiratory droplets and aerosols (Wang et al. 2021). Once a person acquires SARS-CoV-2, it may take 2–14 days to show symptoms, if shown at all (Rabadan 2021; Bar-On et al. 2020; CDC 2021d). Symptoms of SARS-CoV-2 infection include loss of smell (anosmia) and taste, dry cough, tiredness, and/or gastrointestinal symptoms, among others (Christakis 2020). It is estimated that 50% of infected persons have no symptoms, meaning that they are "asymptomatic," but can still transmit the virus to others (Christakis 2020; Bar-On et al. 2020). Studies also indicate that young people are less likely to be symptomatic than older individuals are (Davies et al. 2020). Researchers have also looked to data from COVID-19 outbreaks in environments where people were isolated from the rest of the population to study virus transmission. For example, scientists determined that just under 50% of people on an aircraft carrier that suffered a COVID-19 outbreak were asymptomatic yet positive for the virus (Kasper et al. 2020). In addition, researchers using passenger data from a 2020 cruise ship outbreak proposed an even higher estimate of 74% of infected people showing no symptoms based on their modeling data (Emery et al. 2020). One can imagine the difficulty in identifying and tracking individuals infected with SARS-CoV-2 if members of the entire population are not routinely tested. Many people spread this virus without ever knowing they had it. There is a lot of variability in the type and severity of symptoms of COVID-19 as well, and scientists do not completely understand why this is the case.

Researchers have found that if a person has a mild cold-like illness, it may take up to two weeks to recover, but if the illness is more severe, recovery could take six weeks or longer (Bar-On et al. 2020). The symptoms of temporary loss of smell and taste help set COVID-19 apart from the common cold in many cases. It was reported in fall 2020 that up to 80% of COVID-19 patients suffer from anosmia (Whelan 2020). Other related symptoms affecting the nervous system include parosmia, where things smell differently than expected or as they should, and "brain fog," where people experience a sense of confusion or loss of concentration. Researchers are trying to figure out what is responsible for the loss of smell and have zeroed in on a type of "support cell" around the olfactory neurons known as sustentacular cells. When the virus affects these support cells, inflammation ensues, and then the olfactory neurons themselves are damaged. As the olfactory neurons regenerate, parosmia may result as the neuronal pathways are restructured (Whelan 2020).

SARS-CoV-2 can infect the upper respiratory tract, like cold-causing viruses do, but also the lungs. Severe illness can result from a phenomenon known as "cytokine storm," in which the immune system's attempt to stop the virus can cause quite a bit of damage to the body's organs, such as the lungs (Cyranoski 2020). Some patients develop acute respiratory distress syndrome (ARDS) and may require a ventilator to breathe (Rabadan 2021). Patients with COVID-19 can have a host of symptoms beyond respiratory illness, including the prevalence of blood clots, as well as the phenomenon of "long COVID," "long-haul COVID," or "post-acute COVID-19 syndrome" for some patients who recovered from even mild illness. Symptoms of long COVID involve tiredness and achiness, among other respiratory symptoms like dry cough and shortness of breath that can persist for months (Marshall 2021). Other clinical scientists have expanded the range of post-acute COVID-19 symptoms to include cardiovascular symptoms such as heart palpitations and chest pain, mental health disorders such as anxiety and depression, and renal or endocrine system dysfunction, among others (Nalbandian et al. 2021). A study done in the United Kingdom indicates that as many as 10% of people positive for SARS-CoV-2 may have long COVID, and that women and middle-aged people in general are at slightly higher risk of getting long COVID over others in the population. The reasons for the extended period with symptoms are not understood, but some researchers think that the symptoms are a long-term reaction to a lingering viral protein or possibly an autoimmune reaction (Marshall 2021).

Cardiovascular complications have been associated with COVID-19. These patients may have a range of symptoms including myocarditis (inflammation of the muscle of the heart), shortness of breath, chest pain, irregular heartbeat, or even a sudden heart attack. It is not known why the cardiovascular system specifically would be affected, but it may be due to viral infection of cardiac cells or a side effect of cytokine storm. Physicians have noted that COVID-19 may make the diagnosis of other disease conditions difficult because it may "mask" these other conditions (Giyanani et al. 2021; Wright 2021).

Unlike seasonal influenza, which has a "U-shaped" curve in terms of the number of deaths at different ages (more in the very young and very old), COVID-19 has an "L-shaped" curve in the sense that the number of deaths is highest in older individuals. Males are at greater risk of death than females (Christakis 2020; Petrilli et al. 2020). In addition to sex, having co-morbidities such as heart failure increases the chance of serious illness and death (Petrilli et al. 2020).

6.2.1 Testing and Treatment

Like with other viruses, one can either perform a nucleic acid–based test to detect the viral genome, look for the viral antigen itself, or look for the presence of antibodies against the virus in the patient's blood (Christakis 2020; Daley 2020). The initial tests used by the CDC and WHO were known as reverse transcriptase polymerase chain reaction (RT-PCR) tests (Daley 2020). As mentioned in other chapters, PCR allows for rapid amplification of a DNA sequence of interest, like a gene copier machine. Because the SARS-CoV-2 genome is RNA-based, the reverse transcriptase is needed to make a DNA copy of the genome to use as a template in the PCR reaction. Rapid PCR tests are now available, as are ones that detect viral antigens (Daley 2020). When comparing rapid tests, rapid PCR tests are said to be more sensitive than rapid antigen tests because they can pick up the virus earlier (Guglielmi 2021). Another way of testing is to look for the presence of antibodies in the person's blood, indicating that they had been exposed to SARS-CoV-2 (Daley 2020; Guglielmi 2021).

As more and more people recovered from COVID-19, their convalescent plasma containing antibodies against COVID-19 became a treatment tool for other people. Early in the pandemic in New York City, the Orthodox Jewish community was hard-hit by the virus. However, many members of their community who recovered made significant convalescent plasma donations to treat people in New York and around the United States (Christakis 2020). However, it has been noted that a survivor's immune protection after infection varies widely and is typically better if the person had symptoms (Jagannathan and Wang 2021). More recent clinical studies have indicated that it is unclear if convalescent antibodies are useful against severe disease and are not currently recommended for use by the WHO (WHO 2021e).

However, scientists can select for the best survivors' antibodies and purify them to use for monoclonal antibody therapy, or they can screen for or engineer new monoclonal antibodies in the laboratory, based on the ability of the antibody to bind viral proteins (Du, Yang, and Zhang 2021). Neutralizing antibodies, which include monoclonal antibodies or antibody fragments, work by interfering with the receptor-binding domain of the viral spike protein, preventing it from binding to the ACE2 receptor and getting into cells (Jiang, Hillyer, and Du 2020). The National Institutes of Health (NIH), along with the Food and Drug Administration (FDA), recommends the use of monoclonal antibody therapy to treat patients who have COVID-19 symptoms or who have been exposed to the virus and are at risk of developing more severe illness (NIH 2021).

In addition to monoclonal antibody therapy, antiviral drugs specific to SARS-CoV-2 are starting to be developed. In late 2021, successful clinical trials were completed on two antiviral drugs given in the form of a pill to fight SARS-CoV-2: Molnupiravir and Paxlovid. Molnupiravir works by causing errors in the viral genome during replication, and Paxlovid works by interfering with the maturing of certain viral proteins to stop SARS-CoV-2 (Jayk Bernal et al. 2021; Gordon et al. 2021; Mahase 2021; Ledford 2021).

Researchers are working hard to identify animal models for SARS-CoV-2 to better understand the virus and develop new treatments in the future. When looking at commonly used laboratory animals, researchers have found that mice are not that useful because their ACE2 receptor does not bind to the virus in the same way that a human receptor does, although the mice could be modified to mimic human cells. Ferrets, such as with influenza, are good models for recreating the clinical symptoms, as are hamsters. Nonhuman primates like rhesus macaques may also be used. However, in the future, researchers may rely on *in vitro* cell culturing methods that can substitute for animal organs such as lung organoid or organ-on-chips systems (Muñoz-Fontela et al. 2020). Target organs of SARS-CoV-2 could be studied using organoids to better understand how the virus causes disease. Lung and intestinal organoids of bats or other animals could even be used to compare what happens in different animal hosts (Clevers 2020). Many of these options are already being used to study COVID-19, including for vaccine development.

6.3 Examine the Historical Factors Leading to the Development and Continuation of the COVID-19 Pandemic

6.3.1 First Six Months

For a more detailed account of the first six months of COVID-19, one can look at several other books focusing on the early days of the pandemic, including those used as references here (Christakis 2020; Wright 2021). When cases of COVID-19 first began appearing in the United States, many people thought that the pandemic would play out like a seasonal flu outbreak and that stay-at-home restrictions were an overreaction by the government.

"Flatten the curve" became a mantra of public health officials to try to keep people at home, so new COVID-19 patients did not flood hospitals all at one time (Christakis 2020).

People living in the New York metropolitan area (like the author of this textbook) noted that on several occasions in the spring of 2020 during the first wave of the pandemic in the United States, a number of major hospitals in the region were diverting patients to other medical centers because of new patient volume. It was difficult to find a hospital bed if you needed it for any reason. Elective surgeries and procedures were canceled, and physicians switched to virtual "telehealth" appointments when they could. The COVID-19 pandemic would not play out like the seasonal flu after all, with many people spreading SARS-CoV-2 without even knowing they had the virus due to lack of readily available testing and vulnerable populations like the elderly and disabled living in group housing situations being dramatically and swiftly affected by the disease if even one case came into their home (Wright 2021). One of the first major outbreaks in a long-term care facility happened in King County, Washington (McMichael et al. 2020).

So how did SARS-CoV-2 first contact humans and begin spreading among them? Well, the first cases of COVID-19 occurred in Wuhan, China, in 2019 among people who worked at the Huanan Seafood Market (about two-thirds of the cases) (Rabadan 2021; Christakis 2020). However, the first confirmed case of COVID-19 was on December 1, 2019, in a person who did not go to the market. The Wuhan Center for Disease Control and Prevention and the Wuhan Institute of Virology were also not far from the market, and some people feared that the virus could have come from one of these locations as well. As of fall 2021, the origins of the virus were still unclear, according to U.S. government reports (Barnes 2021). However, genomic analysis done in spring 2020 seems to indicate that humans did not alter the genomic sequence, so it came from a natural source (Andersen et al. 2020).

Physicians in the Wuhan region began seeing patients with an unusual kind of pneumonia, and an ophthalmologist named Dr. Wenliang Li started talking to colleagues and friends over a messaging application about his concerns that a SARS-like virus was spreading among people. He got in trouble with police for spreading rumors. (Dr. Li eventually died of COVID-19 in February 2020 (Christakis 2020; Zakaria 2020; Wright 2021)). However, the case cluster in Wuhan continued to increase in size, and details of the severe respiratory illness seen in 41 patients in Wuhan caused by a novel coronavirus were published in a medical journal in January 2020 (Huang et al. 2020). At the same time, millions of people around China were traveling to see family in celebration of the Lunar New Year. Nevertheless, China ended up shutting down most of the country by January 25, 2020 (Christakis 2020).

Scientists around the world had heard that a virus was spreading in China by early January but had no sequence information, which was critical. The SARS-CoV-2 sequence was released to the world on January 11, 2020, thanks to the Chinese researcher, Zhang Yongzhen, and his colleagues (Cyranoski et al. 2020). One can think of a virus's sequence as like its birth certificate and passport all rolled into one. Some have described the mutations that a virus accumulates regularly over time as being like the "stamps in a passport" (Christakis 2020). A scientist can look at a viral sequence and compare it to others, determining its last common ancestor with other related viruses, what animal it may have spilled over from, and how long it potentially has been circulating in an area. Geographic data combined with the sequence information can help one track the path of the virus and where it might be headed. As mentioned in the last chapter, this type of sequence analysis is based on the "molecular clock" idea of viral evolution (Holmes 2003; Ho 2008). Other critical scientific articles were published in late January/early February 2020, in which a novel coronavirus was described as the cause of the Wuhan epidemic of respiratory illness.

Sequence analysis indicated the virus was 88%–96% identical to a virus isolated from bats, and almost 80% identical to the original SARS-CoV. These researchers also identified the ACE2 receptor as the binding site for the novel coronavirus (Zhou et al. 2020; Lu et al. 2020).

The Centers for Disease Control announced the first case of a person in the United States with COVID-19 in Washington State in January 2020. Sequence analysis of this sample (WA1) determined that this patient's variant or version of the virus could be traced back as related to the viral variant seen in one of the first 41 Wuhan patients (Christakis 2020). Dr. Helen Chu, one of the investigators who was a part of the Seattle Flu Study, began analyzing her samples for the presence of SARS-CoV-2. She found that a teenager in the Seattle area was positive for the virus, with no link to travel to China. He had shown mild respiratory symptoms in late February 2020. In addition, the viral variant seen in the teenager was different from the one found in the first U.S. patient noted by the CDC, indicating that the virus was more widespread in the area than initially realized (Christakis 2020). Researchers who analyzed samples of the SARS-CoV-2 virus taken from community transmission samples in Washington State from late February to early March found that most viral variants were derived from the original Wuhan strain found in China, but some variants were related to the virus circulating in Europe at the time. SARS-CoV-2 had been circulating in Washington State for at least three to six weeks (late January 2020 to early February 2020) according to their sequence analysis (Bedford et al. 2020). The timing of the introduction of the virus to Washington State is confirmed by others (Worobey et al. 2020). The novel coronavirus was officially named SARS-CoV-2 in March 2020 (Coronaviridae Study Group of the International Committee on Taxonomy of 2020). We will talk more about the viral variants that arose during the pandemic later in the chapter.

Outbreaks of note in the first three months were also seen on the Grand Princess and Diamond Princess cruise ships, as well as the aircraft carrier USS *Theodore Roosevelt*. Crowded workplaces such as meatpacking plants were also sources of major outbreaks (Figure 6.3) (Christakis 2020).

While the world was focused on SARS-CoV-2 in China, the virus had apparently already started to spread in Europe, experiencing sustained transmission in Italy, beginning in late January, early February. Sequence analysis indicated that the virus came directly from China to Italy at that time, and that viral variants from Italy did show up in New York after that (Worobey et al. 2020). However, a group of physicians in Italy screened their lung cancer patient samples and found that antibodies against SARS-CoV-2 were present much earlier, perhaps as early as September 2019, although further analysis could be done (Apolone et al. 2021; Sozzi et al. 2021). Other researchers also supported a much earlier timeline, indicating that SARS-CoV-2 could have first shown up in China as early as October 2019 (Roberts, Rossman, and Jarić 2021). Clearly, more research needs to be pursued in this area, but the emergence of SARS-CoV-2 could have happened months earlier than previously stated.

The beautiful town of Bergamo, in the Lombardy region of Italy, was one of the towns that suffered the most COVID-19 deaths, losing approximately one in 200 residents (Sylvers 2020). Many people remembered the images that circulated worldwide when military trucks had to be brought into the city to transport coffins to crematoriums outside the overwhelmed city in March 2020 (Sylvers 2020; Wright 2021). A study that tested blood samples isolated from Bergamo residents from April to June 2020 indicated that 57% of the samples had antibodies against COVID-19 (Amante 2020).

Meanwhile, on the East Coast of the United States, the first official case of SARS-CoV-2 was reported in New York City on March 1 (Christakis 2020). The World Health

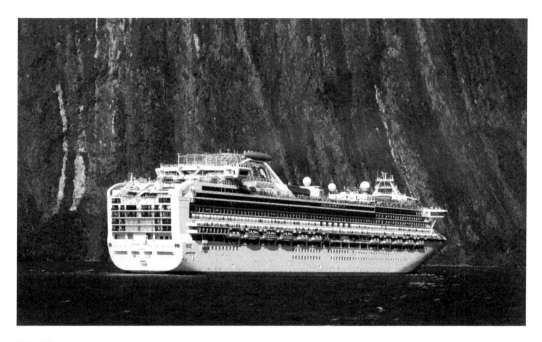

FIGURE 6.3
Photograph of Diamond Princess cruise ship.

This cruise ship was the site of a major COVID-19 outbreak in spring 2020.

Source: "Diamond Princess. Milford Sound. NZ" by Bernard Spragg is licensed under CC0 1.0, in the public domain (https://wordpress.org/openverse/photos/2e9978f1-980f-48fa-9c1d-181f64f58f6e?referrer=creativecom mons.org)

Organization declared COVID-19 a pandemic on March 11, 2020 (Christakis 2020). On that same day, Americans, like the author, heard a presidential address indicating for the first time that the virus was a real threat to the United States, and major news outlets reported that the actor Tom Hanks and his wife Rita Wilson had gotten COVID-19 in Australia.

Public health officials, like Dr. Anthony Fauci, also started relaying stories about the delay between when a person was infected and when they actually knew they had COVID-19, emphasizing the importance of testing. One rather ominous story was the case of a Chinese businessperson who traveled to Germany in January 2020 and was experiencing mild symptoms that she chalked up to jet lag. While on her business trip, she passed SARS-CoV-2 to a bunch of co-workers, most likely in the lunchroom. Then she returned to China where she tested positive for the virus. However, German officials quickly did contact tracing and testing to find everyone affected by this case (Poltz and Carrel 2020).

Before any drugs were available to treat COVID-19, public health officials relied on pushing "non-pharmaceutical interventions," or NPIs, to reduce the number of new COVID-19 cases arising in the early days of the pandemic, or "flatten the curve." These interventions included things like masking, washing hands, social distancing, and staying at home (Christakis 2020). Public health officials may have known at the time, even if the public did not realize it, that many people would still get COVID-19 in the coming months. However, using these interventions prevented the cases from spiking all at once, so that they would instead rise at a more gradual level over a longer period. With this public health approach, officials hoped that medical personnel would not burn out as quickly as they otherwise might and resources like hospital beds and respirators could be utilized by more patients in the end. Although many Americans avoided getting COVID-19, the economic cost of effectively shutting down the country led to 33 million Americans losing their jobs (along with their health insurance) (Christakis 2020).

Another reason that public health officials were encouraging the "flatten the curve" idea was their knowledge of the growth of a virus as it spreads from one person to another, with each of those people giving the virus to someone else, and then each of those people giving the virus to someone else, et cetera, as the number of infected individuals can eventually explode due to exponential growth (Christakis 2020). This type of growth is a concept well known to students of mathematics or microbiology. There are tutorials available on how to study and predict exponential growth (Young-Saver 2021).

One can examine state public health measures side by side with case counts using data available through the Johns Hopkins University and Medicine Coronavirus Resource Center. Here is an example looking at public health measures put into place during the first wave of the COVID-19 pandemic in the State of New Jersey. As of March 16, 2020, New Jersey had 176 COVID-19 cases. On that day, Governor Murphy instituted a voluntary curfew from 8PM to 5AM and closed public places like gyms and restaurants (except for takeout). Cases continued to rapidly rise with 2,844 cases in total by March 23 and 75,317 cases in total by April 16. These case counts illustrate the concept of exponential growth, which had already started before public health restrictions were put into place. The number of new cases per day in New Jersey did not start to decline until late April as New Jersey came out of the first wave. The state started to lift restrictions by early summer 2020, with outdoor dining allowed as of June 15, for example. Cases stayed low all summer and into early fall, so the lifting of restrictions in this case seemed to be well-timed (Center 2021d). One can speculate as to how many new cases would have occurred in New Jersey in spring 2020 without the implementation of NPIs when it did happen, but this example illustrates the importance of the timing of NPIs, just as it had been a factor with the 1918 influenza A pandemic.

Perhaps acting even earlier in the pandemic could have prevented a skyrocketing of cases as seen in New Jersey. For example, some states outside of the northeastern United States, like California, were able to avoid a huge first wave of COVID-19 in spring 2020 since lockdowns were put into place before cases started to climb in those areas (Center 2021c). Another approach, taken by Sweden, involved avoiding lockdowns altogether for most people. However, by late 2020, it had already appeared like there were many more COVID-19 deaths in Sweden when compared to its neighbors Norway and Finland (Christakis 2020).

The United States locked down public venues and schools but was not able to ramp up testing to gather the critical data needed to determine the number of cases that had occurred and in what communities. The United States was slower than other countries at doing widespread testing for several reasons. First, the CDC allowed the release of a faulty PCR test kit, which slowed down initial testing until that could be resolved. Second, the FDA did not approve the creation of tests by individual hospitals, even ones that were readily able to do so. Finally, commercial tests were slow to be released. All these errors meant that we really did not know how many Americans had the virus during the first wave in spring 2020 (Christakis 2020; Wright 2021).

6.3.2 After the First Wave in the United States

Like elsewhere in the United States, New Jersey suffered a second wave of COVID-19 that seemed to be linked to the seasonality of a respiratory virus, with cases gradually rising beginning in late October 2020 and not dropping off until vaccines became readily available in spring 2021 (Center 2021d). However, for some states like California, the wave of cases in winter 2021 was much worse than anything seen in spring 2020 (Center 2021c). The vaccines could not come soon enough for most people.

6.4 Follow the Race to Develop a COVID-19 Vaccine

As mentioned previously, there are many possible approaches in vaccine design. For example, one can use the virus itself in a vaccine, in an inactivated or attenuated form, as was the case with the polio vaccine. In another method, a different virus itself (such as an adenovirus) can be used as a vector to deliver a specific viral protein into cells to invoke an immune response. Nucleic acid–based vaccines such as mRNA-based vaccines may be used. Finally, one can make a protein-based vaccine that introduces one or more of the viral proteins directly to the body for the immune response as well. There are other possible vaccine designs, too (Callaway 2020; Krammer 2020).

Some people wonder how researchers were able to develop a COVID-19 vaccine so quickly. Developing a vaccine before COVID-19 was known to take 15 years or more, involving steps such as research using animal models first, then three different phases of clinical trials, each taking one to three years or longer for each step. However, in the case of SARS-CoV-2, researchers already knew a lot about coronaviruses because of SARS and MERS. In addition, work had previously been conducted on using an mRNA-based platform for a vaccine. Finally, U.S. government agencies and other regulatory bodies had allowed for overlapping clinical trials, so that different phases of the clinical trial could be run simultaneously (Krammer 2020). One may have also noted that, given the climate in 2019–2020, many people were at high risk for infection around the world, so obtaining enough test subjects was not a problem.

As of October 2020, at least 180 COVID-19 vaccines were being developed around the world (Krammer 2020). Nine vaccines started to receive more attention than others given their clinical trial results (Corum and Zimmer 2021b). Vaccines that ended up coming to market most quickly included the Pfizer (also called Comirnaty) and Moderna/BioNTech mRNA vaccines in the United States, the Johnson & Johnson/Janssen vaccine in the United States, and the Oxford-Astra Zeneca (also called Covishield) vaccine in Brazil and many other countries (Krammer 2020; Corum and Zimmer 2021b). Both the Pfizer and Moderna/BioNTech vaccines received emergency use authorization in December 2020 (CDC 2021a) (Figure 6.4).

Other prominent vaccines include the Sputnik V (Gam-Covid-Vac) vaccine used in Russia and other countries, Sinopharm (BBIBP-CorV) used in China and other countries, Sinovac (CoronaVac) also used in China and other countries, and Covaxin used in India and other countries (Krammer 2020; Corum and Zimmer 2021b). Novavax (NVX-CoV2373), a recombinant protein-based vaccine also known as Covovax, which was developed in the United States, received an emergency authorization from the WHO and a conditional approval

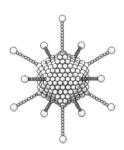

Type:

liponanoparticle (LNP)
containing mRNA

Companies:

Moderna/BioNTech
and Pfizer

Type:

Modified adenoviral vector with
DNA insert

Companies:

Johnson&Johnson/
Janssen and Oxford/Astra Zeneca

FIGURE 6.4
Three major vaccines approved for use in United States as of December 2021.

In the United States, two vaccines based on modified mRNA packaged into a liponanoparticle (LNP) are widely available as of December 2021. These include the Moderna/BioNTech and the Pfizer vaccines. The Johnson & Johnson/Janssen vaccine, based on a modified adenoviral vector, is also widely used in the United States. The Oxford/Astra Zeneca vaccine, used in other places in the world, is also based on this same system.

Source: Adenovirus image from Servier Medical Art (CC BY 3.0); https://smart.servier.com/?s=adenovirus

for use in Europe at the end of December 2021 (Corum and Zimmer 2021b; Krammer 2020; Heath et al. 2021; Dunkle et al. 2021; Novavax 2021).

Both the Oxford-AstraZeneca and the Johnson & Johnson/Janssen vaccines rely on an adenovirus-based vector to deliver the viral protein to the patient's cells to induce an immune response. An altered chimpanzee adenoviral vector is used for AstraZeneca, and an altered human adenoviral vector (Ad26) for Johnson & Johnson, although in both cases the virus has been disabled so it cannot make copies of itself inside the patient's cells (Krammer 2020; Corum and Zimmer 2021b). At first, many Americans were excited about the prospect of the Johnson & Johnson vaccine since it only needed to be given in one dose (also called Ad26.COV2.S, clinical trial number NCT04505722) (Barouch et al. 2021; Sadoff et al. 2021; NLM 2021). The FDA approved the vaccine for emergency use authorization in February 2021 (CDC 2021a). However, the Johnson & Johnson vaccine did face some controversy, since one of its manufacturing partners for the vaccine, Emergent, contaminated millions of doses of the vaccine at its facility in Baltimore (LaFraniere, et al. 2021). In addition, a type of rare blood clot has been seen in one in 100,000 individuals receiving the vaccine, prompting the CDC to indicate that the Pfizer or Moderna vaccines are preferred over the Johnson & Johnson vaccine (Robbins and Jewett 2021). Additional details of the Johnson & Johnson vaccine can also be found through an interactive feature with *The New York Times* (Corum and Zimmer 2021c). In the United States, the most widely used vaccine has been an mRNA-based vaccine, either the Pfizer or Moderna/BioNTech versions. In the next section, we will discuss how the mRNA vaccine platform came about, an exciting new direction in vaccinology.

6.4.1 mRNA Vaccines

Before the COVID-19 pandemic occurred, mRNA had long been studied as a potential therapeutic molecule to treat disease and had been under investigation as a possible vaccine approach. Dr. Katalin Karikó and Dr. Drew Weissman, who worked on developing the modified mRNA technology used in the mRNA-based vaccines, were recently acknowledged for their work with the 2021 Dr. Paul Janssen Award, among other awards (Johnson&Johnson 2021). One might argue that the use of mRNA technology in the COVID-19 vaccines is one of most important breakthroughs in molecular biology since the discovery of the central dogma itself!

When describing her research, Dr. Karikó emphasizes that there was a long road involving many scientists to bring the mRNA-based vaccines to fruition (Karikó 2021; Kwon 2020; Dolgin 2021). The discovery of mRNA in 1961, the understanding of its modifications, and learning how to synthesize mRNA outside the cell in a test tube all contributed to our understanding of mRNA and how to manipulate it (Cobb 2015; Karikó 2021; Sahin, Karikó, and Türeci 2014). Then, researchers introduced mRNA directly into a mouse's muscle and found that a protein was translated. This finding opened the possibility of using mRNA for therapeutic purposes (Wolff et al. 1990; Sahin, Karikó, and Türeci 2014; Pardi et al. 2018). Karikó and colleagues moved the field forward when they were able to transfect mRNA into tissue culture cells and determine that the cells began to make a functional enzyme receptor encoded by the mRNA that they introduced (Karikó, Kuo, and Barnathan 1999). Then, Weismann, Karikó, and their research colleagues introduced mRNA encoding HIV gag into dendritic cells (a major antigen-presenting cell type for the immune system) and found that the gag protein was made in the cells and used by the dendritic cells to elicit a response from the immune system (Weissman et al. 2000). In a critical 2005 study, Karikó and others learned how to modify mRNA, using what they learned from tRNA, so that introducing the mRNA itself did not invoke an immune response, clearing the path for the mRNA to bring a code to the cells to translate into a usable protein to counteract or prevent disease. More specifically, introducing the modified nucleosides found more commonly in tRNA and rRNA, like pseudouridine, dampened the mRNA stimulation of the immune system (Karikó et al. 2005; Karikó et al. 2008; Kwon 2020; Dolgin 2021).

In addition to making the modified mRNA for the vaccine itself, scientists had to figure out a way to package the mRNA so the body could use it. This is where the lipid nanoparticles (LNPs) come into play, providing a packaging that brings the mRNA into the cells. The LNPs are sometimes described as molecular delivery workers, delivering the mRNA to the cells while preventing the mRNA from being degraded. Research on artificial lipids and then specifically cationic lipids (positively charged lipids) to deliver mRNA (naturally negatively charged) into cells began in the 1970s and continued to be optimized into the 1990s (Malone, Felgner, and Verma 1989; Conry et al. 1995; Ostro et al. 1978; Dimitriadis 1978; Chaudhary Weissman, and Whitehead 2021; Hou et al. 2021; Dolgin 2021).

When the mRNA and lipids are combined to make a vaccine, researchers found that the lipids self-assemble around the mRNA, making 60–100 nm particles. When the particles are introduced into the bloodstream, they bind to apolipoprotein E and go to the liver for translation. If introduced through intramuscular injection, the protein can be made from the mRNA template near the injection site itself (Pardi et al. 2018). Researchers have described the systemic introduction of mRNA vaccines as a way to turn the liver into a "bioreactor" making the protein of interest (Horejs 2021). The LNPs may also potentially act as an adjuvant, helping to encourage an immune response to the spike protein (Wadman 2020). Both the Moderna and Pfizer/BioNTech COVID-19 vaccines use modified mRNA (uridines replaced by pseudouridines) packaged into LNPs (Dolgin 2021). Anyone who has received one of these vaccines also knows that the vaccine is introduced intramuscularly. As one can see from the over 50 years of scientific research mentioned in this section, landing upon this vaccine approach did not happen overnight.

When describing the advantages of mRNA-based vaccine technology even over other nucleic acid–based approaches, scientists point out, for example, that mRNA does not need to go to the nucleus of the cell to work; it can be translated by the ribosomes in the cytoplasm. In addition, mRNA is inherently unstable, so it is only in the cells transiently, and researchers can control the mRNA half-life through modification of its cap and tail. In addition to the use of mRNA technology in other viral vaccines such as against Zika virus, this same method is being used to develop new cancer therapies and even approaches for gene editing (Sahin, Karikó, and Türeci 2014; Pardi et al. 2017; Pardi et al. 2018). The mRNA-based vaccine approach is an easy-to-adapt platform where one can just alter the code of the mRNA produced to make a different drug (Kwon 2020). When compared to delivering a protein as a therapy, mRNA-based drugs are also easier to make. These mRNA-based drugs avoid the expense of making the protein in the laboratory and turn to the cells to have them make the protein on their own (Kwon 2020). In the future, it will not be uncommon for mRNA to be used as a drug for disease prevention or treatment.

Once the sequence of SARS-CoV-2 was released in January 2020, both Pfizer and Moderna began developing their mRNA-based vaccines. They were able to create their vaccine candidates and test them in 11 months (Chaudhary, Weissman, and Whitehead 2021; Hou et al. 2021). On December 11, 2020, the Pfizer vaccine crossed the finish line first with emergency use authorization by the FDA, becoming the first mRNA-based vaccine that was approved as a drug. The Moderna vaccine followed a week later (CDC 2021a; Chaudhary, Weissman, and Whitehead 2021). The Pfizer vaccine is called bNT162b2, and this version of the vaccine contains the mRNA encoding the SARS-CoV-2 spike protein, with two changes that make the protein stay in a prefusion shape. The Moderna vaccine, called mRNA-1273, also encodes a modified version of the spike protein (Chaudhary, Weissman, and Whitehead 2021). The clinical trial results for both the Pfizer/BioNTech vaccine and the Moderna vaccine have been published, and it should be noted that both drugs are given as a two-dose regimen (Baden et al. 2021; Anderson et al. 2020; Polack et al. 2020). The clinical trials overview for each study is also publicly available through ClinicalTrials.gov, under the number NCT04470427 for the Moderna study and under the number NCT04368728 for the Pfizer/BioNTech study (Hou et al. 2021; NLM 2021). Interactive articles summarizing the makeup of both the Moderna and Pfizer vaccines and how they work can be found in *The New York Times* (Corum and Zimmer 2021a, 2021d).

Mass-producing a vaccine formulation includes steps such as transcribing the mRNA *in vitro* in mass quantities, purifying the mRNA, and then combining it with lipids to make the LNPs (Chaudhary, Weissman, and Whitehead 2021). Pfizer has made a large part of their procedure public with an interactive feature in *The New York Times* (Cott, deBruyn, and Corum 2021). In a process involving multiple facilities, one can follow the steps of making the vaccine, from pulling the plasmid DNA containing the code for the SARS-CoV-2 spike protein out of the freezer to packaging the lipid and mRNA together to make the vaccine. One facility primarily does the work of mass-producing the DNA code for the spike protein, another transcribes the mRNA and purifies it, and finally another brings together the lipid and mRNA and produces the vials of vaccine. Completing all the steps takes 60 days, not including the four weeks of sample testing for the different batches (Cott, deBruyn, and Corum 2021).

Long-term studies of the effectiveness of both vaccines are underway, but Pfizer formed a unique partnership with the Israel Ministry of Health in which they exclusively made their vaccine available to all adults 16 years of age and older in Israel in December 2020, and ever since then have been collecting data on the efficacy of their vaccine during the pandemic. Researchers estimated that the number of COVID-19-related hospitalizations and deaths reported in Israel would have been three times higher during the wave of the pandemic that happened between December 2020 and April 2021 without the vaccine (Haas et al. 2021).

6.4.2 Vaccine Equity

It is important to note that many people in the world are still waiting for a COVID-19 vaccine. As COVID-19 vaccines were beginning to be developed, the WHO took an interest in creating a program to support the development of new vaccines and ensure equitable distribution of vaccine throughout the world, emphasizing that vaccinating all the people of the world against SARS-CoV-2 will be necessary to keep everyone safe. That program, known as the COVAX program, is a partnership with Gavi, the Coalition for Epidemic Preparedness Innovations (CEPI), and the WHO, and will involve UNICEF for vaccine distribution (WHO 2021b). As of fall 2021, when many vaccinated adults in the United States started seeking out booster shots of the COVID-19 vaccine, the WHO urged caution in distributing booster shots, considering all the people of the world who still needed their first dose (WHO 2021c). As of December 2021, 58.4% of the people of the world had received at least one dose of the vaccine, although there are many countries in the world, including in Africa, Eastern Europe, and Central Asia, where the percentage was much lower (Holder 2021). In Chapter 8 on public health and viruses, we will discuss how a plan to equitably distribute a vaccine in a population can be created.

6.5 Differentiate the Course of the Pandemic before and after Mass Vaccination Campaigns Begin in the United States

Although vaccines have been available in the United States since spring 2021 for adults, approximately 27% of Americans are not taking advantage of the opportunity to get vaccinated even with one dose as of December 2021 (Holder 2021). As continued waves of SARS-CoV-2 infection sweep the world into 2022, people have begun to experience one of two different pandemics: one experienced by the vaccinated, and one experienced by the unvaccinated. Even though vaccinated persons can experience a "breakthrough" case caused by factors such as waning immunity or exposure to a new variant, these cases overwhelmingly are milder than those experienced by the unvaccinated (Lipsitch et al. 2021). In summer 2021, the United States even went ahead to start vaccinating children 5–11 years of age (CDC 2021a). (In contrast to the polio vaccine, adults were given the COVID-19 vaccine before young children due to differences in risk, among other reasons.) As mentioned earlier, adults started receiving their booster shots in the United States in fall 2021 (CDC 2021a). Although access to vaccines and even booster shots is not hard to find, the number of cases in the United States has not dropped off dramatically since vaccinations began. With some counties in the United States having under 50% of their population vaccinated, we have not yet reached herd immunity through vaccination (Holder 2021).

As of the end of December 2021, the rest of the world was still dealing with the COVID-19 pandemic as well. In total there have been 280,738,431 cases and 5,404,167 deaths worldwide as of December 27, 2021 (Center 2021a) (Figure 6.5). When one looks at the United

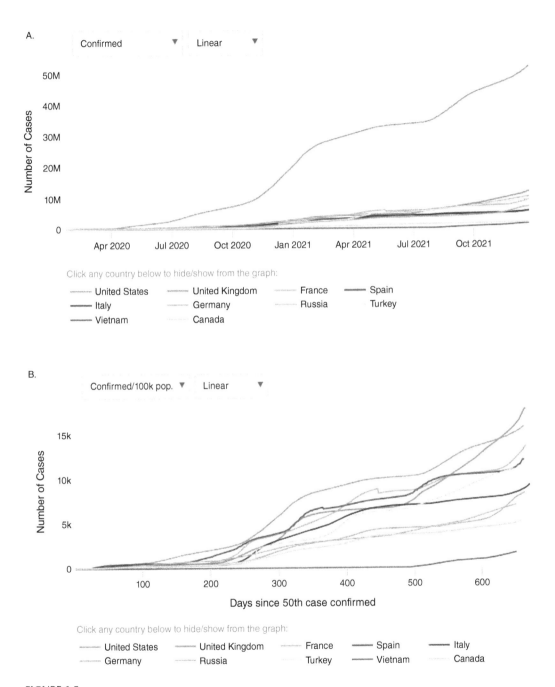

FIGURE 6.5

Cumulative number of COVID-19 cases in United States and nine other countries as of December 2021.

Shown in (A) are the total number of confirmed cases of COVID-19 in ten countries. In (B) are the cases per 100,000 people for those same ten countries.

Used with permission from the Johns Hopkins University and Medicine Coronavirus Resource Center; https://coronavirus.jhu.edu/data/cumulative-cases

States and nine other countries that reported many deaths such as the United Kingdom, Germany, France, Italy, and Vietnam, the United States clearly leads in the total number of cases. When cases are expressed per 100,000 people in the population, the United States was only recently passed by the United Kingdom within the last 100 days before December 27, 2021 (Center 2021b).

6.5.1 SARS-CoV-2 Variants

The World Health Organization (WHO), Centers for Disease Control (CDC), and government agencies around the world track SARS-CoV-2 over time to see if different viral variants or versions emerge. We know that viruses mutate when they multiply, and those changes are incorporated into the genome of the virus going forward as it replicates. If enough mutations accumulate, the mutations may cumulatively or suddenly change certain key characteristics of the virus such as how effectively it binds cells, how effectively it is transmitted, the range of hosts it effects, and so on. When a new version of the virus emerges, this is known as a viral variant (CDC 2021e; WHO 2021d). The WHO will identify what they describe as variants under monitoring (VUM), variants of interest (VOI), and variants of concern (VOC) over time and track their geographic spread. A virus would move into the concern category once a fundamental characteristic as to how it spreads, the severity of disease it causes, or if it bypasses measures put in place to slow the spread becomes apparent (WHO 2021d). As an example of how quickly things can change, as of November 22, 2021, there were four variants of concern around the world, according to the WHO site. Those included alpha (first documented in the United Kingdom), beta (South Africa), gamma (Brazil), and delta (India). However, the omicron variant began to be officially monitored on November 24 and was declared a VOC on November 26. The omicron variant was detected in many countries around the same time through genomic surveillance (WHO 2021d).

Websites such as GISAID help in genome surveillance efforts to track new viral variants and then see how they are related to each other. Also, all variants can be compared to the original reference sequence for SARS-CoV-2, WIV04 (GISAID 2021) (Figure 6.6). Additional analysis and visualization of the GISAID sequence data can be found at Nextstrain or Pango (Hadfield et al. 2018; O'Toole et al. 2021). Although the WHO uses a Greek letter shorthand naming system for variants, it also recognizes an official nomenclature for the viral lineage created in 2020 (Rambaut et al. 2020).

Countries vary a lot in terms of how much genomic surveillance they conduct, related to the government funding and sometimes political pressure needed to make it a priority. The percent of samples sequenced by the United States (3.83%) is lower than the genomic surveillance done by countries like Iceland (5.38%). However, many countries are sequencing between 1% and 15% of their samples, with the United Kingdom for example sequencing 12.3% of their samples and Canada sequencing 8.95%, as reported in April 2022 (JHU&M 2022). In genomic surveillance, scientists monitor the genome of the virus isolated from affected individuals using RT-PCR, which can be followed up with sequencing, or scientists can do sequencing alone. For example, if a PCR test is designed to amplify the sequence one of the virus's genes using specific primers, if that target sequence changes too much through mutation, the PCR will no longer work. The PCR can provide the first clue that the sequence of the virus has changed quite a bit. Such was the case with the discovery of the omicron variant (WHO 2021a). This variant carries about 30 mutations in the sequence encoding the spike protein (Callaway 2021). Although not every corner of the globe is being monitored for new variants, broad genomic surveillance

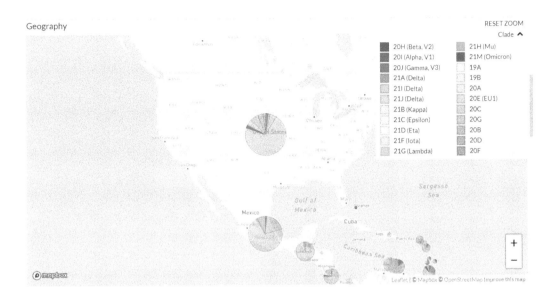

FIGURE 6.6
Mapping emerging variants using NextStrain.

Shown in this image is the distribution of the various novel coronavirus variants in the United States and neighboring countries, based on genomic surveillance data that was available through GISAID as of December 26, 2021.

Screenshot is available under a CC BY 4.0 license, from Nextstrain.org (https://nextstrain.org/sars-cov-2/).

efforts have assisted government agencies in recommending the appropriate public health measures when a new variant, perhaps one with higher transmissibility, is detected in an area (Cyranoski 2021).

6.5.2 Superspreading Phenomenon

One other curious circumstance that played an important role in the spread of SARS-CoV-2 was the superspreading phenomenon. Some believe this includes events such as the one held in the Rose Garden for the Supreme Court nominee in fall 2020 (Wright 2021). Large superspreader events in one part of the world can drive forward a new viral variant to prominence around the world as well. For example, the delta variant of SARS-CoV-2 first became a VOI in April 2021, and then a VOC in May, even though the variant was first documented in India back in October 2020 (WHO 2021d). Some people believe that a religious festival in India called Kumbh Mela, held only once every 12 years and involving millions of people, was at least partly to blame for the spread of the delta variant. In spring 2021, India experienced a huge second wave of the pandemic involving the delta variant (Khare 2021). By August 2021, the delta variant was the "predominant variant" in the United States (CDC 2021c).

However, superspreading also includes the idea that certain single individuals may be able to spread the virus to many more people than other infected individuals can. The superspreader type of infected person is not well understood, but it may involve a person with mild symptoms continuing their normal activities (Wright 2021). For example, there is the infamous choir practice that took place in Washington State, in which 87% of the

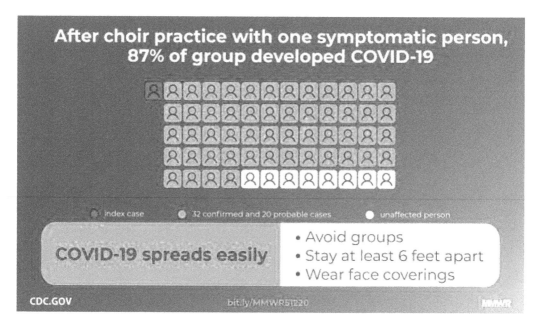

FIGURE 6.7
Spread of SARS-CoV-2 infection at a choir practice.

Shown in this graphic are the number of cases that resulted from a choir practice in Skagit County, Washington, in March 2020 where one individual came to the practice with SARS-CoV-2, and the rest were uninfected at the start of practice.

Hamner, L., P. Dubbel, I. Capron, A. Ross, A. Jordan, J. Lee, J. Lynn, et al. 2020. "High SARS-CoV-2 attack rate following exposure at a choir practice—Skagit County, Washington, March 2020." Morbidity and Mortality Weekly Report 69:606–10. doi: http://dx.doi.org/10.15585/mmwr.mm6919e6

Credit: CDC, Material in the public domain (www.cdc.gov/mmwr/about.html).

people at the practice became newly infected by the one person who came to the practice with COVID-19 (Wright 2021; Hamner et al. 2020) (Figure 6.7). Transmission in this case was most likely facilitated by people being in proximity and singing (Hamner et al. 2020). Superspreading situations include not only choir practices, but also family gatherings, gym classes, and any place where many people are crowded into a space with poor ventilation. If an individual speaks loudly or in general releases more aerosol particles containing virus than another person, then that person could spread the virus to more people than other individuals could (Lewis 2021). Researchers will try to get a better handle on ways to control superspreading in the future, because in the case of both SARS and COVID-19, there were circumstances where a few individuals helped the virus spread to large numbers of people as documented by contact tracing of the situation (Lewis 2021; Normile 2013a).

It is yet to be determined if widespread vaccination in the United States and the world can defeat the march of new SARS-CoV-2 variants emerging as the virus continues to replicate largely in the unvaccinated.

6.5.3 How Many Waves?

Many people in the world are now wondering, will the COVID-19 pandemic ever end? One early estimate of the R_0 value for SARS-CoV-2 was 3.0, meaning that each affected individual on average gave the virus to three people (Christakis 2020). Others provide a range for the R_0 value as between two and four (Bar-On et al. 2020). Using the first estimated R_0 value, one could calculate the number of people who needed to have immunity in the population, through vaccination against COVID-19 or recovery from the illness, using a formula used by epidemiologists. Following that formula, $(R_0 - 1)/R_0$, 67% of the population must be immune for herd immunity. However, this is just an estimate (Christakis 2020). Also, this number does not take into account new viral variants with different properties, such as transmissibility, when compared to the original strain (Wright 2021). Reaching herd immunity is also complicated by uneven vaccination rates in neighboring communities and the emergence of variants that challenge existing vaccines.

In the book *Apollo's Arrow* by Nicholas Christakis released in October 2020, the author comments on possible endings for the pandemic including that SARS-CoV-2 becomes endemic or we reach herd immunity. SARS-CoV-2 would be relegated to causing minor outbreaks in pockets of people who had not gotten COVID-19 or were unvaccinated. He comments, "By 2022 or so, we will reach this outcome naturally or via vaccination" (Christakis 2020, p. 305). However, the ongoing emergence of new viral variants seems to have slowed this resolution of the pandemic.

When looking at the possibility of SARS-CoV-2 of becoming an endemic virus, scientists have used other coronaviruses like OC43 as an example, which causes minor upper respiratory tract illness, although it most likely caused more severe illness when it was first seen in the human population over 100 years ago (Cyranoski 2020; Krammer 2020). All four coronaviruses causing mild illness are endemic, so many scientists surveyed by the journal *Nature* think SARS-CoV-2 will go down that same road and will never be fully eradicated (Phillips 2021). We are not there yet, and there are many possible reasons for this outcome. We will discuss the idea of pandemic prevention and what we learned in the next section.

6.6 Discuss Whether the COVID-19 Pandemic Could Have Been Prevented and What the World Learned from the COVID-19 Pandemic

Since the start of the pandemic, many people have gone back to look at a 2015 TED talk given by Bill Gates on pandemic preparedness (TED 2015; Zakaria 2020). Gates seemed to foreshadow the exact difficulties and hardships that the world would face if a respiratory virus pandemic ever occurred. At the time, Gates called for greater investment in equal access to good healthcare in poorer countries around the world, war-like preparation to quickly mobilize healthcare teams and resources if needed, and greater investment in research and medical diagnostic tools to deal with the virus (TED 2015). When a pandemic response did hit the world four years later, it seemed like there were many missteps in mobilizing our healthcare response, and in the United States, local and state communities were left to scramble for resources. A tremendous burden was placed on healthcare workers to care for the sick and dying. However, private and public investment in biomedical research did pay off, given that vaccines were created and tested quickly, perhaps saving the world from millions of deaths if SARS-CoV-2 had continued to spread completely unchecked.

Some may also wonder that if we only knew that SARS-CoV-2 was coming our way, the United States could have done more to prepare for a pandemic. The WHO has a pandemic warning system and declared a "public health emergency of international concern (PHEIC)" on January 30, 2020, because of the novel coronavirus epidemic. Most countries except those affected by SARS basically ignored the warning (Maxmen 2021b). When looking at the missed opportunities by the U.S. federal government to slow the spread of SARS-CoV-2, one can point out at least three major events. The first would be the lack of transparency on the part of the Chinese government, preventing the CDC from sending a team to China in January. The second is the failure of adequate testing in the United States as mentioned earlier, and finally is the lack of clear consistent messaging on the value of masking in protecting individuals from a respiratory virus, especially one that spread at least half the time through individuals without any symptoms (Wright 2021).

Countries around the world also varied greatly in their use of shutdowns and other public health measures. As mentioned earlier, some countries, like Sweden, decided initially not to do shutdowns like other countries. When the number of deaths from March to July 2020 were compared to previous years, a number known as "excess deaths," there were many more deaths in Sweden relative to other nearby European countries like Germany, but not more than seen in England and Wales. However, 7% of Stockholm's nursing home residents died due to COVID-19 as of October 2020. Sweden has decided to institute policies more like neighboring countries as of fall 2020 (Vogel 2020).

Two years on, where SARS-CoV-2 came from is still not clear. A spring 2021 report by the WHO supports the theory that the virus came from an animal market (Maxmen 2021a). However, researchers doing genomic analysis think that the virus may have crossed from animals to human more than once before it gained a foothold in the human population with sustained human-to-human transmission. They estimate that the virus began being transmitted between people sometime from mid-October to mid-November 2019 somewhere in Hubei Province where Wuhan is located (Pekar et al. 2021).

6.6.1 What We Learned

Realizing that although we have emphasized the biological reasons for the spread of a viral pathogen in this textbook, there are many other things that humans do individually and collectively that can affect the trajectory of a pandemic. We need to also think of pandemics as "sociological phenomena" (Christakis 2020).

When Dr. Deborah Birx, one of the doctors in charge of leading the U.S. COVID-19 pandemic effort, was asked about the initial response by the government, she mentioned that President Trump and his advisors were being given conflicting advice from physicians and scientists around him, which affected the consistency of the messaging going to the American people. While some scientific advisors talking to the White House officials argued for greater protection of the most vulnerable in the population, others argued to let the pandemic go on unchecked (Alfonso III 2021; Becket 2021). However, certain public health officials outside of the White House indicated that they thought Birx could have done more to push her point of view. Birx ended up doing a lot of traveling around the country to bring the public health message directly to people in affected areas at a certain point, rather than trying to make an impact in the White House (Wright 2021). It has been reported that Dr. Anthony Fauci pointed out certain aspects of American culture that all contributed to the poor response in the United States to the pandemic, based on the number of deaths and cases when compared to other countries. These cultural elements included lack of trust of experts including scientists, lack of trust in authority figures, lack of desire to follow masking guidelines, and lack of a unified public health message and response around the country due to political divisions (Wright 2021). The Pew Research Center surveyed people in 17 "advanced economies" including the United States to ask their opinion about their societies before and after the COVID-19 pandemic. Most respondents said their society was "more divided" than before COVID-19. However, 40% agreed with the public health measures put into place in their country, and even 56% of Americans thought there should have been more public health restrictions. Overall, 73% of Americans felt that their lives had changed "a great deal/fair amount" because of the pandemic (Devlin, Fagan, and Connaughton 2021). It is unclear how to address the political and cultural factors that can affect pandemic response and recovery in the future. However, when writers at *The New York Times* asked a group of scientists, public officials, and community leaders about what the United States could do better for the next pandemic, about one year into the current pandemic, they received a variety of answers. Responses included "put science first" and "unified message on masks" as well as the need for investment in public health, to deal with health disparities and to focus on better preparation from the community level on up (Desk 2021).

6.7 Recognize the Impact of the COVID-19 Pandemic on the United States and the World, and What Our Societies Will Look Like Post-Pandemic

6.7.1 How Society Changed in United States

Although the pandemic is not yet over at the time this book was written, politicians, social scientists, physicians, and scientists alike are all wondering what the world will be like once the pandemic is over. Some speculate that the COVID-19 pandemic will be "the hinge event of modern history," while others think the world may eventually return to how it was before the pandemic. One could also take the position that the pandemic merely will speed up societal changes that were happening anyway (Zakaria 2020). Also, if you consider the COVID-19 pandemic an "inflection point" for society, we do not know yet if the changes on the other side of the pandemic will make our society better or worse (Wright 2021).

Both healthcare and education delivery were greatly affected by the pandemic, with many aspects of both transferred online where possible in countries where high-speed internet was readily accessible (Christakis 2020; Zakaria 2020). College students were not only concerned about getting COVID-19 themselves, but also concerned for the people around them, in addition to their fears about being able to successfully complete their courses using remote learning. Students also felt that their workload was increased, and it was harder to determine if they were completing the work as they should. Researchers have found a correlation between increased student concerns over academics and increased feelings of frustration and boredom (Tasso, Hisli Sahin, and San Roman 2021).

Overall, many Americans, with the means, were able to switch over to living a "digital life" during the pandemic (Zakaria 2020). This internet-dependent lifestyle included purchasing groceries and other goods online, finding entertainment in the form of streaming movies and television shows, ordering food takeout and delivery, having telehealth visits with their healthcare providers, and even watching instructional videos for cooking, exercising, flower arranging, and other hobbies online. Now that people have lived this way, will they want to go back to in-person experiences for all these aspects of their lives or will they perform a mixture of both kinds of activities?

The New York Times recently examined the results from "The American Time Use Survey" conducted by the U.S. Labor Department, looking at data from May to December 2020 versus the same time in 2019. Parents spent much more time juggling activities in 2020, including keeping an eye on their children while they were doing other things. As many as one-third of workers worked from home. However, White and Asian workers were more likely to work from home than Black and Hispanic workers (Casselman and Koeze 2021). As of the end of 2021, many workers who moved to remote work are still working that way. This situation has been described as a "massive and unplanned remote-work experiment" (Sinatra Ayres 2021). As workers become accustomed to working outside the office, employers will be asked to be more flexible, giving workers more say in how they structure their workday and when workers will be required to be in the workplace versus working remotely (Sinatra Ayres 2021).

The COVID-19 pandemic has had an impact on the mental health of individuals around the world. Researchers have speculated that there are an additional 53.2 million cases of "major depressive disorder" and an additional 76.2 million cases of "anxiety disorders" worldwide during 2020 (Santomauro et al. 2021) (Figure 6.8).

Early in the COVID-19 pandemic, many people died alone, saying goodbye to loved ones over a phone or tablet because loved ones could not be with them in the hospital (Christakis 2020). People of all ages in the U.S. on average spent more time alone in 2020, especially seniors (Casselman and Koeze 2021). Drug overdoses have dramatically increased in the United States, with the CDC reporting 100,306 drug overdose deaths from April 2020 to April 2021, a 28.5% increase from the previous annual period (Statistics 2021). We as a society will need to address the increased need for substance abuse counseling and general mental health counseling as a part of our healthcare system going forward. In the future, Americans may want to reevaluate the benefits and risks of delivering healthcare using a for-profit system, looking at using certain aspects of socialized medicine in the future (Zakaria 2020). Other aspects of the social safety net, such as the possibility of a universal basic income, have also seen their support increase during the pandemic (Nettle et al. 2021).

The United States will also need to make greater investment in health security to protect its citizens from future threats caused by emerging pathogens or by people seeking to harm others with biological agents. Certainly, the government can seek to partner with the many scientists who have participated in the COVID-19 pandemic to develop new testing methods and treatments (Gronvall 2020). Clearly, the United States did not meet expectations in terms of response to the pandemic based on their previous Global Health Security Index rating (Zakaria 2020; Wright 2021).

6.7.2 Popular Culture

There were over 49 million cases of COVID-19 in the United States alone as of December 10, 2021 (CDC 2021b). This means there are millions of COVID-19 survivors, some of whom had mild or no symptoms and others who are still dealing with recovery. One aspect of COVID-19 recovery culture is how to deal with the loss or change in taste and smell. A cookbook has become available that helps a person create dishes that help enhance flavor sensations related to umami tastes, while downplaying flavors like onion that may be distorted in survivors with taste difficulties (Rothman 2021). This is one small example of how people are trying to support survivors, and certainly the abundance of in-person and online support groups will help survivors cope in other ways, including those with life-threatening complications. Artists have started incorporating their personal stories

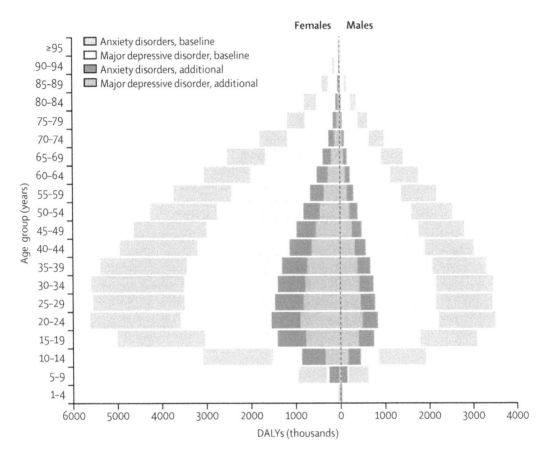

FIGURE 6.8
Cases of anxiety and depression worldwide during the COVID-19 pandemic.

Shown in this figure are the baseline cases per age group and sex for major anxiety disorder (green) and major depressive disorder (teal). The additional cases of major anxiety disorder (orange) and major depressive disorder (lavender) that occurred during the pandemic were determined using analysis of data published from January 1, 2020, to January 29, 2021. Numbers are expressed in disability-adjusted life-years (DALYs).

Source: Figure 4 from Santomauro, D.F., A.M. Mantilla Herrera, J. Shadid, P. Zheng, C. Ashbaugh, D.M. Pigott, C. Abbafati, et al. 2021. "Global prevalence and burden of depressive and anxiety disorders in 204 countries and territories in 2020 due to the COVID-19 pandemic." *The Lancet* 398 (10312):1700–12. doi: 10.1016/S0140-6736(21)02143-7. Epub 2021 Oct 8. PMID: 34634250; PMCID: PMC8500697.

Article was published under a CC BY 4.0 license (www.thelancet.com/journals/lancet/article/PIIS0140-6736(21)02143-7/fulltext).

and stories of others related to COVID-19 into their work. For example, one project known as "COVID Dreams" is "a collection of abstract art in mixed media that capture some mixed feelings related to the pandemic" (Patnala 2021). Another is entitled "New Ways of Living" involving all kinds of media like sculpture, illustrations, and animation, representing artists from different countries around the planet (Artists 2021). In fall 2021, an artist, with help from the public, installed "In America: Remember" which consisted of 660,000 flags set up on the National Mall in Washington, D.C., representing the number of COVID-19 deaths in the United States at the time (Brennan Firstenberg 2021). From fall

2021 until February 2023, the Cooper Hewitt Museum in New York City will run an exhibit entitled "Design and Healing: Creative Responses to Epidemics" looking at many aspects of design including architecture, art, clothing, and other objects that have reflected upon or considered characteristics of diseases such as COVID-19 (Museum 2021). As we adapt and move forward as a society, we will find ways to cope with our experience individually and collectively.

The experience of the COVID-19 pandemic will also potentially cause us to revisit past works of art with a new perspective. In the past, when I talked about emerging viruses with my students and showed clips from the movie *Contagion* in class, we focused on how a virus might emerge from a new interaction between an animal and people (Soderbergh 2011). However, we did not discuss what might really happen six months, one year, or two years later if that virus were to be transmitted unchecked through the human population and then thrive. Even though we are now experiencing it, it was hard to imagine how we, as a society, would deal with the fallout from such a catastrophic event.

Considering what we just experienced in the pandemic and the overwhelming feeling of powerlessness that is created for many people, I hope that future local, state, and national leaders will start routine pandemic preparation as a part of education and job training for all Americans. However, preparedness can be subjective, and we need to take the lead from health professionals as to how to prepare for challenges in the future. In addition, there is no guarantee that future viruses causing pandemics will spread in the same way as previous ones.

6.7.3 How the World Changed

In a United Nations Children's Fund (UNICEF) briefing for World Children's Day 2020, the agency presented a plan for how to address and then creatively deal with life after the pandemic for all the children of the world (UNICEF 2020). Not only are children and/ or their family members getting COVID-19, but they also are impacted by indirect effects such as changes in the accessibility of education and healthcare. For example, there is a concern that children are not getting their necessary immunizations (UNICEF 2020). The COVID-19 pandemic is also affecting the fight against other diseases such as tuberculosis, malaria, and HIV/AIDS (Roberts 2021).

Aside from diseases caused by pathogens, the mental health of children is being affected as well. In addition, poverty, inequality issues, and even the physical safety of children in areas of the world experiencing war or conflict are being exacerbated by the pandemic. UNICEF singles out South Asia, the Middle East, and Latin America as regions of great concern for the welfare of children during and after the pandemic. The report stresses the importance of keeping schools open wherever possible, since switching over to doing school over the internet is an option for only 24% of the world's children (UNICEF 2020). The plan calls on the world's leaders to make internet more accessible to children for applications such as attending school, in addition to increasing access to healthcare and good food, especially if schools are not opened to provide these basic services along with education. Finally, the report calls on the world's leaders to turn their attention to children's concerns and include children when they make decisions in the future (UNICEF 2020). The challenges facing many children in the world certainly makes adjusting to a digital life seem minor in comparison.

To end on a positive note, the organization Global Citizen developed a plan for recovery of the world post-COVID, and asked 18 world leaders to comment on their plan (May 2021). If one takes their quotes, removing terms specific to their own countries, one sees several

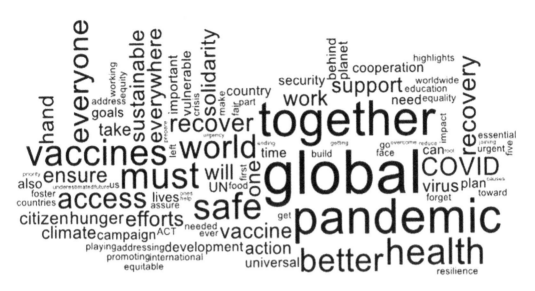

FIGURE 6.9
Word cloud of popular words used in world leaders' comments on a COVID-19 recovery plan.

Shown here is a word cloud generated using the words of encouragement from 18 world leaders posted on the Global Citizen website in February 2021 in response to their proposed recovery plan. Country- or region-specific words were removed before generating the word cloud.

Source: Word cloud created by the author based on quotes from the Global Citizen website (www.globalcitizen. org/en/content/recovery-plan-world-leaders-inspiring-quotes/).

common threads emerge (expressed in the form of a word cloud in Figure 6.9). Words like access, safety, recovery, support, and togetherness come up often. To beat COVID-19, the world needs to work together to provide better healthcare and access to vaccines, especially for children, and support each other so that everyone has an equal chance to thrive in the future.

6.8 Summary

The coronavirus SARS-CoV-2 is responsible for the COVID-19 pandemic. The virus first emerged in China in fall 2019, eventually spread worldwide, and was labeled a pandemic in March 2020 by the WHO. SARS-CoV-2 is a respiratory virus, causing a range of symptoms including coughing, shortness of breath, loss of taste or smell, or no symptoms at all. SARS-CoV-2 is most closely related to a bat coronavirus and is thought to have made the leap from bats to humans, or first through an intermediary animal such as a civet or pangolin. The United States experienced the first wave of cases in spring 2020, and cases continue to climb to this day. Vaccines against SARS-CoV-2 were developed within 11 months of the release of the viral genome, with mRNA vaccines from Pfizer and Moderna/ BioNTech receiving emergency use authorization in December 2020 in the United States. Other vaccines followed, and over half of the world's population was vaccinated as of

December 2021, although large regions of the world still have very limited vaccine access. SARS-CoV-2 variants continue to emerge, causing new waves of infection, beyond the seasonality of a respiratory virus. Future efforts will focus on increasing the number of vaccinated individuals worldwide and working to improve health equity and health security for all.

Discussion Questions:

1. Compare and contrast the 1918 influenza pandemic and the COVID-19 pandemic.
2. Do you think the goal of eradicating SARS-CoV-2 from the earth is attainable? Explain why or why not.
3. Are SARS-CoV-2 mutations necessarily bad for human health? Why or why not?
4. What is the best way to improve confidence in vaccine safety for government-approved vaccines? If you had to design a COVID-19 vaccination poster to be displayed in public and on social media, what words and images would you use to encourage more people to get vaccinated? (See activity: Designing a COVID-19 vaccination poster for examples of other vaccination posters [Garden 2021].)
5. What do you think are two to three of the most important lessons learned from the COVID-19 pandemic?
6. What does it mean to have a flexible workplace, and how has the COVID-19 helped or hindered workplace flexibility?
7. What is one positive thing you have done during the COVID-19 pandemic that you would not have done ordinarily or were putting off completing?

References

Abdelrahman, Z., M. Li, and X. Wang. 2020. "Comparative review of SARS-CoV-2, SARS-CoV, MERS-CoV, and influenza a respiratory viruses." *Frontiers in Immunology* 11:552909. doi: 10.3389/fimmu.2020.552909.

Ackermann, H.-W., L. Berthiaume, and M. Tremblay. 1998. *Virus Life in Diagrams.* Boca Raton, FL: CRC Press, Taylor & Francis Group.

Alfonso III, F. 2021. "Pandemic doctors speak out." *Cable News Network (Warner Media).* Accessed 22 December 2021. www.cnn.com/health/live-news/covid-pandemic-doctors-cnn-special/index.html.

Amante, A. 2020. "Over half of people tested in Italy's Bergamo have COVID-19 antibodies." In *Reuters.* Toronto, Canada: Thomson Reuters.

Andersen, K.G., A. Rambaut, W.I. Lipkin, E.C. Holmes, and R.F. Garry. 2020. "The proximal origin of SARS-CoV-2." *Nature Medicine* 26 (4):450–2. doi: 10.1038/s41591-020-0820-9.

Anderson, E.J., N.G. Rouphael, A.T. Widge, L.A. Jackson, P.C. Roberts, M. Makhene, J.D. Chappell, et al. 2020. "Safety and immunogenicity of SARS-CoV-2 mRNA-1273 vaccine in older adults." *New England Journal of Medicine* 383 (25):2427–38. doi: 10.1056/NEJMoa2028436.

Apolone, G., E. Montomoli, A. Manenti, M. Boeri, F. Sabia, I. Hyseni, L. Mazzini, et al. 2021. "Unexpected detection of SARS-CoV-2 antibodies in the prepandemic period in Italy." *Tumori* 107 (5):446–51. doi: 10.1177/0300891620974755.

Artists, C.S. 2021. "New ways of living." *Center for Computational Structural Biology, The Scripps Research Institute*. Accessed 16 December 2021. https://ccsb.scripps.edu/new-ways-of-living/cellspace-2020-artists/.

Baden, L.R., H.M. El Sahly, B. Essink, K. Kotloff, S. Frey, R. Novak, D. Diemert, et al. 2021. "Efficacy and safety of the mRNA-1273 SARS-CoV-2 vaccine." *New England Journal of Medicine* 384 (5):403–16. doi: 10.1056/NEJMoa2035389.

Baltimore, D. 1971. "Expression of animal virus genomes." *Bacteriological Reviews* 35 (3):235.

Barnes, J.E. 2021. "Intelligence review yields no firm conclusion on origins of coronavirus." In *The New York Times*. New York, NY: The New York Times.

Bar-On, Y.M., A. Flamholz, R. Phillips, and R. Milo. 2020. "SARS-CoV-2 (COVID-19) by the numbers." *Elife* 9:e57309. doi: 10.7554/eLife.57309.

Barouch, D.H., K.E. Stephenson, J. Sadoff, J. Yu, A. Chang, M. Gebre, K. McMahan, et al. 2021. "Durable humoral and cellular immune responses 8 months after Ad26.COV2.S vaccination." *New England Journal of Medicine* 385 (10):951–3. doi: 10.1056/NEJMc2108829.

Becket, S. 2021. "Dr. Deborah Birx on the Trump White House, the politics of the epidemic, retirement and more." *ViacomCBS*. Accessed 22 December 2021. www.cbsnews.com/news/dr-deborah-birx-interview-highlights-face-the-nation/.

Bedford, T., L. Greninger Alexander, P. Roychoudhury, M. Starita Lea, M. Famulare, M.-L. Huang, A. Nalla, et al. 2020. "Cryptic transmission of SARS-CoV-2 in Washington state." *Science* 370 (6516):571–5. doi: 10.1126/science.abc0523.

Brennan Firstenberg, S. 2021. "In America: Remember." In *America Flags and Suzanne Brennan Firstenberg*. Accessed 16 December 2021. www.inamericaflags.org/.

Callaway, E. 2020. "The race for coronavirus vaccines: A graphical guide." *Nature* 580:576–7.

———. 2021. "Heavily mutated Omicron variant puts scientists on alert." *Nature* 600 (7887):21. doi: 10.1038/d41586-021-03552-w.

Casselman, B., and E. Koeze. 2021. "The pandemic changed how we spent our time." *The New York Times*. Accessed 16 December 2021. www.nytimes.com/interactive/2021/07/27/business/economy/covid-parenting-work-time.html?smid.

CDC, Center for Disease Control and Prevention. 2021a. "CDC museum COVID-19 timeline." *Health and Human Services*. Accessed 27 December 2021. www.cdc.gov/museum/timeline/covid19.html.

———. 2021b. "COVID data tracker weekly review." *Health and Human Services*. Accessed 16 December 2021. www.cdc.gov/coronavirus/2019-ncov/covid-data/covidview/index.html.

———. 2021c. "Delta variant: What we know about the science." *Health and Human Services*. Accessed 17 December 2021. www.cdc.gov/coronavirus/2019-ncov/variants/delta-variant.html.

———. 2021d. "Symptoms of COVID-19." *Health and Human Services*. Accessed 28 December 2021. www.cdc.gov/coronavirus/2019-ncov/symptoms-testing/symptoms.html.

———. 2021e. "Understanding variants." *Health and Human Services*. Accessed 17 December 2021. www.cdc.gov/coronavirus/2019-ncov/variants/understanding-variants.html.

Center, Coronavirus Resource. 2021a. "COVID-19 dashboard." *Johns Hopkins University & Medicine*. Accessed 27 December 2021. https://coronavirus.jhu.edu/map.html.

———. 2021b. "Cumulative cases." *Johns Hopkins University & Medicine*. Accessed 27 December 2021. https://coronavirus.jhu.edu/data/cumulative-cases.

———. 2021c. "Impact of opening and closing decisions by state: California." *Johns Hopkins University & Medicine*. Accessed 27 December 2021. https://coronavirus.jhu.edu/data/state-timeline/new-confirmed-cases/california.

———. 2021d. "Impact of opening and closing decisions by state: New Jersey." *Johns Hopkins University & Medicine*. Accessed 27 December 2021. https://coronavirus.jhu.edu/data/state-timeline/new-confirmed-cases/new-jersey/0.

Chaudhary, N., D. Weissman, and K.A. Whitehead. 2021. "mRNA vaccines for infectious diseases: Principles, delivery and clinical translation." *Nature Reviews Drug Discovery* 20 (11):817–38. doi: 10.1038/s41573-021-00283-5.

Christakis, N.A. 2020. *Apollo's Arrow: The Profound and Enduring Impact of Coronavirus on the Way We Live*. 1st ed. New York, NY: Little, Brown Spark.

Clevers, H. 2020. "COVID-19: Organoids go viral." *Nature Reviews Molecular Cell Biology* 21 (7):355–6. doi: 10.1038/s41580-020-0258-4.

Cobb, M. 2015. "Who discovered messenger RNA?" *Current Biology* 25 (13):R526–R32. doi: 10.1016/j.cub.2015.05.032.

Conry, R.M., A.F. LoBuglio, M. Wright, L. Sumerel, M.J. Pike, F. Johanning, R. Benjamin, D. Lu, and D.T. Curiel. 1995. "Characterization of a messenger RNA polynucleotide vaccine vector." *Cancer Research* 55 (7):1397–400.

Coronaviridae Study Group of the International Committee on Taxonomy of, V. 2020. "The species severe acute respiratory syndrome-related coronavirus: Classifying 2019-nCoV and naming it SARS-CoV-2." *Nature Microbiology* 5 (4):536–44. doi: 10.1038/s41564-020-0695-z.

Corum, J., and C. Zimmer. 2021a. "How Moderna's vaccine works." *The New York Times Company*. Accessed 17 December 2021. www.nytimes.com/interactive/2020/health/moderna-covid-19-vaccine.html.

———. 2021b. "How nine Covid-19 vaccines work." *The New York Times Company*. Accessed 21 December 2021. www.nytimes.com/interactive/2021/health/how-covid-19-vaccines-work.html?action=click&module=RelatedLinks&pgtype=Article.

———. 2021c. "How the Johnson & Johnson vaccine works." *The New York Times Company*. Accessed 17 December 2021. www.nytimes.com/interactive/2020/health/johnson-johnson-covid-19-vaccine.html.

———. 2021d. "How the Moderna vaccine works." *The New York Times Company*. Accessed 17 December 2021. www.nytimes.com/interactive/2020/health/moderna-covid-19-vaccine.html?searchResultPosition=1.

Cott, E., E. deBruyn, and J. Corum. 2021. "How Pfizer makes its COVID-19 vaccine." In *The New York Times*. New York, NY: The New York Times Company.

Cyranoski, D. 2020. "Profile of a killer: The complex biology powering the coronavirus pandemic." *Nature* 581 (7806):22–7.

———. 2021. "Alarming COVID variants show vital role of genomic surveillance." *Nature* 589 (7842).

Cyranoski, D., E. Dolgin, N. Gaind, S. Hall, H. Ledford, D. Lewis, S. Mallapaty, E. Rodríguez Mega, and N. Subbaraman. 2020. "Nature's 10: Ten people who helped shape science in 2020." *Nature* 588 (7839):563–76. doi: 10.1038/d41586-020-03435-6.

Daley, J. 2020. "Here's how coronavirus tests work—and who offers them." In *Scientific American*. New York, NY: Springer Nature America.

Davies, N.G., P. Klepac, Y. Liu, K. Prem, M. Jit, C.A.B. Pearson, B.J. Quilty, et al. 2020. "Age-dependent effects in the transmission and control of COVID-19 epidemics." *Nature Medicine* 26 (8):1205–11. doi: 10.1038/s41591-020-0962-9.

Desk, H.a.S. 2021. "14 lessons for the next pandemic." *The New York Times*. Accessed 22 December 2021. www.nytimes.com/interactive/2021/03/15/science/lessons-for-the-next-pandemic.html.

Devlin, K., M. Fagan, and A. Connaughton. 2021. "People in advanced economies say their society is more divided than before the pandemic." *Pew Research Center*. Accessed 22 December 2021. www.pewresearch.org/global/2021/06/23/people-in-advanced-economies-say-their-society-is-more-divided-than-before-pandemic/.

Dimitriadis, G.J. 1978. "Translation of rabbit globin mRNA introduced by liposomes into mouse lymphocytes." *Nature* 274 (5674):923–4. doi: 10.1038/274923a0.

Dolgin, E. 2021. "The tangled history of mRNA vaccines." *Nature* 597 (7876):318–24. doi: 10.1038/d41586-021-02483-w.

Du, L., Y. Yang, and X. Zhang. 2021. "Neutralizing antibodies for the prevention and treatment of COVID-19." *Cellular & Molecular Immunology* 18 (10):2293–306. doi: 10.1038/s41423-021-00752-2.

Dunkle, L.M., K.L. Kotloff, C.L. Gay, G. Áñez, J.M. Adelglass, A.Q. Barrat Hernández, W.L. Harper, et al. 2021. "Efficacy and safety of NVX-CoV2373 in adults in the United States and Mexico." *New England Journal of Medicine*. doi: 10.1056/NEJMoa2116185.

Emery, J.C., T.W. Russell, Y. Liu, J. Hellewell, C.A. Pearson, G.M. Knight, R.M. Eggo, et al. 2020. "The contribution of asymptomatic SARS-CoV-2 infections to transmission on the Diamond Princess cruise ship." *Elife* 9:e58699. doi: 10.7554/eLife.58699.

Enserink, M. 2013. "War stories." *Science* 339 (6125):1264–8. doi: 10.1126/science.339.6125.1264.

Garden, Dr. Jenner's House Museum and. 2021. "Learning activities." Accessed 28 December 2021. https://jennermuseum.com/learning/activities.

GISAID. 2021. "Official hCoV-19 reference sequence." *Freunde of GISAID e.V.* Accessed 2 December 2021. www.gisaid.org/references/hcov-19-reference-sequence/.

Giyanani, N., J. Petro, T. Prol, A. Longo, M. Gioia, L. Alalawi, and S. Rajaram. 2021. "Cardiovascular manifestations of COVID-19." In *COVID-19 by Cases: A Pandemic Review,* edited by S.S. Rajaram, A. Darcey, A Longo and N. Burak, 63–74. New York, NY: Nova Science Publishers.

Gordon, C.J., E.P. Tchesnokov, R.F. Schinazi, and M. Götte. 2021. "Molnupiravir promotes SARS-CoV-2 mutagenesis via the RNA template." *Journal of Biological Chemistry* 297 (1). doi: 10.1016/j.jbc.2021.100770.

Gronvall, G.K. 2020. "The scientific response to COVID-19 and lessons for security." *Survival* 62 (3):77–92.

Guglielmi, G. 2021. "Rapid coronavirus tests: A guide for the perplexed." *Nature* 590 (7845):202–5.

Haas, E.J., J.M. McLaughlin, F. Khan, F.J. Angulo, E. Anis, M. Lipsitch, S.R. Singer, et al. 2021. "Infections, hospitalisations, and deaths averted via a nationwide vaccination campaign using the Pfizer-BioNTech BNT162b2 mRNA COVID-19 vaccine in Israel: A retrospective surveillance study." *The Lancet Infectious Diseases.* doi: 10.1016/s1473-3099(21)00566-1.

Hadfield, J., C. Megill, S.M. Bell, J. Huddleston, B. Potter, C. Callender, P. Sagulenko, T. Bedford, and R.A. Neher. 2018. "Nextstrain: Real-time tracking of pathogen evolution." *Bioinformatics* 34 (23):4121–3. doi: 10.1093/bioinformatics/bty407.

Hamner, L., P. Dubbel, I. Capron, A. Ross, A. Jordan, J. Lee, J. Lynn, et al. 2020. "High SARS-CoV-2 attack rate following exposure at a choir practice—Skagit County, Washington, March 2020." *Morbidity and Mortality Weekly Report* 69:606–10.

Heath, P.T., E.P. Galiza, D.N. Baxter, M. Boffito, D. Browne, F. Burns, D.R. Chadwick, et al. 2021. "Safety and efficacy of NVX-CoV2373 Covid-19 vaccine." *New England Journal of Medicine* 385 (13):1172–83. doi: 10.1056/NEJMoa2107659.

Ho, S. 2008. "The molecular clock and estimating species divergence." *Nature Education* 1 (1):168.

Holder, J. 2021. "Tracking coronavirus vaccinations around the world." *The New York Times.* Accessed 21 December 2021. www.nytimes.com/interactive/2021/world/covid-vaccinations-tracker.html.

Holmes, E.C. 2003. "Molecular clocks and the puzzle of RNA virus origins." *Journal of Virology* 77 (7):3893–7. doi: 10.1128/jvi.77.7.3893-3897.2003.

Horejs, C. 2021. "From lipids to lipid nanoparticles to mRNA vaccines." *Nature Reviews Materials* 6 (12):1075–6. doi: 10.1038/s41578-021-00379-9.

Hou, X., T. Zaks, R. Langer, and Y. Dong. 2021. "Lipid nanoparticles for mRNA delivery." *Nature Reviews Materials*:1–17. doi: 10.1038/s41578-021-00358-0.

Huang, C., Y. Wang, X. Li, L. Ren, J. Zhao, Y. Hu, L. Zhang, et al. 2020. "Clinical features of patients infected with 2019 novel coronavirus in Wuhan, China." *Lancet* 395 (10223):497–506. doi: 10.1016/s0140-6736(20)30183-5.

Irving, A.T., M. Ahn, G. Goh, D.E. Anderson, and L.F. Wang. 2021. "Lessons from the host defences of bats, a unique viral reservoir." *Nature* 589 (7842):363–70. doi: 10.1038/s41586-020-03128-0.

Jagannathan, P., and T.T. Wang. 2021. "Immunity after SARS-CoV-2 infections." *Nature Immunology* 22 (5):539–40. doi: 10.1038/s41590-021-00923-3.

Jayk Bernal, A., M.M. Gomes da Silva, D.B. Musungaie, E. Kovalchuk, A. Gonzalez, V. Delos Reyes, A. Martín-Quirós, et al. 2021. "Molnupiravir for oral treatment of Covid-19 in nonhospitalized patients." *New England Journal of Medicine.* doi: 10.1056/NEJMoa2116044.

Jiang, S., C. Hillyer, and L. Du. 2020. "Neutralizing antibodies against SARS-CoV-2 and other human coronaviruses." *Trends in Immunology* 41 (5):355–9. doi: 10.1016/j.it.2020.03.007.

Johnson & Johnson. 2021. "Eureka moments: Vaccine science superheroes." Accessed 4 December 2021. www.youtube.com/watch?v=OJyUdbGFrFI.

Karikó, K. 2021. "Development of mRNA for therapy—not at light speed." *New York Academy of Sciences.* Accessed 19 November 2021. www.nyas.org/events/2021/the-2021-dr-paul-janssen-award-symposium/?tab=agenda.

Karikó, K., M. Buckstein, H. Ni, and D. Weissman. 2005. "Suppression of RNA recognition by Toll-like receptors: The impact of nucleoside modification and the evolutionary origin of RNA." *Immunity* 23 (2):165–75. doi: 10.1016/j.immuni.2005.06.008.

Karikó, K., A. Kuo, and E. Barnathan. 1999. "Overexpression of urokinase receptor in mammalian cells following administration of the in vitro transcribed encoding mRNA." *Gene Therapy* 6 (6):1092–100. doi: 10.1038/sj.gt.3300930.

Karikó, K., H. Muramatsu, F.A. Welsh, J. Ludwig, H. Kato, S. Akira, and D. Weissman. 2008. "Incorporation of pseudouridine into mRNA yields superior nonimmunogenic vector with increased translational capacity and biological stability." *Molecular Therapy* 16 (11):1833–40. doi: 10.1038/mt.2008.200.

Kasper, M.R., J.R. Geibe, C.L. Sears, A.J. Riegodedios, T. Luse, A.M. Von Thun, M.B. McGinnis, et al. 2020. "An outbreak of Covid-19 on an aircraft carrier." *New England Journal of Medicine* 383 (25):2417–26. doi: 10.1056/NEJMoa2019375.

Khare, V. 2021. "India's Kumbh festival attracts big crowds amid devastating second covid wave." *BBC Hindi*, Delhi. Accessed 17 December 2021. www.bbc.com/news/world-asia-india-56770460.

Krammer, F. 2020. "SARS-CoV-2 vaccines in development." *Nature* 586 (7830):516–27. doi: 10.1038/s41586-020-2798-3.

Kwon, D. 2020. "The promise of mRNA vaccines." In *The Scientist*. Midland, ON, Canada: LabX Media Group.

LabXchange. 2021a. "Life cycle of a coronavirus." *The President and Fellows of Harvard College.* Accessed 23 November 2021. www.labxchange.org/library/items/lb:LabXchange:45dc3c12:html:1.

———. 2021b. "Zoonosis: Animal viruses affecting humans." *The President and Fellows of Harvard College.* Accessed 23 November 2021. www.labxchange.org/library/items/lb:LabXchange:da9562b1:html:1.

LaFraniere, S., S.G. Stolberg, and C. Hamby. 2021. "Federal inspectors fear more vaccines were exposed to contamination." *The New York Times.* Accessed 17 December 2021. www.nytimes.com/2021/04/21/us/politics/emergent-johnson-johnson-covid-vaccine.html.

Lam, T.T.-Y., N. Jia, Y.-W. Zhang, M.H.-H. Shum, J.-F. Jiang, H.-C. Zhu, Y.-G. Tong, et al. 2020. "Identifying SARS-CoV-2-related coronaviruses in Malayan pangolins." *Nature* 583 (7815):282–5. doi: 10.1038/s41586-020-2169-0.

Ledford, H. 2021. "COVID antiviral pills: What scientists still want to know." *Nature* 599 (7885):358–9. doi: 10.1038/d41586-021-03074-5.

Lewis, D. 2021. "Superspreading drives the COVID pandemic-and could help to tame it." *Nature* 590:544–6.

Lipsitch, M., F. Krammer, G. Regev-Yochay, Y. Lustig, and R.D. Balicer. 2021. "SARS-CoV-2 break-through infections in vaccinated individuals: Measurement, causes and impact." *Nature Reviews Immunology* 22:57–65. doi: 10.1038/s41577-021-00662-4.

Lu, R., X. Zhao, J. Li, P. Niu, B. Yang, H. Wu, W. Wang, et al. 2020. "Genomic characterisation and epidemiology of 2019 novel coronavirus: Implications for virus origins and receptor binding." *Lancet* 395 (10224):565–74. doi: 10.1016/s0140-6736(20)30251-8.

Mahase, E. 2021. "Covid-19: Pfizer's paxlovid is 89% effective in patients at risk of serious illness, company reports." *BMJ* 375:n2713. doi: 10.1136/bmj.n2713.

Mallapaty, S. 2021. "The search for animals harbouring coronavirus—and why it matters." *Nature* 591 (7848):26–8.

Malone, R.W., P.L. Felgner, and I.M. Verma. 1989. "Cationic liposome-mediated RNA transfection." *Proceedings of the National Academy of Sciences of the United States of America* 86 (16):6077–81. doi: 10.1073/pnas.86.16.6077.

Marshall, M. 2021. "The four most urgent questions about long COVID." *Nature* 594 (7862):168–70. doi: 10.1038/d41586-021-01511-z.

Maxmen, A. 2021a. "WHO report into COVID pandemic origins zeroes in on animal markets, not labs." *Nature* 592 (7853):173–4.

———. 2021b. "Why did the world's pandemic warning system fail when COVID hit?" *Nature* 589:499–500.

May, C. 2021. "18 inspiring quotes from world leaders in support of the 'recovery plan for the world'." *Global Citizen*. Accessed 27 December 2021. www.globalcitizen.org/en/content/recovery-plan-world-leaders-inspiring-quotes/.

McMichael, T.M., S. Clark, S. Pogosjans, M. Kay, J. Lewis, A. Baer, V. Kawakami, et al. 2020. "COVID-19 in a long-term care facility—King County, Washington, February 27-March 9, 2020." *Morbidity and Mortality Weekly Report* 69 (12):339–42. doi: 10.15585/mmwr.mm6912e1.

Medicine, Johns Hopkins University & (JHU&M). 2022. "The search for COVID-19 variants." *Johns Hopkins University & Medicine*. Accessed 16 April 2022. https://coronavirus.jhu.edu/data/variant-data.

Medicine, U.S. National Library of (NLM). 2021. "ClinicalTrials.gov." *Health and Human Services*. Accessed 17 December 2021. https://clinicaltrials.gov/.

Muñoz-Fontela, C., W.E. Dowling, S.G.P. Funnell, P.S. Gsell, A.X. Riveros-Balta, R.A. Albrecht, H. Andersen, et al. 2020. "Animal models for COVID-19." *Nature* 586 (7830):509–15. doi: 10.1038/s41586-020-2787-6.

Museum, Cooper Hewitt Smithsonian Design. 27 Dec 2021. "Design and healing: Creative responses to epidemics." Accessed 2021. www.cooperhewitt.org/channel/design-and-healing/.

Nalbandian, A., K. Sehgal, A. Gupta, M.V. Madhavan, C. McGroder, J.S. Stevens, J.R. Cook, et al. 2021. "Post-acute COVID-19 syndrome." *Nature Medicine* 27 (4):601–15. doi: 10.1038/s41591-021-01283-z.

Nettle, D., E. Johnson, M. Johnson, and R. Saxe. 2021. "Why has the COVID-19 pandemic increased support for universal basic income?" *Humanities and Social Sciences Communications* 8 (1):79. doi: 10.1057/s41599-021-00760-7.

News, Eyewitness. 2020. "Coronavirus news: 4 more tigers, 3 lions test positive for COVID-19 at Bronx Zoo." *ABC 7 NY, WABC-TV*. Accessed 23 November 2021. https://abc7ny.com/bronx-zoo-tiger-with-coronavirus-tigers-lions/6122810/.

NIH, National Institutes of Health. 2021. "Updated COVID-19 treatment guidelines panel's statement on the prioritization of anti-SARS-CoV-2 monoclonal antibodies for the treatment or prevention of SARS-CoV-2 infection when there are logistical or supply constraints." *Health and Human Services*. Accessed 20 December 2021. www.covid19treatmentguidelines.nih.gov/therapies/updated-statement-on-the-prioritization-of-anti-sars-cov-2-mabs/.

Normile, D. 2013a. "The metropole, superspreaders, and other mysteries." *Science* 339 (6125):1272–3. doi: 10.1126/science.339.6125.1272.

———. 2013b. "Understanding the enemy." *Science* 339 (6125):1269–73. doi: 10.1126/science.339.6125.1269.

Novavax. 2021. *World Health Organization Grants Second Emergency Use Listing for Novavax COVID-19 Vaccine*. Gaithersburg, MD: Novavax. Accessed 20 December 2021. https://ir.novavax.com/2021-12-20-World-Health-Organization-Grants-Second-Emergency-Use-Listing-for-Novavax-COVID-19-Vaccine.

Ostro, M.J., D. Giacomoni, D. Lavelle, W. Paxton, and S. Dray. 1978. "Evidence for translation of rabbit globin mRNA after liposome-mediated insertion into a human cell line." *Nature* 274 (5674):921–3. doi: 10.1038/274921a0.

O'Toole, Á., E. Scher, A. Underwood, B. Jackson, V. Hill, J.T. McCrone, R. Colquhoun, et al. 2021. "Assignment of epidemiological lineages in an emerging pandemic using the pangolin tool." *Virus Evolution* 7 (2):veab064. doi: 10.1093/ve/veab064.

Pardi, N., M.J. Hogan, R.S. Pelc, H. Muramatsu, H. Andersen, C.R. DeMaso, K.A. Dowd, et al. 2017. "Zika virus protection by a single low-dose nucleoside-modified mRNA vaccination." *Nature* 543 (7644):248–51. doi: 10.1038/nature21428.

Pardi, N., M.J. Hogan, F.W. Porter, and D. Weissman. 2018. "mRNA vaccines—a new era in vaccinology." *Nature Reviews Drug Discovery* 17 (4):261–79. doi: 10.1038/nrd.2017.243.

Patnala, R. 2021. "COVID dreams." *Sci-Illustrate*. Accessed 16 December 2021. www.sci-illustrate.com/covid-dreams.

Pekar, J., M. Worobey, N. Moshiri, K. Scheffler, and O. Wertheim Joel. 2021. "Timing the SARS-CoV-2 index case in Hubei province." *Science* 372 (6540):412–7. doi: 10.1126/science.abf8003.

Petrilli, C.M., S.A. Jones, J. Yang, H. Rajagopalan, L. O'Donnell, Y. Chernyak, K.A. Tobin, R.J. Cerfolio, F. Francois, and L.I. Horwitz. 2020. "Factors associated with hospital admission and critical illness among 5279 people with coronavirus disease 2019 in New York City: Prospective cohort study." *BMJ* 369:m1966. doi: 10.1136/bmj.m1966.

Phillips, N. 2021. "The coronavirus is here to stay—here's what that means." *Nature* 590 (7846):382–4. doi: 10.1038/d41586-021-00396-2.

Polack, F.P., S.J. Thomas, N. Kitchin, J. Absalon, A. Gurtman, S. Lockhart, J.L. Perez, et al. 2020. "Safety and efficacy of the BNT162b2 mRNA Covid-19 vaccine." *New England Journal of Medicine* 383 (27):2603–15. doi: 10.1056/NEJMoa2034577.

Poltz, J., and P. Carrel. 2020. "Pass the salt: The minute details that helped Germany build virus defenses." *Reuters World News*, April 9.

Rabadan, R. 2021. *Understanding Coronavirus*. New York, NY: Cambridge University Press.

Rambaut, A., E.C. Holmes, Á. O'Toole, V. Hill, J.T. McCrone, C. Ruis, L. du Plessis, and O.G. Pybus. 2020. "A dynamic nomenclature proposal for SARS-CoV-2 lineages to assist genomic epidemiology." *Nature Microbiology* 5 (11):1403–7. doi: 10.1038/s41564-020-0770-5.

Robbins, R., and C. Jewett. 2021. "C.D.C. Recommends other covid vaccines over J&J's shots." *The New York Times*. Accessed 17 December 2021. https://www.nytimes.com/2021/12/16/health/johnson-and-johnson-vaccine-blood-clots.html.

Roberts, D.L., J.S. Rossman, and I. Jarić. 2021. "Dating first cases of COVID-19." *PLoS Pathogens* 17 (6):e1009620. doi: 10.1371/journal.ppat.1009620.

Roberts, L. 2021. "How COVID is derailing the fight against HIV, TB and malaria." *Nature* 597 (7876):314. doi: 10.1038/d41586-021-02469-8.

Rothman, S. 2021. "Lost taste and smell from COVID-19? A new cookbook aims to help." *ABC News Internet Ventures*. Accessed 16 December 2021. https://abcnews.go.com/Health/loss-taste-smell-covid-19-cookbook-aims/story?id=76887711.

Sadoff, J., G. Gray, A. Vandebosch, V. Cárdenas, G. Shukarev, B. Grinsztejn, P.A. Goepfert, et al. 2021. "Safety and efficacy of single-dose Ad26.COV2.S vaccine against Covid-19." *New England Journal of Medicine* 384 (23):2187–201. doi: 10.1056/NEJMoa2101544.

Sahin, U., K. Karikó, and Ö. Türeci. 2014. "mRNA-based therapeutics—developing a new class of drugs." *Nature Reviews Drug Discovery* 13 (10):759–80. doi: 10.1038/nrd4278.

Santomauro, D.F., A.M. Mantilla Herrera, J. Shadid, P. Zheng, C. Ashbaugh, D.M. Pigott, C. Abbafati, et al. 2021. "Global prevalence and burden of depressive and anxiety disorders in 204 countries and territories in 2020 due to the COVID-19 pandemic." *The Lancet* 398 (10312):1700–12. doi: 10.1016/S0140-6736(21)02143-7.

Sinatra Ayres, A. 2021. "COVID-19 changed the way we work. Will office life every be the same?" In *USA Today*. McLean, VA: Gannett Satellite Info Network LLC.

Soderbergh, S. (director). Shamberg, M., Sher, S., Jacobs, G. (producers). 2011. "*Contagion*." [Film]. 1 hr 46 min. Burbank, CA: Warner Bros. Pictures.

Sozzi, G., A. Manenti, M. Boeri, F. Sabia, E. Montomoli, U. Pastorino, and G. Apolone. 2021. "Reply to comments on: Unexpected detection of SARS-CoV-2 antibodies in the prepandemic period in Italy." *Tumori* 107 (5):472–3. doi: 10.1177/03008916211009688.

Statistics, CDC/National Center for Health. 2021. "Drug overdose deaths in the U.S. top 100,000 annually." *Health and Human Services*. Accessed 18 December 2021. www.cdc.gov/nchs/pressroom/nchs_press_releases/2021/20211117.htm.

Streicker, D.G., and A.T. Gilbert. 2020. "Contextualizing bats as viral reservoirs." *Science* 370 (6513):172–3. doi: 10.1126/science.abd4559.

Sylvers, E. 2020. "Fearful and wary, Italian city ravaged by coronavirus slowly re-emerges." In *Wall Street Journal*. New York, NY: Dow Jones and Company.

Tasso, A.F., N. Hisli Sahin, and G.J. San Roman. 2021. "COVID-19 disruption on college students: Academic and socioemotional implications." *Psychological Trauma: Theory, Research, Practice, and Policy* 13 (1):9–15. doi: 10.1037/tra0000996.

TED. 2015. "Bill Gates: The next outbreak? We're not ready." Accessed 22 December 2021. www.youtube.com/watch?v=6Af6b_wyiwI.

UNICEF, United Nations Children's Fund. 2020. "Averting a lost COVID generation: A six point plan to respond, recover and reimagine a post-pandemic world for every child." Accessed 22 November 2021. https://www.unicef.org/reports/averting-lost-generation-covid19-world-childrens-day-2020-brief.

Vogel, G. 2020. "Sweden's gamble." *Science* 370 (6513):159–63. doi: 10.1126/science.370.6513.159.

Wadman, M. 2020. "Fever, aches from Pfizer, Moderna jabs aren't dangerous but may be intense for some." *Science* 371:6529.

Wang, C.C., K.A. Prather, J. Sznitman, J.L. Jimenez, S.S. Lakdawala, Z. Tufekci, and L.C. Marr. 2021. "Airborne transmission of respiratory viruses." *Science* 373 (6558). doi: 10.1126/science.abd9149.

Wardeh, M., M. Baylis, and M.S.C. Blagrove. 2021. "Predicting mammalian hosts in which novel coronaviruses can be generated." *Nat Communications* 12 (1):780. doi: 10.1038/s41467-021-21034-5.

Weissman, D., H. Ni, D. Scales, A. Dude, J. Capodici, K. McGibney, A. Abdool, S.N. Isaacs, G. Cannon, and K. Karikó. 2000. "HIV gag mRNA transfection of dendritic cells (DC) delivers encoded antigen to MHC class I and II molecules, causes DC maturation, and induces a potent human in vitro primary immune response." *Journal of Immunology* 165 (8):4710–7. doi: 10.4049/jimmunol.165.8.4710.

Whelan, R. 2020. "Sense of smell offers Covid research clues." In *Wall Street Journal*. New York, NY: Dow Jones and Company.

WHO, World Health Organization. 2021a. "Classification of Omicron (B.1.1.529): SARS-CoV-2 variant of concern." *World Health Organization*. Accessed 17 December 2021. www.who.int/news/item/26-11-2021-classification-of-omicron-(b.1.1.529)-sars-cov-2-variant-of-concern.

———. 2021b. "COVAX: Working for global equitable access to COVID-19 vaccines." *World Health Organization*. Accessed 21 December 2021. www.who.int/initiatives/act-accelerator/covax.

———. 2021c. "Interim statement on booster doses for COVID-19 vaccination." Accessed 21 December 2021. www.who.int/news/item/04-10-2021-interim-statement-on-booster-doses-for-covid-19-vaccination.

———. 2021d. "Tracking SARS-CoV-2 variants." Accessed 22 November 2021 and 16 December 2021. www.who.int/en/activities/tracking-SARS-CoV-2-variants/.

———. 2021e. "WHO recommends against the use of convalescent plasma to treat COVID-19." Accessed 22 December 2021. https://www.who.int/news/item/07-12-2021-who-recommends-against-the-use-of-convalescent-plasma-to-treat-covid-19#:~:text=WHO%20has%20updated%20its%20living,and%20critical%20COVID%2D19%20patients.

Wolff, J.A., R.W. Malone, P. Williams, W. Chong, G. Acsadi, A. Jani, and P.L. Felgner. 1990. "Direct gene transfer into mouse muscle in vivo." *Science* 247 (4949 Pt 1):1465–8. doi: 10.1126/science.1690918.

Worobey, M., J. Pekar, B.B. Larsen, M.I. Nelson, V. Hill, J.B. Joy, A. Rambaut, M.A. Suchard, J.O. Wertheim, and P. Lemey. 2020. "The emergence of SARS-CoV-2 in Europe and North America." *Science* 370 (6516):564–70. doi: 10.1126/science.abc8169.

Wright, L. 2021. *The Plague Year: America in the Time of Covid*. New York, NY: Alfred A. Knopf.

Young-Saver, D. 2021. "The math of ending the pandemic: Exponential growth and decay." *The New York Times*. Accessed 27 December 2021. www.nytimes.com/2021/05/14/learning/the-math-of-ending-the-pandemic-exponential-growth-and-decay.html.

Zakaria, F. 2020. *Ten Lessons for a Post-pandemic World*. 1st ed. New York, NY: W.W. Norton and Company.

Zhang, T., Q. Wu, and Z. Zhang. 2020. "Probable pangolin origin of SARS-CoV-2 associated with the COVID-19 outbreak." *Current Biology* 30 (7):1346–51.e2. doi: 10.1016/j.cub.2020.03.022.

Zhou, P., X.L. Yang, X.G. Wang, B. Hu, L. Zhang, W. Zhang, H.R. Si, et al. 2020. "A pneumonia outbreak associated with a new coronavirus of probable bat origin." *Nature* 579 (7798):270–3. doi: 10.1038/s41586-020-2012-7.

7

Recombinant DNA Technology and Gene Therapy Using Viruses

Learning Outcomes:

7.1 Extend Your Understanding of Viruses beyond Viruses Just as Pathogens

7.2 Examine the Uses of Viruses as a Potential Molecular Delivery System

7.3 Understand the Concept of Recombinant DNA Technology and How Viruses Are Involved

7.4 Discover the Use of Viruses for Gene Therapy

7.5 Discuss the Use of Viruses in Vaccines and Other Drugs

7.1 Extend Your Understanding of Viruses beyond Viruses Just as Pathogens

In this textbook, we have mainly talked about viruses as agents of disease. However, viruses are a part of our world, and they have other roles to play on the planet. For example, we know that viruses can form in a "symbiotic relationship" with their organismal host, which can result in mutualism where both the virus and host gain some benefit (Mietzsch and Agbandje-McKenna 2017; Roossinck 2011). In addition, scientists have harnessed the power of viruses to use them to treat disease, including using viruses to fight cancer, as was mentioned in Chapter 1 (Mietzsch and Agbandje-McKenna 2017; Brown 2020). Scientists also can use modified viruses for gene therapy and vaccines. Any time a virus is used to treat a disease, it is known as virotherapy (Mietzsch and Agbandje-McKenna 2017).

In the area of regenerative medicine, scientists have developed induced pluripotent stem cells, which are adult cells conditioned to behave like stem cells, with the help of a virus to induce certain gene expression changes (Alberts et al. 2019; Clarke and Frampton 2020). In this case, a virus is being used to alter the nature of the cell, making the cell usable to regenerate tissues. Either directly or indirectly, in the natural world or after modification in the laboratory, humans can use viruses to improve the world around them.

Many organisms have relationships with viruses. One of the best-understood examples of a mutualistic type of relationship is between the parasitoid wasp and a polydnavirus. The virus depends on the wasp for replication, and the virus expresses genes that allow wasp eggs laid in an insect larva to survive (Roossinck 2011). As mentioned briefly in Chapter 1, humans carry the remnants of retroviruses in their genome, and some of these integrated genes were thought to have a positive effect on evolution. For example, the syncytin genes, derived from ancient retroviruses that integrated into the genome, are

DOI: 10.1201/9781003172260-7

expressed in a specialized cell type of the human placenta. Expression of these genes allows for cell fusion events that are critical to the structure of the placenta (Roossinck 2011; Roberts et al. 2021). Other scientists are studying what is known as the human virome, the portion of the human microbiome made up of viruses—all the viruses that inhabit the cells of the body. Although some viruses in our virome infect our cells, even without us knowing it, in most cases, most of the viruses in our virome are infecting the bacteria that inhabit our bodies. These viruses are known as bacteriophages or phages. More research still needs to be done as to how the kind and number of viruses in our virome affect our general health (Pride 2020; Liang and Bushman 2021). Given that viruses do many things and are all around us, some say that life on the planet would not work without viruses (Nuwer 2020). Now that we have recognized the importance of viruses, how are scientists exploiting the characteristics of viruses for our own medicinal purposes?

7.2 Examine the Uses of Viruses as a Potential Molecular Delivery System

Viruses can enter the human body and potentially cause dramatic changes. However, scientists have long considered the possibility of using viruses for our own purposes as a type of molecular delivery system, called viral vectors, to treat diseases. As we have seen, viruses tend to infect certain cell types of the body, based on the receptors displayed on those cells. Knowing what we know now, one can examine viruses that infect humans already and find those that can be weakened or altered in some manner, and then they can be used to express a beneficial gene in the body in those places that they normally infect. However, before we can understand how this is accomplished, we must go back to the beginnings of genetic engineering, when genes could first be manipulated and placed into a virus in the first place. For this to happen, the discovery of restriction enzymes and vectors for gene cloning were critical first steps, as the following describes (Colavito 2007).

7.3 Understand the Concept of Recombinant DNA Technology and How Viruses Are Involved

Recombinant DNA technology, also known as genetic engineering, is the idea that a gene or stretch of DNA from one biological source can be transferred to another source where it can be expressed in that new organism (Alberts et al. 2019; Kurreck and Stein 2016; Mukherjee 2016; Colavito 2007; Minkoff and Baker 2004). The transfer of genetic material into the new organism is a kind of genetic modification, resulting in a genetically modified organism (LabXChange 2022). The genetically modified organism (GMO) can also be called a transgenic organism, meaning that it is an organism containing a transgene or newly introduced gene (Pray 2008).

When one first isolates the gene, it is called gene or DNA cloning (Figure 7.1). The ability to do a cut and paste, where one removes a gene from one source, the "cut" part, and then places it in a vector to be expressed in a new organism, the "paste" part, critically depends on enzymes known as restriction enzymes (Pray 2008). These are enzymes, identified first in bacteria, that reliably cut the DNA at a particular short nucleotide sequence. Restriction

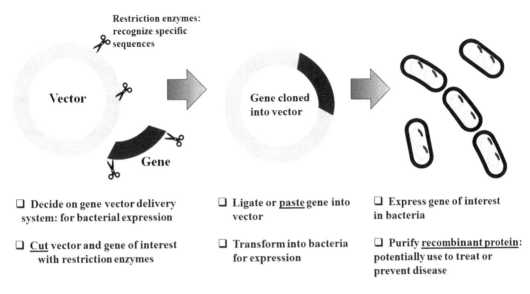

FIGURE 7.1
Steps of Gene Cloning

The first step of gene cloning is to identify the vector you want to use to transfer the gene of interest into a new organism. In this image, a vector for bacterial expression is chosen. Then both the vector and gene of interest are cut with restriction enzymes. Restriction enzymes recognize specific nucleic acid sequences and allow a gene to be tailored to fit into a particular vector. Then, the gene is ligated, or pasted, into the vector. Next, the vector is transformed into bacteria for expression. Then, the expressed protein can be purified from the bacteria and used as a treatment for a disease or a preventative tool such as a vaccine. The protein is called a recombinant protein because the gene encoding the protein came from another organism.

enzyme sites can be mapped out in any gene sequence and used to cut the DNA strategically (Kurreck and Stein 2016; Alberts et al. 2019; Minkoff and Baker 2004; Mukherjee 2016).

Once the DNA is removed from one source, it is placed in a vector. A vector is the intermediary that allows the transfer of the gene from one organism to the other. Vectors may be artificial pieces of DNA known as plasmids, based on circular DNAs first found in bacteria (Alberts et al. 2019; Kurreck and Stein 2016; LabXChange 2022). The first viral vectors used were bacteriophages (Kurreck and Stein 2016; Pray 2008). It is important to note that the discovery of polymerase chain reaction (PCR) in the 1980s became an important tool used for DNA cloning as well, allowing researchers to make millions of copies of a gene of interest before putting it into a vector (Alberts et al. 2019).

After the gene of interest is inserted into the vector, the vector is then transferred to another organism, typically bacteria or yeast, to express the recombinant protein (LabXChange 2022; Minkoff and Baker 2004). In 1977, the human hormone somatostatin was expressed in *E. coli* bacteria using recombinant DNA technology (Kurreck and Stein 2016; Mukherjee 2016).

Recombinant DNA technology has been used to make many drugs. In 1982, the FDA approved the use of recombinant human insulin (Kurreck and Stein 2016; Minkoff and Baker 2004; Mukherjee 2016). In the past 40 years, there have been over 250 drugs made using recombinant technology (Kurreck and Stein 2016). Many of these products include recombinant protein vaccines like the vaccines against human papilloma virus and hepatitis B (Kurreck and Stein 2016). The recently approved SARS-CoV-2 vaccine, Novavax, is a recombinant protein vaccine (Heath et al. 2021; Novavax 2021; Corum and Zimmer 2021).

In summary, recombinant DNA technology is used to express a gene from one source in a new way, using a vector. Viruses have been used as vectors in the past and are an important delivery system used in many applications, including gene therapy and vaccine development. It is important to note that scientists recognized the significance of conducting genetic modification of an organism and helped establish guidelines for using recombinant DNA technology at a famous conference in the 1970s known as the Asilomar Conference. These guiding principles are still used by the National Institutes of Health in the United States (Mukherjee 2016) (Collins and Gottlieb 2019).

7.4 Discover the Use of Viruses for Gene Therapy

After the development of recombinant DNA technology, scientists began investigating how to use cloned genes to treat disease. Gene therapy involves using some type of gene transfer method, usually a virus, to deliver a gene for expression in a person's cells to treat a disease (Colavito 2007; Kurreck and Stein 2016). The therapy may be designed so that the new gene substitutes for a defective gene (a type of gene editing), or that the new gene inactivates another gene. In addition, gene therapy can work by adding another gene to the patient's genome to treat a disease, rather than replacing or inactivating a gene (FDA 2022b; Anguela and High 2019). Gene therapy was first explored as a type of disease treatment for individuals with a monogenic disease, meaning that the disease or disorder was caused by a change in a single gene (Colavito 2007).

Examples of monogenic diseases include sickle cell disease and cystic fibrosis. The idea was that gene therapy could correct the single gene defect in a targeted manner, whether it was defective in one copy or both copies of the gene in the patient's cells. If a monogenic genetic disorder is caused by an "autosomal recessive" mutation, this means that an individual needs to inherit a defective copy of the gene from both their mother and their father to have the disorder. However, if a gene is "autosomal dominant," one defective copy from either parent is enough to causes the disease. "Autosomal" refers to the 22 non-sex chromosomes (not X or Y) in humans. There are some monogenic disorders that are found on the X chromosome, for example, but most are recessive. If a person has one copy of the X chromosome, then that person has the disease, but it is masked if one has two X chromosomes (Kurreck and Stein 2016).

To treat a person for a disease using gene therapy, one needs to obtain the correctly functioning gene, through gene cloning, and then find a way to express it in the patient's cells. Then, a virus or other method is used to deliver the gene to the patient's cells. Gene therapy is typically aimed at somatic cells, meaning the adult cells of the body, not the germline cells like sperm or egg. With this approach, the therapy is not meant to be passed onto the next generation (Colavito 2007; Kurreck and Stein 2016).

There are different gene therapy approaches. For example, a patient's cells may be removed, modified using the viral vector with the gene insert (therapeutic transgene), and then reintroduced into the body. This is known as the *ex vivo* approach. Alternatively, the viral vector with the gene insert could be introduced directly to an organ or systemically to modify the target cells within the patient's body. This is known as the *in vivo*

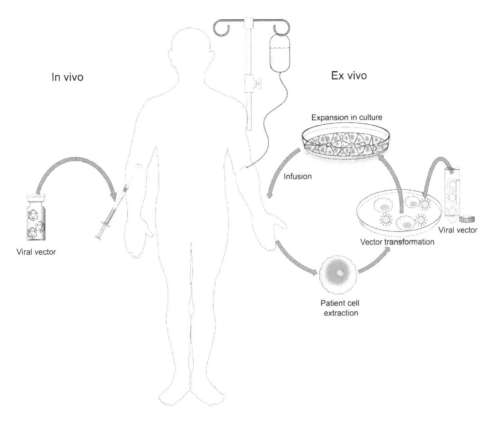

FIGURE 7.2
In vivo versus ex vivo approaches to delivering gene therapy.

Shown here are two ways of delivering gene therapy to a patient. In the *in vivo* method shown on the left, the vector with the gene of interest (therapeutic transgene) is introduced directly into the patient through the bloodstream. In the *ex vivo* approach shown on the right, the patient's cells are removed and the vector carrying the gene of interest is introduced into the patient's cells using a cell culturing method. Then, the patient's cells are allowed to grow in culture, before being transferred back into the patient.

Source: Figure 1 in the article: Bulcha, J.T., Y. Wang, H. Ma, P.W.L. Tai, and G. Gao. 2021. "Viral vector platforms within the gene therapy landscape." *Signal Transduction and Targeted Therapy* 6 (1):53. https://doi.org/10.1038/s41392-021-00487-6

approach (Figure 7.2). (Mietzsch and Agbandje-McKenna 2017; Colavito 2007; Minkoff and Baker 2004; Kurreck and Stein 2016). It should be recognized that the *ex vivo* gene therapy approach is built on knowledge gained from successful bone marrow transplants using patient-matched hematopoietic (blood) stem cell donors. This is known as allogeneic bone marrow transplantation. With gene therapy, now the patient's own cells can be modified and given back to them in an approach known as an autologous bone marrow transplantation (Dunbar et al. 2018).

Different viral vectors are used for in *ex vivo* versus *in vivo* approach. For example, an integrating virus like a lentivirus might be used in the *ex vivo* approach. On the other hand, a non-integrating virus like an adeno-associated virus (AAV) might be used for the *in vivo* approach (Anguela and High 2019; Li and Samulski 2020). The different kinds of viruses used for gene therapy are described in the next section.

7.4.1 Viruses Commonly Used for Gene Therapy

Since gene therapy was first done in the 1990s, scientists have tried to optimize viral vectors by modifying them specifically for their use in gene therapy. A few classes of viruses are more commonly used than others, including adenoviruses, parvoviruses, and retroviruses. Adenovirus, a double-stranded DNA virus (Class I, Baltimore classification) has been used because it can carry a large gene insert and it does not readily recombine into a host chromosome. Parvoviruses, a small ssDNA virus (Class II, Baltimore classification) can carry a small gene insert but also does not recombine into the host chromosome. Retroviruses, including lentiviruses, are ssRNA viruses (Class IV, Baltimore classification) that can carry an insert bigger than a parvovirus but smaller than an adenovirus, but by their nature integrate into the host cell's chromosome (Lostroh 2019; Kurreck and Stein 2016; Lee et al. 2017; Bulcha et al. 2021). In some cases, a viral promoter (gene regulatory element) from another virus, like cytomegalovirus (CMV), can also be used in gene therapy. The CMV promoter can be used to drive high expression of a gene insert (Lostroh 2019). If the viral vector can integrate into the genome, it's a way that the delivered gene can permanently be expressed in the cell, but it does carry the risk of something called insertional mutagenesis, in which the delivered gene may alter expression of a gene already in the genome, such as one controlling cell growth (Lostroh 2019).

Over the years, scientists have found new ways to tailor viral vectors to their gene therapy needs, making what are known as second and third generation technology. For example, retroviruses have been altered to become replication defective. Then, researchers began working with lentiviruses as a type of retroviral vector because this virus can integrate into cells that are not dividing but leave alone cells in a dormant state called quiescence. In addition, if a lentivirus does integrate into the genome, it tends to do so within a gene, rather than going into a DNA regulatory element where there was a greater risk of activating a cancer-causing gene (Dunbar et al. 2018). Scientists have created what are known as "gutless" adenoviral vectors, removing almost all the viral genes to make more room for an insert, but this change does render the adenovirus unable to make complete viral particles without a helper virus. Thus, certain specialized cell lines are needed for these gutless vectors, which help with the processing of the final gene therapy product (Lostroh 2019; Kurreck and Stein 2016; Colavito 2007; Bulcha et al. 2021; Lee et al. 2017). Using a viral vector derived from viruses that are commonly found in the human population like the parvovirus AAV might be an issue. Scientists are working to modify AAVs, for example, so that the capsid of the virus is something that has not been seen before by the patient's immune system. (A micrograph of AAV was shown in Figure 1.5.) Scientists can use a viral capsid from a nonhuman primate or even engineer new capsids in the laboratory that can be systematically tested (Wang, Tai, and Gao 2019; Li and Samulski 2020). Many humans have been exposed to adenoviruses as well, and scientists have started focusing on using uncommon adenovirus serotypes such as Ad2 or Ad5 as viral vectors. Scientists are making many advances to tailor viral vectors for gene therapy to the disease and to the patient, making viruses a part of personalized medicine (Lee et al. 2017).

Some common characteristics to consider when picking a viral vector for gene therapy include how long and where you want the virus to drive expression of a gene, whether the virus can replicate inside the cell, what the risk is of causing a change in the genome if it is an integrating virus, and what the likelihood is that the virus itself will activate the immune system (Kurreck and Stein 2016). Different applications favor different characteristics. In some cases, you may not want the virus to replicate if your goal is to correct a monogenic disease, but replication might be all right if are trying to create an oncolytic virus to go after the rogue dividing cells (Kurreck and Stein 2016). Sometimes a viral vector is chosen based on its "tissue tropism." For example, many types of AAVs target different organs ranging from the liver, heart, and skeletal muscle to other organs (Kurreck and Stein 2016). For example, AAV9 can cross the blood-brain barrier, meaning that potentially it can be used to treat neurological disorders (Wang, Tai, and Gao 2019). However, it should be noted that AAVs are not found to cause human disease on their own and are not capable of their own replication (Dunbar et al. 2018; Wang, Tai, and Gao 2019; Li and Samulski 2020).

Although gene therapy was initially targeted at monogenic diseases, researchers are now trying this approach to treat other more complex diseases including cancer and cardiovascular disease (Kurreck and Stein 2016; Colavito 2007; Anguela and High 2019; Shahryari et al. 2019). The number of gene therapy clinical trials involving anti-cancer treatments outnumber all others (Anguela and High 2019).

In the next section, I will describe some notable gene therapy examples as well as the key gene therapies that are currently approved for use in the United States. Developing a new gene therapy approach is a huge undertaking, and before human clinical trials are done, scientists work out many of the conditions using animal models. However, improvements continue to be made in this stage of the process as well, with the development of "humanized" mice and three-dimensional cell culturing methods as popular new preclinical trial approaches (Li and Samulski 2020).

7.4.2 Examples of Gene Therapies Involving Viruses

Starting 30 years ago, researchers explored the use of gene therapy to treat severe combined immunodeficiency (SCID), a disorder in which the patient's immune system never fully develops making the person prone to acquiring life-threatening infections. Researchers focused on two forms of SCID, caused by different genes. For adenine deaminase–severe combined immunodeficiency (ADA-SCID), a retroviral vector was used to replace the defective ADA gene, using an *ex vivo* approach where the patient's T cells were modified and then transplanted back into the body. It is believed that the therapy worked, but patients were receiving an enzyme-based treatment during the entire gene therapy course. Another form of SCID involving a mutation in a gene on the X chromosome (X-SCID) was also treated using a retroviral vector. However, several children in the trial developed leukemia a few years after treatment, most likely due to a viral integration event affecting cell growth regulation (Minkoff and Baker 2004; Lostroh 2019; Colavito 2007; Kurreck and Stein 2016; Anguela and High 2019; Dunbar et al. 2018). An adverse outcome was also seen with a gene therapy trial to treat a deficiency in the metabolic enzyme ornithine transcarbamylase in 1999. One patient died and the trial was halted (Lostroh 2019; Colavito 2007; Mukherjee 2016; Minkoff and Baker 2004). This tragedy prompted a period of basic research into new viral vector delivery systems and more oversight of gene therapy trials that continues to this day (Collins and Gottlieb 2019). Since that time, new technologies have been used to tackle SCID. Strimvelis is a type of gene therapy product using an updated viral vector delivery system to treat ADA-SCID patients. However, demand for this new therapy is quite low due to the small number of patients with the disease, and it is unclear how long the product will be marketed (Anguela and High 2019; Li and Samulski 2020; Aiuti, Roncarolo, and Naldini 2017; Dunbar et al. 2018). Another gene therapy product, alipogene tiparvovec, also known as Glybera, is used to treat familial lipoprotein lipase deficiency using an AAV vector. It was approved for use in Europe in 2012 (Lostroh 2019; Kurreck and Stein 2016; Wang, Tai, and Gao 2019; Li and Samulski 2020). However, the treatment is quite expensive, costing over a million dollars a treatment (Kurreck and Stein 2016). Glybera is no longer being marketed in Europe (Shahryari et al. 2019). Rexin-G is an anti-cancer gene therapy that works by blocking cell cycle progression by expressing a modified version of a gene called cyclin G using a retroviral vector. It is being tested right now in clinical trials of people with advanced pancreatic cancer (Lostroh 2019; Shahryari et al. 2019). Although the development of gene therapy treatments is a long road with many possible setbacks, several gene therapy products are approved for use in the United States right now, as described next.

7.4.3 Key Gene Therapy Products Approved in the United States

Many gene therapy trials have been attempted over the past 30 years, and many approaches have run into difficulty due to the complex nature of the treatment. Others were too expensive and targeted at too few patients. Currently, there are 20 FDA-approved cellular and gene therapy products in the United States (FDA 2022a). Of the gene therapy products on the list, we will focus on five therapies that involve viruses in the gene therapy delivery system (FDA 2022a; Anguela and High 2019; Shahryari et al. 2019).

LUXTURNA is a type of gene therapy used for patients with "retinal dystrophy" caused by mutations in RPE65. The specific disease involved is also known as Leber congenital amaurosis, which causes a deterioration of the retina leading to blindness. The drug was approved for use in 2017 and was the first *in vivo* gene therapy approved using an AAV vector (AAV2) in the United States (Anguela and High 2019; Russell et al. 2017; Ledford 2015; Wang, Tai, and Gao 2019; Dunbar et al. 2018; Li and Samulski 2020; Shahryari et al. 2019).

ZOLGENSMA is a gene therapy product that has been developed using an AAV-based vector (AAV9) to treat spinal muscular atrophy in children. In this therapy, a wildtype copy of the survival motor neuron 1 (SMN1) gene is delivered systemically through intravenous injection. It was approved for use in the United States in 2019 (Dunbar et al. 2018; Li and Samulski 2020; Shahryari et al. 2019).

IMLYGIC, also known as talimogene laherparepvec, is a melanoma treatment that uses a modified herpesvirus (Lostroh 2019; Anguela and High 2019; Lee et al. 2017; Shahryari et al. 2019). It should be noted that IMLYGIC was the first oncolytic virus treatment approved in the United States back in 2015 (Anguela and High 2019).

KYMRIAH and YESCARTA are a type of cancer immunotherapy called CAR-T therapy. In CAR-T therapy, T cells are modified (using a retrovirus or another approach) so that they express special receptors on their surface to recognize and bind to tumor proteins. This type of gene therapy is delivered using the *ex vivo* approach. Both treatments can be used for non-Hodgkin's lymphoma, and KYMRIAH is also used to treat chronic lymphocytic leukemia (CLL) (Figure 7.3) (Anguela and High 2019; Dunbar et al. 2018; Li and Samulski 2020; Shahryari et al. 2019; NCI 2022).

7.4.4 Future of Gene Therapy

Although a small number of gene therapy products have been approved in the United States, many are being tested right now, including potential treatment for monogenic disorders that have been studied for many years. As mentioned earlier, both cystic fibrosis

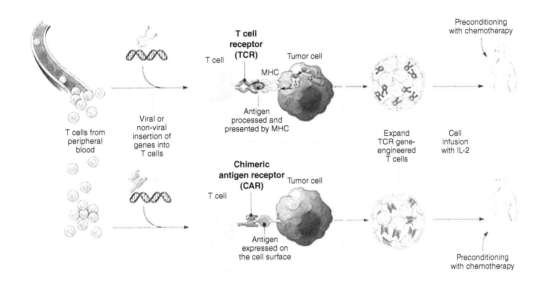

FIGURE 7.3
Steps of CAR-T therapy.

The first step is to remove T cells from the blood of the patient. T cells display certain receptors on their surface known as T cell receptors or TCRs. In the second step, using either a viral- or a nonviral-based method, the T cells are modified to display a new kind of receptor on their surface called a chimeric antigen receptor (CAR). This new kind of receptor can be engineered to recognize tumor cells in the patient. The modified T cells are grown in culture and transplanted back into the patient to find and kill the cancer cell expressing a particular antigen on its cell surface.

Credit: National Cancer Institute. Original figure can be found (in 2021) at www.cancer.gov/about-cancer/treatment/research/car-t-cells

"Graphics explicitly credited to NCI are copyright-free and may be used without our permission" (www.cancer.gov/policies/copyright-reuse).

(CF) and sickle cell disease (SCD) are well-known monogenic disorders. Cystic fibrosis involves a defective chloride ion transporter causing mucus buildup in the lungs, making patients prone to infections, among other issues. Other organs, such as parts of the digestive system, are also affected in CF. Physicians and scientists have been working on gene therapy approaches to treat CF for many years. So far, there are no approved gene therapy treatments, although several approaches are being tested in clinical trials. Since CF can affect more than one organ, determining where to deliver the therapy is one challenge, in addition to providing a treatment that is long lasting (Foundation 2022; Colavito 2007). Sickle cell disease (also known as sickle cell anemia) involves the loss of functional adult hemoglobin for oxygen transport in the blood due to a defective beta-globin gene. Clinical trials in SCD patients are underway to use a lentivirus-based vector to restore a normal copy of the beta-globin gene. A second treatment approach for SCD involves using gene therapy to reactivate expression of the gamma-globin gene, a component of fetal hemoglobin, to substitute for the defective beta-globin in the adult hemoglobin form (Eisenstein 2021; Kunz and Kulozik 2020).

Although many gene therapy challenges have been addressed using optimized viral vectors, certain risks remain, such as the possible complication of mutation from an integrating viral vector (Colavito 2007; Kurreck and Stein 2016; Anguela and High 2019). In addition, gene therapy is a complicated and expensive treatment process, so it is unclear if pharmaceutical companies will continue to make gene therapy drugs for rare disease treatment. However, several therapeutic areas, including cancer treatment, hold great promise for new uses of gene therapy. Aside from using viral vectors for genetic modification, scientists have started using gene editing using CRISPR/Cas9 technology (Lostroh 2019; Dunbar et al. 2018; Doudna 2020). Whether viral-based delivery systems are used or not, gene-based therapies will certainly be a big part of medical treatment in the future.

7.5 Discuss the Use of Viruses in Vaccines and Other Drugs

Like a virus can be used to deliver a therapeutic transgene to treat a disease, viruses can also be used to facilitate an immune response as a part of a vaccine. Several different kinds of viral vectors are used for vaccines, but using modified versions of adenovirus, usually Ad5, is a common approach. When choosing a vector, researchers must look at the ability of the viral vector to induce the desired immune response. In addition, practical considerations include if the proper cell lines are available to produce the vaccine and if they can be scaled up for mass production (Weiner and Nabel 2018). Because many people have been exposed to adenoviruses in the population, scientists may need to use chimeric or hybrid adenoviral vectors for the vaccine (Weiner and Nabel 2018).

Millions of people around the world have been given either the Johnson & Johnson/Janssen or the Oxford/Astra Zeneca COVID-19 vaccines. Both vaccines involve the use of modified adenovirus-based vectors to deliver the gene encoding the SARS-CoV-2 spike protein into the patient's cells so it can be expressed into those cells and provoke an immune response. Both modified adenovirus vectors cannot multiply inside the patient's cells and do not cause disease themselves (Corum and Zimmer 2021; Krammer 2020).

In addition to COVID-19 vaccines, viral vectors have been used in other circumstances such as for candidate Ebola vaccines. Two Ebola vaccines are in clinical trials right now. One uses a recombinant vesicular stomatitis virus (VSV), an animal virus, as a vector. The other uses a modified adenovirus from chimpanzees as a vector (NIAID 2022).

Besides using viruses as vaccines to induce antibody protection in the body, scientists are developing viruses to deliver the antibodies themselves, by expressing broadly neutralizing antibodies for therapy (Mietzsch and Agbandje-McKenna 2017; Lin and Balazs 2018). Bacteriophages, viruses that infect bacteria, are experiencing renewed interest as alternatives to antibiotics or as a treatment in cases of antibiotic resistance (Salmond and Fineran 2015; Lostroh 2019). Other researchers are exploring the use of viruses and virus-like particles (VLPs) derived from viruses to bring drugs to certain areas of the body that cannot be reached through conventional drug delivery methods. For example, scientists are using VLPs derived from a flock house virus to deliver a chemotherapy drug directly to tumor cells (Ghosh and Banerjee 2021). As you can see, modified viruses are being utilized for many different types of therapies to treat all different kinds of diseases, from the preventative stage as a vaccine onward to first-line treatments and beyond.

7.5.1 Other Uses of Viruses to Treat Disease—Regenerative Medicine

As mentioned in the introduction, induced pluripotent stem cells (iPSCs) are a type of stem cell made by reprogramming adult cells to behave like stem cells. Early work on iPSCs involved using a retroviral-based vector to express a set of genes that turn the clock back on the adult cell nucleus, making it behave like a stem cell present back in early development of the organism. (Alberts et al. 2019; Clarke and Frampton 2020; Kurreck and Stein 2016). Researchers are also working to use adenoviral-based vectors to make iPSCs as well (Stadtfeld et al. 2008). Stem cells are important for regenerative medicine due to their potential to form many cell types of the body, not just one specialized kind. The goal of regenerative medicine is to replace tissues that are affected by disease or worn out with age. Future research will involve further fine-tuning of the iPSC approach to see if these cells can be effectively used to treat patients. Beyond making pluripotent stem cells themselves, researchers are also developing adenoviral vectors to express certain growth factors needed in the tissue specialization process, such as to make bone, to make particular tissues for regenerative purposes (Lee et al. 2017).

7.6 Summary

Viruses do not just cause disease. Naturally or through genetic engineering, viruses can be used to help humans. Genetic engineering, also known as recombinant DNA technology, was developed about 50 years ago as a method to bring together DNA from different organisms. This technology has revolutionized biomedical research, allowing scientists to express any gene of interest in a new organism, including producing recombinant proteins such as human insulin outside of the body. Recombinant DNA technology includes the use of viruses as one type of vector to deliver a gene for expression in a new organism, and these viral vectors have been used in both gene therapy treatments and vaccines, among other applications. Gene therapy treatments involving viral vectors are being used to treat all different kinds of diseases, including cancer. Viral vectors are also used in vaccines, including COVID-19 vaccines. Undoubtedly, viruses will be a part of many therapeutic applications to prevent or treat diseases in the future.

Discussion Questions:

1. What are the benefits of genetic engineering for humankind?
2. What do you think are the risks of genetic modification of organism? How should scientific research involving genetic modification be regulated?
3. If you were born with a life-threatening metabolic disease, would you consider doing gene therapy to permanently correct your condition? Why or why not?
4. Summarize the challenges and benefits of using a viral vector-based vaccine.
5. What are the safety considerations to consider when introducing a new virus into a human for any purpose?

References

Aiuti, A., M.G. Roncarolo, and L. Naldini. 2017. "Gene therapy for ADA-SCID, the first marketing approval of an ex vivo gene therapy in Europe: Paving the road for the next generation of advanced therapy medicinal products." *EMBO Molecular Medicine* 9 (6):737–40. doi: 10.15252/emmm.201707573.

Alberts, B., D. Bray, K. Hopkin, A.D. Johnson, J. Lewis, M. Raff, K. Roberts, and P. Walter. 2019. *Essential Cell Biology*. 5th ed. New York, NY: W.W. Norton & Company.

Anguela, X.M., and K.A. High. 2019. "Entering the modern era of gene therapy." *Annual Review of Medicine* 70:273–88. doi: 10.1146/annurev-med-012017-043332.

Brown, C. 2020. "Scientists are harnessing viruses to treat tumours." *Nature* 587 (7835):S60-S2.

Bulcha, J.T., Y. Wang, H. Ma, P.W.L. Tai, and G. Gao. 2021. "Viral vector platforms within the gene therapy landscape." *Signal Transduction and Targeted Therapy* 6 (1):53. doi: 10.1038/s41392-021-00487-6.

Clarke, M.L., and J. Frampton. 2020. *Stem Cells: Biology and Application*. Boca Raton, FL: CRC Press, Taylor & Francis Group.

Colavito, M.C. 2007. *Gene Therapy*. Edited by M. Palladino, *Special Topics in Biology*. New York, NY: Pearson Education Benjamin Cummings.

Collins, F.S., and S. Gottlieb. 2019. "The next phase of human gene-therapy oversight." *New England Journal of Medicine* 380 (4):402. doi: 10.1056/NEJMc1815776.

Corum, J., and C. Zimmer. 2021. "How nine Covid-19 vaccines work." *The New York Times*. Accessed 21 December 2021. www.nytimes.com/interactive/2021/health/how-covid-19-vaccines-work.html?action=click&module=RelatedLinks&pgtype=Article.

Doudna, J.A. 2020. "The promise and challenge of therapeutic genome editing." *Nature* 578 (7794):229–36. doi: 10.1038/s41586-020-1978-5.

Dunbar, C.E., K.A. High, J.K. Joung, D.B. Kohn, K. Ozawa, and M. Sadelain. 2018. "Gene therapy comes of age." *Science (New York, N.Y.)* 359 (6372). doi: 10.1126/science.aan4672.

Eisenstein, M. 2021. "Gene therapies close in on a cure for sickle-cell disease." *Nature* 596 (7873): S2–S4. doi: 10.1038/d41586-021-02138-w.

FDA, Food and Drug Administration. 2022a. "Approved cellular and gene therapy products." *Health and Human Services*. Accessed 3 January 2022. www.fda.gov/vaccines-blood-biologics/cellular-gene-therapy-products/approved-cellular-and-gene-therapy-products.

———. 2022b. "What is gene therapy?" Health and Human Services. Accessed 3 January 2022. www.fda.gov/vaccines-blood-biologics/cellular-gene-therapy-products/what-gene-therapy.

Foundation, Cystic Fibrosis. 2022. "Gene therapy for cystic fibrosis." Accessed 5 January 2022. www.cff.org/gene-therapy-cystic-fibrosis.

Ghosh, S., and M. Banerjee. 2021. "A smart viral vector for targeted delivery of hydrophobic drugs." *Scientific Reports* 11 (1):7030. doi: 10.1038/s41598-021-86198-y.

Heath, P.T., E.P. Galiza, D.N. Baxter, M. Boffito, D. Browne, F. Burns, D.R. Chadwick, et al. 2021. "Safety and efficacy of NVX-CoV2373 Covid-19 vaccine." *New England Journal of Medicine* 385 (13):1172–83. doi: 10.1056/NEJMoa2107659.

Krammer, F. 2020. "SARS-CoV-2 vaccines in development." *Nature* 586 (7830):516–27. doi: 10.1038/s41586-020-2798-3.

Kunz, J.B., and A.E. Kulozik. 2020. "Gene therapy of the hemoglobinopathies." *HemaSphere* 4 (5).

Kurreck, J., and C.A. Stein. 2016. *Molecular Medicine: An Introduction*. Berlin, Germany: John Wiley & Sons, Incorporated.

LabXChange. 2022. "What is genetic engineering?" *The President and Fellows of Harvard College*. Accessed 3 January 2022. www.labxchange.org/library/items/lb:LabXchange:8d3ca92b:html:1.

Ledford, H. 2015. "Gene therapy sees early success against progressive blindness: Treatments for inherited eye diseases show promise in clinical trials, but worries linger over how long the beneficial effects will last." *Nature* 526 (7574):487–9.

Lee, C.S., E.S. Bishop, R. Zhang, X. Yu, E.M. Farina, S. Yan, C. Zhao, et al. 2017. "Adenovirus-mediated gene delivery: Potential applications for gene and cell-based therapies in the new era of personalized medicine." *Genes & Diseases* 4 (2):43–63. doi: 10.1016/j.gendis.2017.04.001.

Li, C., and R.J. Samulski. 2020. "Engineering adeno-associated virus vectors for gene therapy." *Nature Reviews Genetics* 21 (4):255–72. doi: 10.1038/s41576-019-0205-4.

Liang, G., and F.D. Bushman. 2021. "The human virome: Assembly, composition and host interactions." *Nature Reviews Microbiology* 19 (8):514–27. doi: 10.1038/s41579-021-00536-5.

Lin, A., and A.B. Balazs. 2018. "Adeno-associated virus gene delivery of broadly neutralizing antibodies as prevention and therapy against HIV-1." *Retrovirology* 15 (1):66. doi: 10.1186/s12977-018-0449-7.

Lostroh, P. 2019. *Molecular and Cellular Biology of Viruses.* 1st ed. Boca Raton, FL: Taylor & Francis Group, LLC.

Mietzsch, M., and M. Agbandje-McKenna. 2017. "The good that viruses do." *The Annual Review of Virology* 4 (1):iii–v. doi: 10.1146/annurev-vi-04-071217-100011.

Minkoff, E.C., and P.J. Baker. 2004. "Chapter 4: Genetic engineering and genomics." In *Biology Today*, 95–122. New York, NY: Garland Science.

Mukherjee, S. 2016. *The Gene: An Intimate History.* New York, NY: Scribner.

NCI, National Cancer Institute. 2022. "CAR T cells: Engineering patients' immune cell to treat their cancers." *Health and Human Services.* Accessed 5 January 2022. www.cancer.gov/about-cancer/treatment/research/car-t-cells.

NIAID, National Institute of Allergy and Infectious Diseases. 2022. "Ebola vaccines." *Health and Human Services.* Accessed 5 January 2022. www.niaid.nih.gov/diseases-conditions/ebola-vaccines.

Novavax. 2021. *World Health Organization Grants Second Emergency Use Listing for Novavax COVID-19 Vaccine.* Gaithersburg, MD: Novavax. Accessed 20 Dec 2021. https://ir.novavax.com/2021-12-20-World-Health-Organization-Grants-Second-Emergency-Use-Listing-for-Novavax-COVID-19-Vaccine.

Nuwer, R. 2020. "Why the world needs viruses to function." *BBC.* Accessed 29 December 2021. www.bbc.com/future/article/20200617-what-if-all-viruses-disappeared.

Pray, L. 2008. "Recombinant DNA technology and transgenic animals." *Nature Education* 1 (1):51.

Pride, D. 2020. "Viruses can help us as well as harm us." In *Scientific American.* New York, NY: Springer Nature America.

Roberts, R.M., T. Ezashi, L.C. Schulz, J. Sugimoto, D.J. Schust, T. Khan, and J. Zhou. 2021. "Syncytins expressed in human placental trophoblast." *Placenta* 113:8–14. doi: 10.1016/j.placenta.2021.01.006.

Roossinck, M.J. 2011. "The good viruses: Viral mutualistic symbioses." *Nature Reviews Microbiology* 9 (2):99–108. doi: 10.1038/nrmicro2491.

Russell, S., J. Bennett, J.A. Wellman, D.C. Chung, Z.F. Yu, A. Tillman, J. Wittes, et al. 2017. "Efficacy and safety of voretigene neparvovec (AAV2-hRPE65v2) in patients with RPE65-mediated inherited retinal dystrophy: A randomised, controlled, open-label, phase 3 trial." *Lancet* 390 (10097):849–60. doi: 10.1016/s0140-6736(17)31868-8.

Salmond, G.P.C., and P.C. Fineran. 2015. "A century of the phage: Past, present and future." *Nature Reviews Microbiology* 13 (12):777–86. doi: 10.1038/nrmicro3564.

Shahryari, A., M. Saghaeian Jazi, S. Mohammadi, H. Razavi Nikoo, Z. Nazari, E.S. Hosseini, I. Burtscher, S.J. Mowla, and H. Lickert. 2019. "Development and clinical translation of approved gene therapy products for genetic disorders." *Frontiers in Genetics* 10 (868). doi: 10.3389/fgene.2019.00868.

Stadtfeld, M., M. Nagaya, J. Utikal, G. Weir, and K. Hochedlinger. 2008. "Induced pluripotent stem cells generated without viral integration." *Science (New York, N.Y.)* 322 (5903):945–9. doi: 10.1126/science.1162494.

Wang, D., P.W.L. Tai, and G. Gao. 2019. "Adeno-associated virus vector as a platform for gene therapy delivery." *Nature Reviews Drug Discovery* 18 (5):358–78. doi: 10.1038/s41573-019-0012-9.

Weiner, D.B., and G.J. Nabel. 2018. "Development of gene-based vectors for immunization." In *Plotkin's Vaccines*, edited by S.A. Plotkin, W.A. Orenstein, P.A. Offit and K.M. Edwards, 1305–19. e8. Amsterdam, Netherlands: Elsevier.

8

Public Health and Viruses

Learning Outcomes:

8.1 Explain the Meaning of Public Health and Epidemiology

8.2 Understand the Critical Parts of Epidemiology Related to Infectious Disease Caused by Pathogens like Viruses

8.3 Explore Social Determinants of Health and How They Are Connected to Infectious Disease

8.4 Examine Major Global Public Health Issues Related to Infectious Disease

8.5 Understand Vaccine Equity

8.1 Explain the Meaning of Public Health and Epidemiology

Public health involves the collective wellness of the population when it comes to disease. At the core of public health is epidemiology, the study of the cause of disease in a community. Those who practice epidemiology, epidemiologists, typically rely heavily on statistical analysis to examine the distribution of disease in a particular geographic area, follow the number of cases as they change over time, as well as calculate the number of cases relative to the entire population. Public health officials seek to prevent disease, keep people healthy if they are healthy, and improve their health, where possible (Rothman 2012). Another key goal of public health is to increase life span, and by its nature, public health focuses on whole populations rather than individuals (Dawson and Verweij 2007). It is important to note that some public health professionals rely on a narrower or broader definition of public health than others, meaning that the exact definition of public health and all the issues it includes is a "contested concept" (Dawson and Verweij 2007).

Public health includes many issues that affect a population, not just diseases caused by pathogens like viruses. Public health first started in communities where humans sought the most basic ways to keep their drinking water clean and remove human waste from the area. Modern public health workers care about these issues, and much more. They work to educate people about all aspects of their health, such as good habits like a healthy diet and avoiding behaviors like smoking. They participate in sexual health education and even help individuals find safe housing, according to some public health definitions (Rothman 2012).

According to the Centers for Disease Control and Prevention, there are ten essential services performed by those in public health, which can be grouped into the categories of "assessment," "policy development," and "assurance," with "equity" at the center (CDC 2022a). Public health officials need to look at the overall health of the population and pursue health issues when they arise by gathering epidemiological data. Effective communication with the public on these matters is essential. Then, public health officials need to work with local leaders to better the health of people in the community. This may involve making new public health policies and/or using existing policies, even if this means using legal means to do so. To improve and maintain public health, public health officials need to work to facilitate the right healthcare infrastructure for all the members of the community as well (CDC 2022a).

Public health ethics as an area of bioethics seeks to address issues related to the implementation of "preventative interventions" on a population level. These issues include persuading individuals to go along with a public health measure implemented for the good of the society. In addition, how far does an individual need to go in their "moral obligation" to follow a public health measure for the good of the population? Finally, issues of health equity also come under the umbrella of public health ethics (Dawson and Verweij 2007). It is critical for public health officials and workers to take these ethical considerations into account when communicating with the public about public health measures.

It is important to note that public health communication has been affected by scientists who abused their public trust in the past, such as unethically conducted medical studies like the syphilis study at Tuskegee. Back in 1974, the United States government passed the "National Research Act" to address the ethics of conducting a research study (Franklin 2019; CDC 2022g). The ethics of research study design have been adopted by scientists and all related fields including science communication. These ethical principles include having an institutional review board evaluate the planned study, making sure that participants have given informed consent, deidentifying participant data to maintain confidentiality, and making sure the organization funding the study is declared (Dijkstra and Cormick 2020). However, mistrust of public health workers and other scientists in certain communities still lingers from past events and cannot be ignored when the public is approached with a new study or public health measure involving their participation.

8.2 Understand the Critical Parts of Epidemiology Related to Infectious Disease Caused by Pathogens like Viruses

When it comes to epidemiology, public health workers are critical in establishing a connection between a particular pathogen or chemical and a particular disease (Rothman 2012). One could say that epidemiology provides the evidence or support to back public health measures (Dawson and Verweij 2007). There are famous criteria known as the "Causal Criteria of Hill" that scientists use to establish a consistent, specific connection between a suspected cause of disease and the disease itself (Rothman 2012). Epidemiological data on who is afflicted in the population, if they were around a suspected causative agent, when they were around the agent, how long were they around the agent, and how much of it they were around are all collected by public health workers and used to root out the cause of a disease (Rothman 2012). Once a suspected agent is identified, public health workers can partner with other aspects of government and other scientists to help control the disease in their community and prevent future issues.

How do public health officials control an infectious disease once it is in a particular community? Outside of molecular biology–related tools, many of the public health measures that we use today have been around a long time, including contact tracing to find all affected individuals, quarantining the affected individuals, and doing surveillance for any new cases (Rothman 2012). Genomic surveillance is also used to follow a disease outbreak, as was mentioned in Chapter 6 in the case of SARS-CoV-2. During the COVID-19 pandemic, scientists around the world started doing whole genome sequencing to look at different strains of the virus and posted that information on websites providing open access for all. Viral sequence information could also be linked to the patient information itself, such as if they suffered from mild or severe symptoms and if they recovered from the disease, among other information (Lo and Jamrozy 2020).

Although we are in the middle of the COVID-19 pandemic now, it is important to remember that there have been many public health success stories in the United States over the years. For example, cholera, a disease caused by a bacterial pathogen spread by contaminated drinking water, was a huge problem in the 1800s in the United States and around the world. For example, there were six cholera pandemics from 1817 to 1923. A physician in Great Britain, John Snow, is famously credited with finding the association between cholera and drinking water contaminated by human waste in the mid-1800s. Modern sanitation helped put an end to cholera epidemics in the United States and many parts of the world. However, millions of people are still affected by cholera in places where access to clean drinking water is disrupted or not available (Harris et al. 2012). Even malaria, a disease caused by mosquitoes carrying a protozoan pathogen associated with tropical areas, was once widespread in the United States, especially on the Gulf and East Coasts. A public health campaign after World War II was able to eliminate malaria from the United States (CDC 2022e). However, we know now that the heavy use of DDT in that project had a negative impact on the environment, especially bird populations (CDC 2022d).

Once a pathogen is discovered, epidemiologists can mobilize to characterize the pathogen and the disease it causes. As mentioned in Chapter 1, several major characteristics govern how pathogens spread, including route of entry, vector, virulence, and environmental conditions (Minkoff and Baker 2004). Epidemiologists keep track of the incidence of the disease, which involves recording the number of new cases. They would also determine the prevalence of the disease, that is, the total number of cases in a population (Minkoff and Baker 2004). For pathogens that can be spread from person to person, epidemiologists typically calculate a basic reproductive number, which is the average number of people who will become infected from one infected person. One can also calculate an effective reproductive number for the virus during a disease outbreak that can change over time. For example, using a public health measure like quarantining can lower this effective number. One can also follow the effective reproductive number as the number of vaccinated individuals increases, if a vaccine is made available (Rothman 2012; Christakis 2020).

As epidemiologists and other scientists gather data during a disease outbreak, they may begin to communicate recommended changes in public health measures to government officials. However, public health recommendations, such as mask wearing, can be confusing to the public if the recommendation changes, even slightly, over time. In addition, it takes a while to change culture, and mask wearing may not be readily adopted by the whole population from the start. Countries in East Asia that have had experience with SARS seemed to have adjusted their culture more quickly to COVID-19 public health measures like masks (Kwon 2020). However, more than two years into the pandemic, and millions of deaths later, somehow the message of mask wearing to prevent the spread of a respiratory virus has not been embraced by all.

One cannot discuss public health and viral pathogens without mentioning the concept of herd immunity. As mentioned in Chapter 1, herd immunity has to do with the number of people in the population who are not likely to get an infectious disease either through preexisting immunity or vaccination (Fine 1993; Piot et al. 2019). Conveying the importance of herd immunity is critical in any kind of disease outbreak when a vaccine campaign is necessary. Herd immunity flies in the face of the personal freedom argument against vaccination, in the sense that the decision to be vaccinated does not only affect one person, but also the quality of life of all individuals in your community, especially the very young and the immunocompromised who cannot be protected by a vaccine. Another way to put herd immunity is that it can break the "chain of infection" in diseases that are transmitted from one person to another, like a respiratory illness. Protection from herd immunity can start to be seen with as few as 40% of the population vaccinated, but for most infectious diseases, 80%–95% of people in the population would need to be vaccinated to see the benefits of herd immunity (Philadelphia 2022). As one can see from this typical high percentage vaccinated requirement, herd immunity requires all or almost all able adults and young adults to be vaccinated, almost like a call to service against a viral pathogen.

With all public health policy, good science communication is critical to explain the measures to the public and get their support for the measures. Researchers have pointed out that public policy makers, politicians, and state and local officials may have a different agenda than the scientists do. A scientist may have gotten into a particular area of research for love of the subject before it even became relevant to the public (as is the case with modified mRNAs and Dr. Karikó, as mentioned in Chapter 6). In addition, a public health crisis may affect the time in which the public expects scientists to react and come to the rescue with a new breakthrough (Kwon 2020). We will talk about the importance of science communication in Chapter 9.

Some public health goals, like supporting smoking cessation programs to help prevent lung cancer, are very straightforward in terms of the direct cause-and-effect relationship. Social and economic factors can also contribute to one's disease risk, even in the case of infectious disease. These risk factors are typically more indirectly correlated with the disease, nonmedical, and more challenging to address, especially for complex diseases. The challenges of the social determinants of health are described in the next section.

8.3 Explore Social Determinants of Health and How They Are Connected to Infectious Disease

Social determinants of health include all the factors in a person's environment that can affect his or her health. These factors include economic status, occupation, educational background, housing situation, access to healthcare providers and facilities, and other aspects of community such as support from friends and family (ODPHP 2022). The Office of Disease Prevention and Health Promotion, a part of the Department of Health and Human Services in the U.S. government, has launched the Healthy People 2030 initiative to reduce health disparities arising from differences in social environment. For example, disparities in access to healthy foods, good healthcare providers, clean water and air, and other factors can contribute to different health outcomes (ODPHP 2022). People of color are more likely to experience health inequities linked to differences in these social determinants (CDC 2022f).

During the COVID-19 pandemic, racial disparities in both cases and deaths have been seen. African Americans have higher rates of acquiring COVID-19 and dying from it than White Americans, relative to their representation in the population (Maness et al. 2021;

Price-Haywood et al. 2020; Mackey et al. 2021). However, this information needs to be put in the context of other variables like socioeconomic status to thoroughly study the major causes of these differences (Chowkwanyun and Reed 2020). One can also single out public health measures such as social distancing and see how factors like housing and occupation affect one's ability to follow this measure (Maness et al. 2021). The American Public Health Association has made health equity one of their priorities and is committed to removing barriers that allow health disparities to exist, making equal access to a healthy environment and healthcare resources a priority for all (APHA 2022).

8.4 Examine Major Global Public Health Issues Related to Infectious Disease

The world has faced other challenges from viral pathogens less than five years before COVID-19, most notably the Zika virus in 2016 and the Ebola virus from 2014 to 2016. Before the 2016 Olympic and Paralympic Games in Brazil, there was a concern that athletes would contract Zika virus during the games. Zika virus is a flavivirus (like West Nile virus) that is spread through mosquito bites but can be sexually transmitted by infected individuals. However, public health officials published a report indicating that for athletes from almost all the countries, the risk of contracting Zika virus was no greater than if they were traveling to a Zika-infected region (other countries in North and South America) for another reason. The researchers also cited evidence that fewer mosquitoes would be around during the winter months in Brazil (August) as well. However, the scientists did recommend taking precautions against getting mosquito bites and taking preventative measures to avoid sexual transmission even in the weeks after returning from the games. Nevertheless, pregnant women were advised not to attend due to the known risk of brain defects for the fetus (Grills et al. 2016). The recommended public health measures seemed to have worked, and no Zika cases were reported after the Olympics as of September 2016 (Tavernise 2016).

In 2014, an Ebola outbreak started in Guinea and spread to two neighboring West African countries of Sierra Leone and Liberia. Ebola causes a hemorrhagic fever and is spread by bodily fluids. Once the Ebola outbreak began to move into more populated areas, the WHO declared it a public health emergency of international concern (an alarm sounded before a pandemic), and scientists and physicians from around the world were mobilized to help in the fight against the virus. International efforts on the ground in these countries were able to stop the virus from spreading worldwide. These efforts included healthcare workers and public health support from other countries, and the implementation of public health measures like increasing awareness of how to handle Ebola patients as well as those who died from the disease. Aggressive contact tracing and quarantining also helped put a stop to the virus in 2016, although 11,325 people died (Zimmer 2011; CDC 2022b).

Scientists were met with a new challenge when the COVID-19 pandemic was declared in March 2020 (Christakis 2020). As described extensively in Chapter 6, that pandemic is ongoing at the time this book was written. In addition, the HIV/AIDS pandemic (Chapter 5) is also in progress. As described in other chapters, viral pathogens will continue to spill over into the human population in the future, and preparing for a pandemic needs to be an ongoing part of any global or national public health plan. Part of that planning may involve a vaccination campaign as described next.

8.5 Understand Vaccine Equity

Aside from working on improving public health on a day-to-day basis, public health officials may also be mobilized in a time of crisis to participate in and organize vaccination
campaigns. Such was the case in spring 2021 when the United States began a mass vaccination campaign against COVID-19. In planning such campaigns, public health officials
must work with community members, politicians, physicians, vaccine manufacturers, and
other stakeholders to plan and execute a vaccination campaign. One of the questions asked
when organizing a vaccination campaign is how to distribute a vaccine equitably in the
population. Given the public's concern already about health disparities in terms of healthcare access, it is critical to achieve buy-in from the public by establishing equitable access
for all.

The National Academies of Science in the U.S. formed a committee to create a model
for COVID-19 vaccine distribution that was released in fall 2020. A well-executed vaccination campaign was critical for the country and eventually the planet. Their report was
released in fall 2020 (National Academies of Sciences 2020). In their report, the committee
provided a vaccine distribution model rolled out in four phases, including certain groups
in each phase as priority populations for receiving the vaccine. Phase 1a included "high
risk" healthcare workers and first responders to keep the health system running. Phase
1b included older adults living in group housing situations like nursing homes as well as
people at very high risk for COVID-19 complications due to conditions like diabetes and
obesity. Phase 2 included teachers, essential workers, people at moderate risk of complications due to certain other health conditions, and people of all ages living in group housing
situations. Phase 3 included young adults, children, and other critical workers. Finally,
phase 4 included everyone else (National Academies of Sciences 2020). In these phases, not
only were age and medical conditions considered, but also circumstances like if a person
was an essential worker, addressing social determinants of health as well.

The recommendations of the National Academies committee were sent to the Advisory
Committee on Immunization Practices (ACIP). This committee is made of physicians, scientists, and public health officials appointed by the Department of Health and Human
Services secretary (CDC 2022c). The ACIP pretty closely followed the recommendations
from the committee. However, the federal government ended up leaving distribution plans
up to each state. Many states largely followed these phases, although some states shifted
members of certain professions like teachers to higher or lower phases, or prioritized vaccination of all seniors. However, unlike the National Academies report, children ended up
being the last to receive the vaccine, due to certain restrictions in the emergency use authorization of the available vaccines. Listings of state-by-state guidelines can be found online,
including through the Kaiser Family Foundation (KFF 2021). As mentioned in Chapter 6,
by late spring 2020, most adults in the United States were able to get the COVID-19 vaccine
because demand was not overwhelming in many areas.

Researchers have also turned their attention to how to distribute COVID-19 vaccine
equitably worldwide. A group of policy experts from institutions around the world developed a model known as the "Fair Priority Model," which includes a three-tiered ranking system for prioritizing vaccine distribution around the world (Emanuel et al. 2020).
The first priority of the model involves maximizing the avoidance of premature deaths,
using a calculation of "standard expected years of life lost" (SEYLL) to see how many
years would be saved with every vaccine dose. The second priority includes limiting

economic and social harm by giving vaccine to countries in which the vaccine would have the most impact in reducing poverty. Last, the third phase would include rapidly decreasing transmission rates by prioritizing countries with high transmission rates (Emanuel et al. 2020). In contrast, the WHO has put forward a strictly population-based distribution model for countries in their COVAX program based on their own advisory committee's plan. Countries then internally prioritize giving vaccine to healthcare workers, seniors, and adults with underlying health conditions putting them at risk for COVID-19 complications (WHO 2022). As of January 2022, the COVAX program has shipped approximately 975 million doses of vaccine to 144 countries (UNICEF 2022). As one can see, there is more than one way to come up with an equitable vaccine distribution plan, and there is ongoing discussion about the best way to distribute the COVID-19 vaccine. Fortunately, governments around the world have sought the advice of public health officials and other experts when developing distribution plans. These plans consider, at least to some extent, those individuals in a population most vulnerable to COVID-19 because of both medical reasons and social determinants of disease. However, one should point out that vaccine nationalism has not been completely eliminated, and the United States and other countries made sure that their citizens had access to vaccines, and even boosters, before some parts of the world even had access to the vaccine (Katz et al. 2021). Hopefully the United States can make a greater commitment to vaccine equity around the world by increasing its commitment to helping to bring the COVID-19 vaccine to everyone on the planet.

8.6 Conclusion

Any public health crisis, especially a pandemic, should force a society to look at how it supports the most vulnerable individuals in its population. Following the 1918 influenza pandemic, many countries, including Russia and Western European nations, began changing their healthcare infrastructure. Major changes were also seen after World War II with the establishment of the National Health Service in the United Kingdom and the World Health Organization through the United Nations (Spinney 2017). Calls for a robust universal healthcare safety net in the United States have increased since the start of the COVID-19 pandemic (Zakaria 2020). The COVID-19 pandemic has also forced our society to confront social and economic factors that contributed to one's chance of getting COVID-19 and even dying from the disease. The pandemic has shined a light on the need to improve health equity in the United States and around the world.

As I mentioned in the beginning of the chapter, one of the goals of public health is to increase life expectancy. Recently, *The New York Times* reported on the doubling of the average human life span from 1920 to 2020. The doubling was largely attributed to vaccines, antibiotics, and the acceptance of the idea that pathogens cause infectious disease (Johnson 2021). These key factors in the significant increase in life span depended on scientific innovation, advances in healthcare, robust public health systems, and the cooperation of the public. There have been many success stories mentioned in this book like the eradication of smallpox and the defeat of polio in the 20th century. Hopefully, communities around the world will find a way to end the COVID-19 pandemic, the HIV/AIDS pandemic, and other public health threats we face today, as well as plan for the next inevitable public health challenge.

8.7 Summary

Public health involves the health of entire populations, not specific individuals. The field of epidemiology involves the data collection and analysis needed to look at population-based trends in disease. In the case of infectious disease, data such as the number of new cases, the total number of cases relative to the total population, and the basic reproductive number of the pathogen are critical to following a disease outbreak. Public health measures can be implemented based on analysis of the transmission of the pathogen gathered from these data. Certain concepts like herd immunity depend on the understanding of how population-based efforts are critical in controlling infectious disease, rather than individual decision-making. Public health also involves the prevention of disease and finding ways to improve health, not just addressing existing health crises. There has been much interest in the public health community in examining social determinants of health and finding ways to improve health equity. Health equity was also considered with the recent distribution of COVID-19 vaccine in the United States. Public health encompasses many factors, and public health officials need to work together with their communities to continue to improve the health of the entire population.

Discussion Questions:

1. How would the response to a viral epidemic be different from the response to an opioid epidemic? How are both important to public health?
2. How would you define the moral obligation of an individual to participate in a public health initiative for the good of the population? What are your personal limits and how do you define them?
3. Why do you think the herd immunity threshold is so high for certain pathogens?
4. What do you think are the top three most important social determinants of health in the United States? In the world? Why?
5. In what order do you think these five individuals should be prioritized to receive a COVID-19 vaccine. Explain your ranking system.
   a. 20-year-old pharmacy technician
   b. 30-year-old lab technician who does COVID-19 PCR tests
   c. 50-year-old with preexisting health conditions who is working from home
   d. 75-year-old in good health
   e. 45-year-old smoker
6. Do you think the standard response to disease epidemics needs to change in your community? What about the response to a pandemic? Assess the public health response to SARS-CoV-2 on all levels, town, county, state, country, and world and comment.

References

APHA, American Public Health Association. 2022. "Health equity." Accessed 10 January 2022. www.apha.org/Topics-and-Issues/Health-Equity.

CDC, Centers for Disease Control and Prevention. 2022a. "10 essential public health services." *Health and Human Services*. Accessed 10 January 2022. www.cdc.gov/publichealthgateway/publichealthservices/essentialhealthservices.html.

———. 2022b. "2014–2016 Ebola outbreak in West Africa." *Health and Human Services*. Accessed 9 January 2022. www.cdc.gov/vhf/ebola/history/2014-2016-outbreak/index.html.

———. 2022c. "ACIP committee members." *Health and Human Services*. Accessed 10 January 2022. www.cdc.gov/vaccines/acip/members/index.html.

———. 2022d. "Dichlorodiphenyltrichloroethane (DDT) factsheet." *Health and Human Services*. Accessed 10 January 2022. www.cdc.gov/biomonitoring/DDT_FactSheet.html.

———. 2022e. "Elimination of malaria in the United States (1947–1951)." *Health and Human Services*. Accessed 10 January 2022. www.cdc.gov/malaria/about/history/elimination_us.html.

———. 2022f. "Racism and health." *Health and Human Services*. Accessed 10 January 2022. www.cdc.gov/healthequity/racism-disparities/index.html.

———. 2022g. "Research implications." *Health and Human Services*. Accessed 10 January 2022. www.cdc.gov/tuskegee/after.htm.

Chowkwanyun, M., and A.L. Reed. 2020. "Racial health disparities and Covid-19—caution and context." *New England Journal of Medicine* 383 (3):201–3. doi: 10.1056/NEJMp2012910.

Christakis, N.A. 2020. *Apollo's Arrow: The Profound and Enduring Impact of Coronavirus on the Way We Live*. 1st ed. New York, NY: Little, Brown Spark.

Dawson, A., and M. Verweij. 2007. *Ethics, Prevention, and Public Health*. Oxford, United Kingdom: Oxford University Press.

Dijkstra, A.M., and C. Cormick. 2020. "Research in science communication." In *Science Communication: An Introduction*, edited by A.M. Dijkstra, L. de Bakker, F. van Dam and E.A. Jensen, 223–51. Hackensack, NJ: World Scientific.

Emanuel, E.J., G. Persad, A. Kern, A. Buchanan, C. Fabre, D. Halliday, J. Heath, et al. 2020. "An ethical framework for global vaccine allocation." *Science* 369 (6509):1309–12. doi: 10.1126/science.abe2803.

Fine, P.E. 1993. "Herd immunity: History, theory, practice." *Epidemiologic Reviews* 15 (2):265–302. doi: 10.1093/oxfordjournals.epirev.a036121.

Franklin, S. 2019. "Ethical research—the long and bumpy road from shirked to shared." *Nature* 574 (7780):627–30. doi: 10.1038/d41586-019-03270-4.

Grills, A., S. Morrison, B. Nelson, J. Miniota, A. Watts, and M.S. Cetron. 2016. "Projected Zika virus importation and subsequent ongoing transmission after travel to the 2016 Olympic and Paralympic games—country-specific assessment, July 2016." *Morbidity and Mortality Weekly Report* 65 (28):711–5. doi: 10.15585/mmwr.mm6528e1.

Harris, J.B., R.C. LaRocque, F. Qadri, E.T. Ryan, and S.B. Calderwood. 2012. "Cholera." *The Lancet* 379 (9835):2466–76. doi: 10.1016/S0140-6736(12)60436-X.

Johnson, S. 2021. "How humanity gave itself an extra life." In *The New York Times*. New York, NY: The New York Times Company.

Katz, I.T., R. Weintraub, L.-G. Bekker, and A.M. Brandt. 2021. "From vaccine nationalism to vaccine equity—finding a path forward." *New England Journal of Medicine* 384 (14):1281–3. doi: 10.1056/NEJMp2103614.

KFF, Kaiser Family Foundation. 2021. "State COVID-19 vaccine priority populations." Accessed 10 January 2022. www.kff.org/other/state-indicator/state-covid-19-vaccine-priority-populations/?currentTimeframe=0&sortModel=%7B%22colId%22:%22Location%22,%22sort%22:%22asc%22%7D.

Kwon, D. 2020. "Science and policy collide during the pandemic." In *The Scientist*. Wilmington, DE: LabX Media Group.

Lo, S.W., and D. Jamrozy. 2020. "Genomics and epidemiological surveillance." *Nature Reviews Microbiology* 18 (9):478-. doi: 10.1038/s41579-020-0421-0.

Mackey, K., C.K. Ayers, K.K. Kondo, S. Saha, S.M. Advani, S. Young, H. Spencer, et al. 2021. "Racial and ethnic disparities in COVID-19-related infections, hospitalizations, and deaths: A systematic review." *Annals of Internal Medicine* 174 (3):362–73. doi: 10.7326/m20-6306.

Maness, S.B., L. Merrell, E.L. Thompson, S.B. Griner, N. Kline, and C. Wheldon. 2021. "Social determinants of health and health disparities: COVID-19 exposures and mortality among African American people in the United States." *Public Health Reports* 136 (1):18–22. doi: 10.1177/0033354920969169.

Minkoff, E.C., and P.J. Baker. 2004. "Chapter 17: New infectious threats." In *Biology Today: An Issues Approach*, 611–40. New York, NY: Garland Press.

National Academies of Sciences, E., and Medicine. 2020. *Framework for Equitable Allocation of COVID-19 Vaccine*. Washington, DC: The National Academies Press. https://www.nap.edu/read/25917/chapter/1.

ODPHP, Office of Disease Prevention and Health Promotion. 2022. "Social determinants of health." *Health and Human Services*. Accessed 10 January 2022. https://health.gov/healthypeople/objectives-and-data/social-determinants-health.

Philadelphia, College of Physicians of. 2022. "Herd immunity." Accessed 9 January 2022. www.historyofvaccines.org/content/herd-immunity-0.

Piot, P., H.J. Larson, K.L. O'Brien, J. N'kengasong, E. Ng, S. Sow, and B. Kampmann. 2019. "Immunization: Vital progress, unfinished agenda." *Nature* 575 (7781):119–29. doi: 10.1038/s41586-019-1656-7.

Price-Haywood, E.G., J. Burton, D. Fort, and L. Seoane. 2020. "Hospitalization and mortality among Black patients and White patients with Covid-19." *New England Journal of Medicine* 382 (26): 2534–43. doi: 10.1056/NEJMsa2011686.

Rothman, K.J. 2012. *Epidemiology: An Introduction*. 2nd ed. New York, NY: Oxford University Press.

Spinney, L. 2017. *Pale Rider: The Spanish Flu of 1918 and How it Changed the World*. New York, NY: PublicAffairs, Hachette Book Group, Perseus Books LLC.

Tavernise, S. 2016. "No Zika cases reported during Rio Olympics." In *The New York Times*. New York, NY: The New York Times Company.

UNICEF, United Nations Children's Fund. 2022. "COVID-19 vaccine market dashboard." Accessed 10 January 2022. www.unicef.org/supply/covid-19-vaccine-market-dashboard.

WHO, World Health Organization. 2022. "Access and allocation: How will there be fair and equitable allocation of limited supplies?" Accessed 10 January 2022. www.who.int/news-room/feature-stories/detail/access-and-allocation-how-will-there-be-fair-and-equitable-allocation-of-limited-supplies.

Zakaria, F. 2020. *Ten Lessons for a Post-pandemic World*. 1st ed. New York, NY: W.W. Norton and Company.

Zimmer, C. 2011. *A Planet of Viruses*. 2nd ed. Chicago, IL: University of Chicago Press.

9

Science Communication and Viruses

As we come to the end of the book, I hope that you have a much greater understanding of viruses than when you started. Once one understands how the world of viruses works, the next step is to promote dialogue between scientists and nonscientists on this topic through science communication. Communication among scientists, between scientists and the public, and among members of the public is critical for scientific knowledge to be able to benefit society. In this chapter, I will provide an overview of science communication from a historical perspective, as well as the current efforts within the scientific community to promote good science communication. I will then discuss how members of the public can be informed citizens when it comes to scientific discoveries and innovations, potentially how to filter through all the information that is available regarding scientific discoveries to find the most reliable sources of information.

Learning Outcomes:

9.1   Understand the Historical Relationship between Science and Society in the U.S. and around the World

9.2   Understand How Science Communication Should Work and in What Form

9.3   Discuss What the Responsibility of Scientists Is to Communicate Their Work

9.4   Discuss What the Responsibility of the Public Is Towards Scientific Issues

9.5   Understand How to Avoid Science Misinformation

9.6   Understand the Urgent Issues of Science Communication in Our Society Today

9.1 Understand the Historical Relationship between Science and Society in the U.S. and around the World

Almost 500 years since the start of the scientific revolution, tensions between scientists and the rest of society still exist. What causes these tensions and how can they be reduced? Historically, scientific explanations for how the world works may have run counter to traditional beliefs based in religious or other cultural ideas. Scientists are often seen as being a part of an insular community with no interest in explaining their complicated experiments to the rest of the public. When you think scientific revolution, you may think of Galileo because of his famous accomplishments and contributions to the scientific method that scientists still use today (Zanatta et al. 2017). However, scientists are participating in ongoing scientific revolutions as we speak. Many scientists cite the *Structure of Scientific Revolutions* by Thomas Kuhn as a work that crystallized how scientists work and new scientific advances emerge (Minkoff and Baker 2004). In this work, Kuhn uses the field of physical science as an example for how scientific

DOI: 10.1201/9781003172260-9

revolutions occur. This book was first published before the emergence of molecular biology as a new field as described in Chapter 1, which some might say is a more recent example of a scientific revolution. Kuhn discusses "normal science" as the way that scientists work on a day-to-day basis. Scientists operate within the boundaries of existing scientific understanding by testing theories and advancing fields within known parameters and using established methods (Kuhn 2012). When these approaches hit a snag where the findings cannot be explained using existing scientific knowledge and articulated theory, then a "paradigm shift" can occur. A paradigm involves an established way of looking at how something in the world works. The paradigm shift is radical, rejecting previous theories and replacing them, and more than just a procedural reinterpretation of data. New methods of experimentation may be used, and different groups of scientists may promote competing theories. When a scientific revolution finally occurs, it often involves many scientists coming to a resolution of the new paradigm over a period (Koster and Kupper 2020; Kuhn 2012). Thomas Kuhn refers to a scientist as being a "puzzle-solver" in conducting normal science (Kuhn 2012). Scientific training is unique in that it has been said that the student undergoes many "transformations of vision" before he or she is finally able to think and act like a scientist—a process which is rarely captured in undergraduate science textbooks (Kuhn 2012). Textbooks are written and rewritten after the revolution, when the community of scientists has agreed upon a set of theories and paradigms communicated through the primary literature, scientific conferences, and internal discussions.

The approach to scientific inquiry emphasizes the scientific method in which a hypothesis is proposed, data are gathered, and then the hypothesis is either supported or refuted. If a hypothesis is rejected, the scientist moves on to the next hypothesis to test. If supported, then other related hypotheses are tested, or the original hypothesis is generalized and tested again. After many hypotheses are tested and supported, one can begin to build a model for how something in the world works, which is molded into a theory. Scientists are trained to operate from a mindset that even well-established ideas could be improved upon and modified, leading to the labeling of even the most supported theories such as gravity and the cell as theories. The 20th-century philosopher Karl Popper popularized the emphasis on a hypothesis as being falsifiable (Minkoff and Baker 2004; Koster and Kupper 2020; Kuhn 2012). For experimental work, the hypothesis also must be carefully defined so it is testable using the investigational tools available to the scientist. Simplicity is key. It is also important to note that for biology in particular, the variability inherent in living systems means that the larger the sample size, the better in testing a hypothesis. In other words, it is impossible to control for all the conditions of a dynamic environment with living things, so studying many samples is the best way to go (Minkoff and Baker 2004).

We know that communication between scientists and the public is critical on many levels. There are economic impacts if scientific and technological advances cannot be fully deployed in a society. People need to understand the impact of science on their health and environment. In addition, from a positive point of view, scientists like Carl Sagan relished the beauty and wonder of science and wanted to share that with everyone around them (Planetary Science Division 2021).

9.2 Understand How Science Communication Should Work and in What Form

Communicating science can be challenging depending on the amount of technical knowledge required to understand the subject matter. Even among scientists, each specialized area of biology, chemistry, physics, or engineering has its own terminology or jargon that can create a barrier in communication. Scientists need to take great care to use simplified language without oversimplifying or talking down to the public. In addition to science, learning from experts in the fields of education, communication studies, political science and sociology, psychology, and other social sciences can be helpful in being an effective science communicator. The study of science communication is a growing field, and communicators are encouraging scientists to apply their knowledge of scientific methods like data collection to analyzing science communication itself (Dijkstra et al. 2020; Jamieson 2017).

The first key steps in effective science communication include identifying your audience and your communication goal (Dijkstra et al. 2020; Aines and Aines 2019). It is important to distinguish between "transmission-oriented activities," in which the goal is to provide information to a group of people, and "transaction-oriented activities," in which an information exchange and dialogue should take place between the speaker and the audience (Dijkstra et al. 2020). Others note the importance of multiple directions of communication with several interested parties (Akin and Scheufele 2017).

Scientists are encouraged to use caution when using persuasion as a goal with nonscientists. Although it is appropriate for a scientist to use persuasion when asking for grant funding or promoting his or her work professionally, this communication approach can backfire with the public. People can accept the expertise of the scientist, but also want the scientist to be honest, upfront about his or her intentions, and clear about sources of funding and the limitations of his or her work (Blastland et al. 2020; Nisbet and Scheufele 2009). Communicating uncertainty is also a challenge for scientists and may require training to explain to those outside of science who treat uncertainty in a different way (Jamieson 2017; Sciences 2014, 2018). Scientists need to make sure that the audience does not mistake expression of an uncertainty for an obscuring of the facts or a lack of confidence in a scientific finding.

Others, like Randy Olson, a tenured science professor who left that position to become a filmmaker, have emphasized training scientists to expressively discuss their work and open dialogue with the public using a storytelling model (Olson 2009). The actor Alan Alda developed a method using improvisation as a communication style to create a connection between the communicator and the audience. He also helped create the Alan Alda Center for Communicating Science at Stony Brook University to promote science communication training for scientists, as well as scholarship in this area. The Alda Center has collaborated with other institutions to help define communication skills, create more training opportunities in the community, and foster collaboration (Aurbach et al. 2019). Other scientists have advocated for reaching students in new ways, such as science comic books, and found that the use of a comic book textbook improved students' attitudes towards biology and helped improve their science literacy as well (Hosler and Boomer 2011).

Written science communication skills are critical as well. In her book, *Writing Science in Plain English*, Anne Greene notes that poor science writing is not only difficult to read, but also can slow scientific progress if other scientists cannot understand your work. Greene also advocates for a storytelling model, with a focus on characters and actions in the writing. Furthermore, Greene recommends using a formatting style on the sentence level, the paragraph level, and eventually the entire document fostering a science communication style consistent with how humans prefer to gather information in a written format (Greene 2013).

One other area where science communication is different from other fields is in the revision of a theory and the self-correcting that takes place within the scientific community. Other research communities do not necessarily follow the same practice or way of speaking about the iterative nature of scientific research, and this can be an area quite prone to being misunderstood (Sciences 2018). In addition, when a scientific paper is retracted, there has been a tendency in the media to create a hook for the story involving the "science is broken" angle (Hilgard and Jamieson 2017). This particular communication approach is problematic for scientists in that it distorts the frequency of mistakes or misconduct in science. It emphasizes the negative side of finding the error versus the positive self-correction that has taken place. Scientists can emphasize how rare such incidents are given the number of scientific papers published in any given year, and then focus on the ongoing nature of the scientific process.

9.2.1 How Are New Forms of Communication, Including Social Media, Affecting Science Communication?

Journalists are critical to informing the public and helping convey the importance of a scientific breakthrough. Although they are not generating scientific data, they are providing an interpretation and framing of the science that is also important for policymaking. Scientists need to work with journalists (Sciences 2014). However, at certain times, the role of the science journalist has changed in society, from celebrating and lauding breakthroughs to helping keep scientists accountable (Dijkstra et al. 2020; Rensberger 2009). Nevertheless, according to the National Association of Science Writers (NASW), the most important source for scientific information for the American public is the media (Blum and Knudson 1997). The definition of media has expanded in recent years—it includes traditional forms of mass media like TV, radio, newspapers, movies, science magazines, and books, but now also other sources such as blogs, podcasts, and social media. Social media has become a critical medium for communication on any issue. Researchers have noted that people are moving away from traditional media to primarily content available in an online environment—a modality rife for misinformation. People are not picking up the daily newspaper to read a featured science article anymore; they are typing questions into search engines leading them to online content (Sciences 2014; Jamieson 2017; Schafer 2017; Brossard and Scheufele 2013; Fleischman and Szalinski 2014). Little is known about the impact of the delivery of science content in this matter. In addition, the context in which a story is read, including input from other readers in a social media environment, may influence a person's opinion on a topic (Brossard and Scheufele 2013). People are also consuming more than one type of media at the same time, such as watching TV and using Twitter (Sciences 2014).

Social media has opened science communication to anyone who wants to set up a Facebook page. In 2019, scientists evaluated the number of Facebook pages devoted to anti-vaccine information versus pro-vaccine information. After labeling pages as for or against vaccines based on their content, the researchers found that there were more pages devoted to anti-vaccine information than pro-vaccine information. The authors indicated that the anti-vaccine pages also had more connections to non-vaccine related pages. However, the pro-vaccine pages, although smaller in number, still had more followers overall (Johnson et al. 2020; Wadman 2020). This is just one example, but it shows how science communication networks can be built in so many ways and in some cases with little or no connection to the scientific community.

What strategies have the U.S.-based and global science agencies and nongovernmental organizations (NGOs) taken to science communication in an online environment? Both the Centers for Disease Control and Prevention (CDC) and World Health Organization (WHO) have an active presence on Facebook and other forms of social media. Major scientific journals such as *Science* and *Nature* have daily briefings, podcasts, and a significant web presence in addition to the journals themselves. Scientists will have to continue to evolve to meet the public where they get their news information.

9.3 Discuss What the Responsibility of Scientists Is to Communicate Their Work

Scientists who mainly work as researchers have an obligation to publish their findings in peer-reviewed scientific journals. With many journals creating an "open access" format or at least an open access option, research reports will potentially be available to an even wider audience than before open publishing. Having fellow scientists evaluate your work and then publishing it is usually the standard way to report new scientific discoveries. However, scientists are often not under any kind of obligation to explain the work and its significance in nontechnical language to an audience outside of their own research community. There is no requirement for engagement with the public. If the research findings represent a new breakthrough directly affecting public health, scientists can work with the communication office or public relations group affiliated with their institution to translate the work for a broader audience. Many science communication researchers and enthusiasts believe that we also need to motivate scientists to become better communicators, perhaps through changing tenure requirements or other ways to incentivize the communication step as part of the job of a working scientist (Sciences 2018). It also cannot be ignored that focusing on communicating science to the public rather than exclusively on scientific research and publication has been looked down upon in academia (Yeo and Brossard 2017). The public wants to feel like they can trust scientists, and scientists need to be aware that their expertise alone is not enough for effective communication (Sciences 2018; Fiske and Dupree 2014).

When scientists write grant proposals for funding using public tax dollars, a broader impacts section is usually required in the application, obligating the scientist to explain, even in the proposal form, why the study is critical for society. Increasingly, scientists at major medical centers are encouraged to do what is known as translational research, where the conversion or path of the scientific knowledge into treatments for disease can more readily occur. The public wants to learn more about scientific innovation, and scientists are encouraged to do so on many levels. However, it is important to note that basic research, research conducted just to understand how a living system works, should be encouraged as well so that a pipeline of translational research foundation work is available many years in the future.

Scientists can also foster scientific communication by engaging in interdisciplinary work with other scientists or even nonscientists to help them adapt to explaining their plans and discoveries to an audience outside of their laboratory. Increasingly, scientists are also called upon to make their work more accessible to others, including marginalized members of the community. A new area of research, inclusive science communication, is taking shape. Researchers working in this area seek acknowledgement of the historic exclusion of marginalized groups from science communication, a problem beginning with the biases, whether explicit or implicit, with the science communicators themselves. Future efforts in science communication can become more inclusive and thus more effective, if as many kinds of people from multiple perspectives as possible are a part of formal and informal science communication (Canfield et al. 2020). From my perspective as a woman, feeling included in the community of cell and molecular biologists did not come easily and is not to be underestimated as an important step in science communication. In addition, some scientists are of the opinion that there are major limitations in science communication that have come with making English the "international language of science." Scientific information and dialogue would be more accessible to non-English speakers if major scientific journals translated their work into other languages, more science journalism was conducted in languages besides English, and scientists tried to reach out to wider audiences to help bring scientific information to members of the public speaking languages besides English (Márquez and Porras 2020).

Major scientific societies also release position statements as new discoveries with broader ethical or societal implications emerge. These same scientific societies are also quite active in promoting science communication. The American Association for the Advancement of Science (AAAS) established the Center for Public Engagement with Science and Technology to provide resources for scientists to promote effective communication. The American Society for Microbiology has an advocacy page for scientists and provides scientific topic information that can be searched based on audience, ranging from clinical scientists to undergraduate students to policy makers.

When a groundbreaking, paradigm-shifting discovery is made, should scientists call for a conference to discuss the impact of the new discovery on society? This happened in 1975 when the International Congress on Recombinant DNA Molecules, a group of molecular biologists, met to discuss the implications of recombinant DNA technology at the Asilomar Conference Center in Pacific Grove, California (often shortened to Asilomar meeting) (Figure 9.1). I should note that this conference was technically Asilomar II, since Paul Berg had organized an earlier smaller conference on the topic at the same location in 1973 (Mukherjee 2016). Researchers had actually stopped their research to consider the implications of their work. The conference attendees ended up narrowing their focus to the immediate issue of safety of using recombinant DNA, including how it should be contained in various situations. At the time, the commercial applications of recombinant DNA were not yet explored although assumed to be numerous (Berg et al. 1975). For many years after the Asilomar conference, no public health issues were linked to the millions of research experiments performed using recombinant DNA technology since the conference (Berg 2008; Berg and Singer 1995).

Twenty-five years after the original conference, a small group of scientists, some from the original Asilomar meeting, met to discuss the value of the "Asilomar process" in which scientists self-reflect on the implications of their work beyond science into society. Although the group deemed the process valuable, many wondered if the public needed to play a bigger role in the process (Barinaga 2000; Davatelis 2000). In addition, safety concerns have been raised regarding advanced applications using recombinant DNA technology such as gene therapy and gene editing. Modification of a human pathogen, the influenza virus, has raised concerns related to bioterrorism (Falkow 2012; Editorials 2015).

Some of the same organizers of the 1975 Asilomar meeting did participate in the 2015 Innovative Genomics Initiative Forum on Bioethics held in Napa, California. They met to discuss the germline modification of organisms, considering the new CRISPR gene-editing tool making such genomic modifications easier to execute. Germline modifications involve genetic changes that are passed onto the next generation, not just an altering of the adult or somatic cells of the body to correct a disease. This group of scientists made a statement discouraging germline modification of the human genome and called for the establishment of bioethical discussion including scientists and nonscientists. They also called

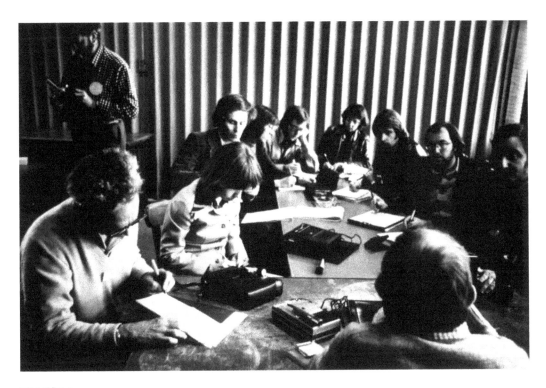

FIGURE 9.1
The Asilomar process.

Photo of Sydney Brenner (lower right corner) talking to the press. Dr. Brenner was an attendee and one of the organizers of the Asilomar Conference.

The original image can be found at https://collections.nlm.nih.gov/catalog/nlm:nlmuid-101441124-img. The image is in the public domain according to U.S. National Library of Medicine.

for more research on the applications of CRISPR-Cas9 technology. Finally, they called for a meeting of international scientists, policy makers, and other leaders in the field to discuss this issue (Baltimore et al. 2015). The International Summit on Human Gene Editing was held the same year, and the group concluded that the needed safety precautions were not yet in place to do germline human gene editing safely. They recommended that a standing international group or committee be created to reexamine gene editing when more research data became available (National Academies of Sciences and Medicine 2015). In the future, can our national and international institutions build more of a framework to accommodate policy dialogue on rapidly emerging technologies? We need to consider as a society how to formalize public engagement with scientists.

Other scientists have organized advocacy groups such as the Union of Concerned Scientists. The Union of Concerned Scientists, founded by scientists at MIT during the Vietnam War, aims to inform the public about scientific issues related to environmental and society, as well as advocating for causes, also calling for less of an emphasis on military innovation among scientists (Scientists 2021).

Recently, a group of scientists and policy makers have come together to develop a rating system to be used to evaluate scientific evidence that is relevant to public policy. The system is called the Theoretical, Empirical, Applicable and Replicable Impact (THEARI) rating system (Kwon 2020; Ruggeri et al. 2020). The rating system is actually laid out in the name, with the first of five levels being when a scientific idea is only theoretical and may be an opinion up to the fifth level where the impact of a scientific idea has clearly been measured and evaluated in detail by multiple scientists. The hope was this rating system could be applied to many scientific disciplines so that misinformation is not perpetuated in the media or in other forms of communication with the public. Given the speed of the release of new scientific information in times of crisis like the COVID-19 pandemic, if people pause to evaluate the information using the rating system, or to examine the rating level designated by scientists themselves, it could help filter out scientific information not based on rigorous scientific examination. The researchers who created the THEARI system have also noted the potential impact of the Foundations for Evidence-Based Policymaking Act of 2018 on evaluation of scientific information in the future (Congress 2017). In this new law, federal agencies will be required to collect data and evaluate it to inform their policies. Protections for privacy, at the same time as making data available for research purposes, are a part of the law as well. This new evidence-based policy evaluation law will affect many areas of the government, not just science policy. Having a method in place to separate out evidence rooted in scientific data from anecdotes and opinion will be critical for this law to be effective.

To conclude this section, I would like to focus on one scientist who is widely seen as an effective science communicator: Anthony Fauci, M.D., director of the National Institute of Allergy and Infectious Disease (NIAID) that is a part of the National Institutes of Health (NIH). Dr. Fauci comes to mind as an example of a scientist who is quite willing to speak to the public and provide recommendations, without judging those who do not take his advice. Having been an infectious disease expert for over 30 years, Dr. Fauci has interacted with advocacy groups as well as the public on a regular basis regarding several infectious disease crises, even before the COVID-19 pandemic. Recently, the initially contentious but eventually friendly relationship between Dr. Fauci and Larry Kramer, who organized the ACT UP group of AIDS activists and the Gay Men's Health Crisis, was put in the spotlight after Kramer died in 2020. Tensions arose between the two men in the 1980s over the distribution of the AIDS drug, AZT. However, they eventually came to a truce and were able to move forward together on this issue. Dr. Fauci indicated in a PBS NewsHour interview upon Kramer's death in 2020 that Kramer changed the relationship between those who have a disease and those who are working to treat it or cure it (NewsHour 2020; McNeil Jr. 2020).

9.4 Discuss What the Responsibility of the Public Is Towards Scientific Issues

When I teach a science course for nonscience majors, my major goal of the course is to help the students understand scientific topics that are relevant or will become relevant to their everyday lives, including health, economic, and government policy-related issues. I hope that when they finish the course, they will have the tools to translate scientific information so that it can be useful in personal decision-making in the future. Fortunately, my institution requires at least one science course for all college of arts and science students. However, many Americans have had limited basic coursework in the sciences even on the K-12 level. So, after schooling is complete, how can one learn more about science and continue to keep up with scientific innovations? People must turn again to the media and their personal networks, including their physician, family, and friends, to understand new scientific discoveries. For those who become science enthusiasts, they can use social media to become active in the "citizen science" movement, in which members of the public contribute data to large-scale scientific projects, including bird counts and other types of biodiversity-related projects, among others (Land-Zandstra, De Bakker, and Jensen 2020). While science literacy is important, other science communicators note the importance of teaching the public to be able to recognize reliable scientific information or seek out experts to help them with the science, rather than taking on the task of learning all the science themselves (Jamieson 2017). A model of science literacy is emerging now that not only requires scientific knowledge itself, but also competence in interpreting media, in particular digital media, to avoid misinformation, coupled with an awareness of how people are influenced by their emotions and other factors when making decisions, not just facts. Science journalists could also benefit from all three of these skills in their training (Howell and Brossard 2021).

9.4.1 What Is the Perception of the Value of Science and Scientists in the Public Domain?

Even when a scientist presents scientific evidence to the public, it may not be accepted by the public and instead criticized, even sometimes with the public questioning the expertise of the scientist (Kahan 2015, 2017a). What is behind the mistrust of scientific expertise? The Pew Research Center published their findings of a survey conducted just before the COVID-19 crisis became a pandemic, from October 2019 to March 2020. In this survey, adults in 20 countries were asked their opinions about trust in institutions, including the scientific community and the media, as well as their opinion on several specific scientific issues (Pew 2020). The survey found that most adults have "some trust in scientists to do what is right," but public trust did depend on personal politics and level of education. Shown in Figure 9.2, one can see public trust in key institutions, with 56% of adults in the United States having a high trust in the military, but only 38% of adults having a high trust in scientists. In the U.S. and other countries, those adults identifying on the "left" politically had a greater trust in scientists than did those on the "right" (Figure 9.3). In addition, those individuals with more education were more likely to trust scientists. Many people valued the opinion of those with "practical experience" in solving problems over those labeled as experts. Interestingly, even though most adults labeled the news media as doing a "good job" on science coverage, most people surveyed are of the opinion that the public does not have enough foundational scientific knowledge to grasp fully what was being covered in the media (Pew 2020). Other organizations, such as the nonprofit ScienceCounts, have conducted surveys in the United States with similar results indicating that most people trust scientists. ScienceCounts also notes that people are hopeful about the future of science (ScienceCounts 2015, 2017).

The need to make science "more relatable" was one of the major takeaways from the 3M Company's Annual State of Science Index Survey conducted in 2019 surveying adults internationally. To help scientists meet this need, 3M created a "Scientists as storytellers guide" featuring advice on how to tell an engaging story about one's research and how to find a way to capture the audience's attention (3M 2019). 3M conducted the survey in two segments in 2020, one before and one after the COVID-19 pandemic started. The COVID-19 pandemic did have an impact on the survey results, according to 3M. Although most people surveyed in 2020 said they rarely think about the impact of science on their daily lives, there was a decrease in skepticism towards science expressed by survey participants after the pandemic began relative to before the pandemic (3M 2021).

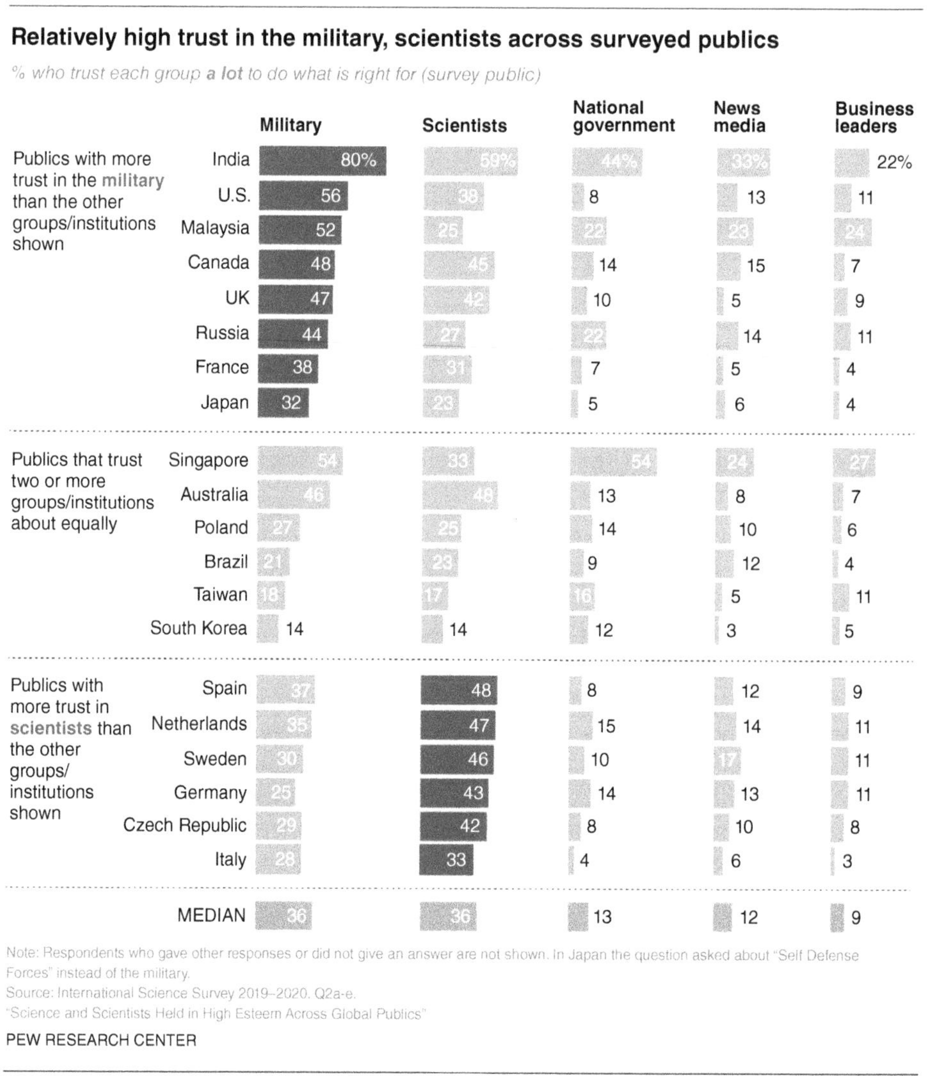

Viruses and Society

Relatively high trust in the military, scientists across surveyed publics

*% who trust each group **a lot** to do what is right for (survey public)*

		Military	Scientists	National government	News media	Business leaders
Publics with more trust in the military than the other groups/institutions shown	India	80%	59%	44%	33%	22%
	U.S.	56	38	8	13	11
	Malaysia	52	25	22	23	24
	Canada	48	45	14	15	7
	UK	47	42	10	5	9
	Russia	44	27	22	14	11
	France	38	31	7	5	4
	Japan	32	23	5	6	4
Publics that trust two or more groups/institutions about equally	Singapore	54	33	54	24	27
	Australia	46	48	13	8	7
	Poland	27	25	14	10	6
	Brazil	21	23	9	12	4
	Taiwan	18	17	16	5	11
	South Korea	14	14	12	3	5
Publics with more trust in scientists than the other groups/institutions shown	Spain	37	48	8	12	9
	Netherlands	35	47	15	14	11
	Sweden	30	46	10	17	11
	Germany	25	43	14	13	11
	Czech Republic	29	42	8	10	8
	Italy	28	33	4	6	3
	MEDIAN	36	36	13	12	9

Note: Respondents who gave other responses or did not give an answer are not shown. In Japan the question asked about "Self Defense Forces" instead of the military.
Source: International Science Survey 2019–2020. Q2a-e.
"Science and Scientists Held in High Esteem Across Global Publics"

PEW RESEARCH CENTER

FIGURE 9.2
Public trust in groups and institutions.

Shown here are the results of a Pew Research Center survey looking at public trust in institutions such as scientists and the military in 20 countries. Percent who trust each particular group a lot were reported for each country, and then percents were grouped based on whether the military is trusted more than other groups, two or more groups are trusted equally, or there is more trust in scientists as a group in than other institutions.

Source: Pew Research Center (Washington, DC), Sept. 2020, "Science and Scientists Held in High Esteem across Global Publics," www.pewresearch.org/science/2020/09/29/science-and-scientists-held-in-high-esteem-across-global-publics/, see "Complete Report PDF" on webpage.
"Pew Research Center bears no responsibility for the analyses or interpretations of the data presented here. The opinions expressed herein, including any implications for policy, are those of the author and not of Pew Research Center" (www.pewresearch.org/about/terms-and-conditions/).

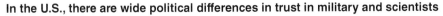

In the U.S., there are wide political differences in trust in military and scientists

% of U.S. adults who trust each group___ to do what is right for the United States

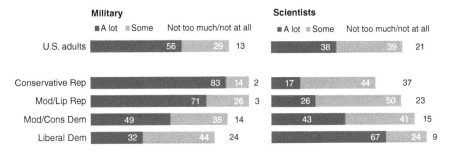

FIGURE 9.3
In the United States, public trust in certain groups/institutions varies depending on one's political affiliation.

Shown in this figure are the results of a Pew Research Center survey asking U.S. adults if they trust the military and scientists to do what is right for the United States. The percent responding "a lot," "some," or "not too much/not at all" are shown, along with the breakdown of these results taking into account the person's political affiliation, if stated.

Source: Pew Research Center (Washington, DC), Sept. 2020, "Science and Scientists Held in High Esteem across Global Publics," www.pewresearch.org/science/2020/09/29/science-and-scientists-held-in-high-esteem-across-global-publics/. see "Complete Report PDF" on webpage.
"Pew Research Center bears no responsibility for the analyses or interpretations of the data presented here. The opinions expressed herein, including any implications for policy, are those of the author and not of Pew Research Center" (www.pewresearch.org/about/terms-and-conditions/).

Based on national and international survey data, one's personal level of science education does play a role in trust of scientists. These survey data seem to fit with a model known as the "deficit model of science communication," which indicates that the more knowledge or awareness that a person has of a scientific topic, the more willing that person will be to accept and support the science. However, many science communication researchers have found that greater acceptance and support of science does not always come with knowledge, and even the opposite can be the case as well, depending on the issue (Akin and Scheufele 2017; Dijkstra et al. 2020; Nisbet and Scheufele 2009; Scheufele 2013).

Science communication researchers have advocated for a focus moving beyond science literacy to careful consideration of how an issue is framed in a science policy discussion, meaning how one organizes an argument and ideas for a particular audience (Nisbet and Scheufele 2009; Druckman and Lupia 2017; Vaidyanathan 2020). Framing involves finding new ways to state why an issue is important to the public, taking into account what different groups of people consider to be important. Examples of ways of framing a scientific issue include helping a society advance and improve lives through a scientific achievement, increasing economic progress, appealing to one's morality and ethics, holding political figures accountable for their actions, and preventing the opening of a "Pandora's box" (Nisbet 2009). Frames can be tailored to the particular values of the audience. Scientific issues can often be framed in more than way, with varying decreases of successful transmission to the public.

Scientists need to choose how to present their research findings, in what order to present, and how to keep the information short enough not to lose the audience's attention to something else, especially a competing frame for the information. Politicized scientific issues are quite challenging to frame, and researchers have found that if there is a scientific consensus on an issue, that can be an effective frame for the topic. Timing is critical, however, with the scientific consensus statement needing to be communicated before the politicized framing of the issue muddies the waters (Druckman and Lupia 2017). This is sometimes called providing "inoculative information" in anticipation of a highly politicized issue (Stroud 2017). In addition, scientists are encouraged to meet people where they are in terms of sources of media, in particular social media. Effective science communication also means using scientific data analysis itself to the see if the communication is working (Nisbet and Scheufele 2009). Other communication researchers are working on understanding how social influence contributes to changing behaviors. For example, someone they like or who is seen as an authority figure, as well as the perception that others around them are following the same path (Sciences 2014; Vaidyanathan 2020; Contractor and DeChurch 2014), influences people.

9.4.2 Skepticism versus Mistrust in Science

Skepticism is often fueled by mistrust in science within a community. Even major scientific discoveries might still be mistrusted by groups within a community. When interacting with the public, scientists may meet skepticism if they are seen as being susceptible to external influences such as political or economic factors. A scientist may think he or she is simply transmitting knowledge, but his or her motives may be questioned if scientists are perceived to be nonobjective by the audience (Koster and Kupper 2020). Not all scientific ideas or issues are equally embraced or rejected because of skepticism by the public. Certain ideas can become "wicked problems" if the idea taps into an area with many opposing viewpoints within the society, such as how to end a pandemic, at the same time being a high-stake evolving topic that urgently needs to be addressed by a society (Verhoeff and Kupper 2020). Wicked problems also may not have one straightforward solution and involve such new science that scientists cannot provide all the answers, and ethicists are pushed to limit of what can be debated and studied within existing societal frameworks (Akin and Landrum 2017).

Skepticism can give way to outright rejection of a scientific concept. Sean Carroll has laid out what he describes as the "denialism playbook," which includes the major steps used by a small group to lead to the rejection of scientific concepts like vaccination or evolution. He notes steps such as starting by questioning the science, and then turning on scientists themselves by emphasizing any small disagreements they may have about the details of the discovery while questioning their motivation. The next steps include emphasizing harm from accepting the scientific concept and then falling back on personal freedom claims before ultimately rejecting the idea (Carroll 2020).

Others have expressed the importance of identifying pseudoscience, which can affect the acceptance of a true scientific idea as well. As described by Atul Gawande in a recent National Academy report, selectively highlighting pieces of data and relying on so-called experts without scientific credentials are some characteristics of those who push pseudoscience. Attempting to counter pseudoscience can backfire for scientists, and it is recommended to lead with facts rather than taking on the pseudoscience directly point for point (Sciences 2018).

9.5 Understand How to Avoid Science Misinformation

Dealing with misinformation can be challenging for scientists. Many scientists feel the urge to call it out when scientific misinformation is put on the same playing field as scientifically supported data in places like social media. Scientists like Neil DeGrasse Tyson, who stated in a tweet, "The good thing about science is that it's true whether or not you believe in it," articulate this reaction (Tyson 2013).

Some science communicators promote the idea of "prebunking," in which the audience is warned of possible sources of misinformation and how to anticipate it (Blastland et al. 2020). Some researchers even developed an online game in which the user can play the role of a producer of fake news, using common techniques to spread misinformation as a part of the game. The game is meant to prepare the user for encounters with misinformation in the real world, and it seems to work according to the researchers (Roozenbeek and van der Linden 2019).

Misinformation emerges along with emerging viruses, such as in the case of the Zika outbreak in 2016. One conspiracy theory arose stating that the microcephaly occurring in newborns was not because of Zika infection during the mother's pregnancy (as supported by peer-reviewed research studies), but instead somehow caused by the genetically modified mosquitoes being used in Brazil at the time to control malaria (Jamieson 2017). One famous instance in which misinformation was perpetuated was the erroneous connection reported between the measles, mumps, and rubella (MMR) vaccine and autism in the 1990s. The initial report, made by Dr. Andrew Wakefield in 1998, was retracted from *Lancet*, and Dr. Wakefield lost his British medical license when it was found that he lied about his results and hundreds of studies failed to show any connection at all (Chan, Jones, and Albarracin 2017). He is reported to have moved to the United States to work on anti-vaccine initiatives (Smith 2017). It can be quite difficult to root out such misinformation, especially when it is repeated in the media and by parents looking for a cause of their child's autism (Li, Stroud, and Jamieson 2017). However, the arguments against vaccination are predictable and pretty well defined but have now been taken up by a group of "influencers" active in social media (Smith 2017). As has been said in many places, vaccines are victims of their own success. Most people have never seen a child with measles, nor have their physicians (Smith 2017; Sciences 2018). If people do not have a good basis to evaluate the harm of children not being vaccinated, this leads some people to incorrectly reason that somehow not being vaccinated is better for their children.

9.6 Understand the Urgent Issues of Science Communication in Our Society Today

9.6.1 Science Communication Issue: Vaccine Hesitancy

Hesitancy to receive a vaccine is a heavily studied area of science communication research. As reported in the news, an anti-vaccination movement in the United States has been present for years. The movement is linked to many societal factors, including the changing nature of the physician-patient relationship, the prevalence of anti-vaccination groups online and in communities influencing parents, as well as the misinterpretation of the risk associated with childhood vaccines due to faulty science communication (Hoffman 2019).

Communication researchers also look to public health officials to encourage them "to protect the vaccine science communication environment" (Kahan 2017b). Despite vocal groups expressing their concerns about childhood vaccines, a 2019–2020 Pew Research Center survey indicated that most adults in 19 of 20 countries see a "high preventative health benefit" from childhood vaccination. However, there is variability in assessment of the risk of side effects in those same countries. Among adults surveyed in the U.S., only 60% indicated that there would be low or no risk of side effects to childhood vaccines (Pew 2020). Nevertheless, in a March 2019 article summarizing parental opinion on childhood vaccines, 82% of U.S. parents surveyed indicated that the MMR vaccination should be required to attend public school (Villa 2019).

Looking beyond parental opinion to parental actions, parents in the United States are vaccinating their children against measles. It should be more widely known that childhood vaccination rates in the United States are consistently high (Kahan 2017b). According to the CDC, as of 2017, 91.5% of children aged 19–35 months have been vaccinated against measles via the MMR vaccine (CDC 2021b). This seems like a high percentage, but measles has a high herd immunity threshold, requiring 92%–95% of the population to be fully vaccinated according to reliable sources (Piot et al. 2019; Strebel et al. 2017). However, data analysis and mathematical modeling in the past have also resulted in estimates ranging from 70% to 96%, depending on the assumptions of the model or analysis (Fine 1993). Nevertheless, there are small clusters of people in several regions of the United States where the vaccination rate is low, and this issue does need to be addressed. Researchers have found geographic clusters of unvaccinated or undervaccinated children in Northern California, for example (Lieu et al. 2015). People in those clusters would be more susceptible to outbreaks of measles and other childhood diseases, typically with the initiation of the outbreak through an individual infected in another country. In fact, geographic clusters with un- or undervaccinated children have been linked to increased measles outbreaks in the United States. The highest number of measles cases in the United States since 1992 were reported from January to October 2019, with two outbreaks occurring in New York State (Patel et al. 2019). In 2000, the World Health Organization declared that measles was eliminated in the United States, and the United States would like to maintain this status (CDC 2021c). Major U.S. outbreaks like those reported recently do threaten this status, and four European countries (United Kingdom, Greece, Albania, and the Czech Republic) have recently lost their measles elimination status (Piot et al. 2019).

Despite these localized outbreaks, we must keep in mind that most of the population is protected by herd immunity because of widespread compliance with vaccination. Vaccinating one's children therefore protects other people's children too and any others in the population who cannot get vaccinated (Kahan 2017b). This contribution to society should be noted and valued. In the case of mass vaccination campaigns against emerging viruses such as against SARS-CoV-2, everyone who is vaccinated is making a great contribution to society to quell a pandemic.

Science communication researchers have found that it is critical for scientists to consider "cultural cognition" when communicating about the benefits and risks of an innovation such as a new vaccine. Nonscience-related cultural factors in a community could have a huge impact on the assessment of risk and need to be anticipated and addressed through science communication research (Kahan, Jenkins-Smith, and Braman 2011; Kahan and Landrum 2017). A big communication misstep occurred in the United States with the initial rollout of the human papilloma virus (HPV) vaccine Gardasil by Merck (Kahan and Landrum 2017; Kahan 2013). The FDA fast-tracked approval of the vaccine for early adolescent girls specifically, due to the serious risk of cervical cancer for women, and this decision ended up being politicized. Certain groups focused in on HPV being sexually transmitted and what vaccination would mean in terms of potentially promoting sexual activity in girls. In contrast, a vaccine for a different sexually transmitted disease, Hepatitis B, did not receive the same political challenges. Science communication researchers have described the failure of the health benefits of the HPV vaccine from being effectively communicated to parents as due to a "polluted science communication environment." Other factors, such as Merck's approach to advocating for legislation to mandate the vaccine, also contributed to the science communication lapse (Kahan 2013; Kahan and Landrum 2017). One cannot underestimate the power of certain cultural factors in affecting the public's assessment of a valuable medical tool that could save so many lives down the road. Presentation of scientific facts is not enough to get the public's acceptance.

Many researchers are actively studying the best ways to counteract vaccine hesitancy for childhood vaccination through specific kinds of messaging. The major myths surrounding vaccine hesitancy, such as fears of certain vaccine components or potential side effects, have been debunked (Geoghegan, O'Callaghan, and Offit 2020). Surprisingly, researchers found in some studies that choosing a message to promote awareness of the science facts behind a vaccine could backfire with people who are very concerned about the vaccine, leading to fewer people choosing vaccination for their children or themselves. Science communication researchers also encourage collaboration with healthcare professionals to gather data on what messaging works (Sciences 2018; Nyhan and Reifler 2015; Nyhan et al. 2014). Some researchers have found positive results in changing vaccination attitudes by focusing on the avoidance of disease by vaccination, rather than in correcting the mistaken link to autism (Horne et al. 2015). More data also needs to be gathered on all the possible reasons behind lack of vaccination, not just misinformation (Sciences 2018). A survey of the vaccine hesitancy literature from 2007 to 2013 indicated that multipronged approaches including science literacy, engaging community leaders, and addressing vaccine access and convenience all have a positive impact on vaccination (Jarrett et al. 2015). Scientists also must consider and address vaccine hesitancy among any healthcare providers (Paterson et al. 2016).

In 2014, officials in the United States decided to look at the health and economic impacts of a 20-year campaign called the Vaccines for Children (VFC) program (Figure 9.4). Astoundingly high numbers of illnesses, hospitalizations, and deaths were prevented in the United States because of this program. For example, over 700,000 deaths and over 300 million illnesses were prevented, not to mention over a trillion dollars in costs (Cohn et al. 2017; CDC 2021a). Scientists must keep in mind that the stakes are high, and we need to pay attention to how we communicate our work. In his book *Don't Be Such a Scientist*, Randy Olson points out that if we do not pay attention to how we communicate, we risk being "drowned out by either the new anti-science movement or just the cacophony of society's noise" (Olson 2009, page 8).

9.6.2 Science Communication Issue: Emerging/Spillover Viruses

One thing that has become even clearer to many people since the COVID-19 pandemic is the risk of emerging/spillover viruses to human health. Viruses are found in all different kinds of species on the planet, and when people encounter other species, there is a risk that a virus will make the leap from an animal to a person and thrive. Many scientists have dedicated their lives to conducting surveillance work using genomics to find new viruses and other pathogens that might emerge in the human population. For example, Project PREDICT run by UC Davis, working with partners in the field like the EcoHealth Alliance,

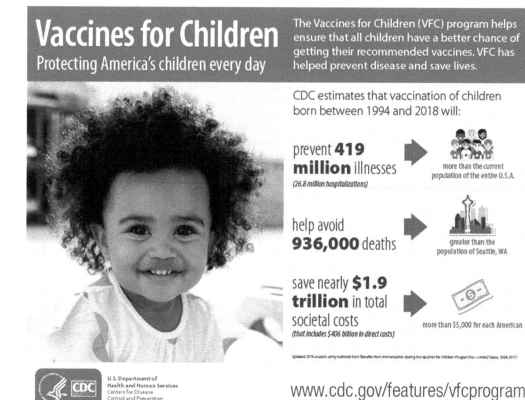

Vaccines for Children
Protecting America's children every day

The Vaccines for Children (VFC) program helps ensure that all children have a better chance of getting their recommended vaccines. VFC has helped prevent disease and save lives.

CDC estimates that vaccination of children born between 1994 and 2018 will:

prevent **419 million** illnesses
(26.8 million hospitalizations)
more than the current population of the entire U.S.A.

help avoid
936,000 deaths
greater than the population of Seattle, WA

save nearly **$1.9 trillion** in total societal costs
(that includes $406 billion in direct costs)
more than $5,000 for each American

U.S. Department of
Health and Human Services
Centers for Disease
Control and Prevention

www.cdc.gov/features/vfcprogram

FIGURE 9.4

Illnesses, hospitalizations, and deaths prevented by the Vaccines for Children program (VFC) in the United States.

Shown here are some statistics from the Vaccines for Children program (VFC) in the United States. Millions of illnesses, thousands of deaths, and over a trillion dollars in costs have been saved because of this program.

Centers for Disease control (CDC) VFC Infographic: Protecting America's children every day. www.cdc.gov/vaccines/programs/vfc/protecting-children.html

Source: "Benefits from Immunization during the Vaccines for Children Program Era—United States, 1994–2013." *Morbidity and Mortality Weekly Report.* 25 Apr 2014. Use of this material in the textbook does not imply endorsement by U.S. Government, Department of Health and Human Services, or Centers for Disease Control and Prevention.

has identified 949 new viruses, including a new strain of Ebolavirus (The Regents of the University of California 2021). Project Predict was shut down by the U.S. government in 2019 but received an extension of funding in 2020 during the COVID-19 pandemic (McNeil Jr. 2019; Burns 2020). Another project, the Global Virome Project, was started in 2016 building on the same principles as PREDICT (Kress, Mazet, and Hebert 2020; Institute 2021). Surveillance programs, like PREDICT, have been cited as useful tools in keeping emerging infectious diseases under control (Morens and Fauci 2012). The Global Health Security Index evaluates a country's ability to prevent a pandemic, but also how a country would respond, assigning an index score (Ravi et al. 2020). It is my hope and belief that scientists and policy makers will successfully advocate for more funding for an effective "pandemic alert system" into the future, and greater emphasis will be placed on the social and economic importance of maintaining health security.

Viruses have the potential to cause infectious disease anytime when wildlife encounters people directly or through livestock. Changes to ecosystems because of deforestation and agriculture increase the likelihood of new wildlife contacts with people (Wolfe, Dunavan, and Diamond 2007; Jones et al. 2013). For example, the EcoHealth Alliance has identified hotspots around the world for "emerging infectious disease (EID) events." They found that tropical areas where humans have changed land use, combined with a high number of different mammalian species in the environment, could create a hotspot (Allen et al. 2017). Others specifically note the "edge" of a tropical forest as being a vulnerable area, where humans are newly interfacing with a deforested area or areas where animal habitat fragmentation has occurred. Protecting forested areas and limiting wildlife trade would reduce the risk of an emerging virus spilling over into a community (Dobson et al. 2020). Scientists need additional funding to work at places in the world where the interface between humans and wildlife makes us most vulnerable. Scientists need to educate the public on the risks of interacting with wildlife or disrupting their habitat.

Some researchers are working on a type of paradigm shift, emphasizing the concept of "One Health" when addressing emerging infectious diseases. This paradigm emphasizes the intersection and interdependence of human health, animal health, and environmental health (Bird and Mazet 2018; Davis et al. 2017; Monath, Kahn, and Kaplan 2010; Zinsstag et al. 2018). It is critical for scientists to communicate the need for this kind of intervention to the public. More work needs to be done to increase awareness of the issue of emerging infectious disease among the general population. Beyond awareness, risk communication researchers indicate that effective communication needs to be done before a pandemic threat, engaging the public in dialogue and understanding that people and institutions can perceive risk in different ways (Holmes 2008). Whatever scientific approach we take going forward in the future, any emerging infectious disease hotspot in the world has the potential to affect all people on the planet, and we cannot forget it.

9.6.3 Recommended Sources for Scientific Information on Viruses and Society (Current in 2022)

It may be challenging to weed through all the media sources available online, especially in social media. Here is a list of reputable scientific societies, science publications or newspapers, and podcasts that may be potential sources of scientific information for you in the future.

Scientific societies and organizations:

American Association for Advancement of Science (AAAS)

National Academies of Sciences, Engineering and Medicine (NAS)

American Society for Microbiology (ASM)

American Society for Cell Biology (ASCB)

American Society for Biochemistry and Molecular Biology (ASBMB)

Science news (print and online):

Scientific American

The New York Times

Science (publication of AAAS)

Nature

www.nobelprize.org/ (official website for Nobel Prize information)

The Scientist

Other media:

National Public Radio—*Science Friday* and *Radiolab* programs

Nature (Magazine) Podcasts

Science (Magazine) Podcasts (AAAS)

ASM podcasts

9.7 Summary

Scientists have always been key participants in society in the United States and around the world. They are united in the method that they use to conduct their work, the scientific method. Scientists historically collaborate to build theories about how the world operates, and occasionally uncover very new approaches to looking at the world, leading to a paradigm shift. Science communication is critical to keeping other members of society informed and engaged in the scientific and technological changes happening around them. Scientists need to work to bring the public into the conversation and help them place their scientific findings in the context of the society around them. The public needs an awakening to how important science is in their lives, including their health and environment. Being well informed about science is critical for life's decisions. No one can understand every new scientific finding, even a scientist, but with the right tools, you can learn to seek out and recognize good science when you see it. Informed citizens can learn to avoid science misinformation, and scientists need to do a better job at guiding the public with transparency and a commitment to good science communication. Some urgent issues in our society right now include vaccine hesitancy and emerging viruses. These critical issues must be addressed now, as we never know when they may directly influence our families or us.

Discussion Questions:

1. When scientists use the scientific method correctly, their results are true and accurate. Is this statement correct? Why or why not?

2. Scientific theories are subject to ongoing testing and revision. Do you agree or disagree with this statement?

3. What form of media has had the biggest impact on your science education? Why?

4. What has been the effect of social media on your understanding of science?

5. Go to www.vaccines.gov/diseases and explore one of the fact sheets on a vaccine. Do you understand the information provided or could it be improved? How? Would you give this vaccine to your child if asked by a pediatrician?

6. Let us explore the concept of "One Health" where human, animal, and environmental health intersect. What would be the impact of the following events on the health of all three if they were to occur in your community?

   a. Natural disaster like a hurricane

   b. The building of a new highway

   c. Human epidemic involving a respiratory virus

   d. Human epidemic involving a virus carried by mosquitoes

   e. Animal epidemic among livestock

References

3M. 2019. "Scientists as storytellers guide." St. Paul, MN. Accessed 27 January 2021. https://multimedia.3m.com/mws/media/1667242O/sosi-3-13-toolkit-pdf.pdf.

———. 2021. "State of science index survey." Accessed 27 January 2021. www.3m.com/3M/en_US/state-of-science-index-survey/.

Aines, R.D., and A.L. Aines. 2019. *Championing Science*. Oakland, CA: University of California Press.

Akin, H., and A.R. Landrum. 2017. "A recap: Heuristics, biases, values, and other challenges to communicating science." In *The Oxford Handbook of the Science of Science Communication*, edited by K.H. Jamieson, D. Kahan and D.A. Scheufele, 455–60. New York, NY: Oxford University Press.

Akin, H., and D.A. Scheufele. 2017. "Overview of the science of science communication." In *The Oxford Handbook of the Science of Science Communication*, edited by K.H. Jamieson, D. Kahan and D.A. Scheufele, 25–34. New York, NY: Oxford University Press.

Allen, T., K.A. Murray, C. Zambrana-Torrelio, S.S. Morse, C. Rondinini, M. Di Marco, N. Breit, K.J. Olival, and P. Daszak. 2017. "Global hotspots and correlates of emerging zoonotic diseases." *Nature Communications* 8 (1):1–10.

Aurbach, E.L., K.E. Prater, E.T. Cloyd, and L. Lindenfeld. 2019. "Foundational skills for science communication: A preliminary framework." In *University of Michigan Library "Deep Blue Documents"*. Ann Arbor, MI: University of Michigan. https://deepblue.lib.umich.edu/handle/2027.42/150489.

Baltimore, D., P. Berg, M. Botchan, D. Carroll, R.A. Charo, G. Church, J.E. Corn, et al. 2015. "Biotechnology. A prudent path forward for genomic engineering and germline gene modification." *Science* 348 (6230):36–8. doi: 10.1126/science.aab1028.

Barinaga, M. 2000. "Asilomar revisited: Lessons for today?" *Science* 287 (5458):1584–5. doi: 10.1126/science.287.5458.1584.

Berg, P. 2008. "Meetings that changed the world: Asilomar 1975: DNA modification secured." *Nature* 455 (7211):290–1. doi: 10.1038/455290a.

Berg, P., D. Baltimore, S. Brenner, R.O. Roblin, 3rd, and M.F. Singer. 1975. "Asilomar conference on recombinant DNA molecules." *Science* 188 (4192):991–4. doi: 10.1126/science.1056638.

Berg, P., and M. Singer. 1995. "The recombinant DNA controversy: Twenty years later." *Biotechnology (N Y)* 13 (10):1132–4. doi: 10.1038/nbt1095-1132.

Bird, B.H., and J.A. Mazet. 2018. "Detection of emerging zoonotic pathogens: An integrated one health approach." *Annual Review of Animal Biosciences* 6:121–39.

Blastland, M., A.L.J. Freeman, S. van der Linden, T.M. Marteau, and D. Spiegelhalter. 2020. "Five rules for evidence communication." *Nature* 587 (7834):362–4. doi: 10.1038/d41586-020-03189-1.

Blum, D., and M. Knudson. 1997. *A Field Guide for Science Writers*. New York, NY: Oxford University Press.

Brossard, D., and D.A. Scheufele. 2013. "Social science. Science, new media, and the public." *Science* 339 (6115):40–1. doi: 10.1126/science.1232329.

Burns, K. 2020. "PREDICT receives extension for COVID-19 pandemic emergency response." *The Regents of the University of California, Davis Campus*. Accessed 27 January 2021. www.ucdavis.edu/coronavirus/news/predict-receives-extension-covid-19-pandemic-emergency-response/.

Canfield, K.N., S. Menezes, S.B. Matsuda, A. Moore, A.N. Mosley Austin, B.M. Dewsbury, M.I. Feliú-Mójer, et al. 2020. "Science communication demands a critical approach that centers inclusion, equity, and intersectionality." *Frontiers in Communication* 5 (2). doi: 10.3389/fcomm.2020.00002.

Carroll, S.B. 2020. "The denialist playbook." In *Scientific American*. New York, NY: Springer Nature America.

CDC, Centers for Disease Control and Prevention. 2021a. "Measles home/measles elimination." Accessed 27 January 2021. www.cdc.gov/measles/elimination.html.

———. 2021b. "National center for health statistics/FastStats/healthcare and insurance/immunization." Accessed 27 January 2021. www.cdc.gov/nchs/fastats/immunize.htm.

———.2021c. "Vaccines for children program (VFC)." Accessed 8 July 2021. www.cdc.gov/vaccines/programs/vfc/index.html.

Chan, M.P., C. Jones, and D. Albarracin. 2017. "Countering false beliefs: An analysis of the evidence and recommendations of best practices for the retraction and correction of scientific misinformation." In *The Oxford Handbook of the Science of Science Communication*, edited by K.H. Jamieson, D. Kahan and D.A. Scheufele, 341–50. New York, NY: Oxford University Press.

Cohn, A., L.E. Rodewald, W.A. Orenstein, and A. Schuchat. 2017. "Immunization in the United States." In *Vaccines E-Book*, edited by S.A. Plotkin, W. Orenstein, P.A. Offit and K.M. Edwards, 1421–40.e4. Saint Louis, MO: Elsevier.

Congress, United States. 2017. "H.R. 4174—foundations for evidence-based policymaking act of 2018." Accessed 26 January 2021. www.congress.gov/bill/115th-congress/house-bill/4174.

Contractor, N.S., and L.A. DeChurch. 2014. "Integrating social networks and human social motives to achieve social influence at scale." *Proceedings of the National Academy of Sciences* 111 (Supplement 4):13650–7.

Davatelis, G.N. 2000. "The Asilomar process: Is it valid?" In *The Scientist*, 51. Wilmington, DE: LabX Media Group.

Davis, M.F., S.C. Rankin, J.M. Schurer, S. Cole, L. Conti, P. Rabinowitz, G. Gray, L. Kahn, C. Machalaba, and J. Mazet. 2017. "Checklist for one health epidemiological reporting of evidence (COHERE)." *One Health* 4:14–21.

Dijkstra, A.M., L. de Bakker, F. van Dam, and E.A. Jensen. 2020. "Setting the scene." In *Science Communication: An Introduction*, edited by A.M. Dijkstra, L. de Bakker, F. van Dam and E.A. Jensen, 1–16. Hackensack, NJ: World Scientific.

Dobson, A.P., S.L. Pimm, L. Hannah, L. Kaufman, J.A. Ahumada, A.W. Ando, A. Bernstein, J. Busch, P. Daszak, and J. Engelmann. 2020. "Ecology and economics for pandemic prevention." *Science* 369 (6502):379–81.

Druckman, J.N., and A. Lupia. 2017. "Using frames to make scientific communication more effective." In *The Oxford Handbook of the Science of Science Communication*, edited by K.H. Jamieson, D. Kahan and D.A. Scheufele, 351–60. New York, NY: Oxford University Press.

Editorials. 2015. "After Asilomar." *Nature* 526 (7573):293–4. doi: 10.1038/526293b.

Falkow, S. 2012. "The lessons of Asilomar and the H5N1 'affair'." *mBio* 3 (5). doi: 10.1128/mBio.00354-12.

Fine, P.E. 1993. "Herd immunity: History, theory, practice." *Epidemiologic Reviews* 15 (2):265–302.

Fiske, S.T., and C. Dupree. 2014. "Gaining trust as well as respect in communicating to motivated audiences about science topics." *Proceedings of the National Academy of Sciences of the United States of America* 111 (Suppl 4):13593–7. doi: 10.1073/pnas.1317505111.

Fleischman, J., and C. Szalinski. 2014. "So you want to be a science writer." *Molecular Biology of the Cell* 25 (13):1938–41. doi: 10.1091/mbc.E14-04-0857.

Geoghegan, S., K.P. O'Callaghan, and P.A. Offit. 2020. "Vaccine safety: Myths and misinformation." *Frontiers in Microbiology* 11:372.

Greene, A.E. 2013. *Writing Science in Plain English*. Chicago, IL: The University of Chicago Press.

Hilgard, J., and K.H. Jamieson. 2017. "Science as 'broken' versus science as 'self-correcting': How retractions and peer-review problems are exploited to attack science." In *The Oxford Handbook of the Science of Science Communication*, edited by K.H. Jamieson, D. Kahan and D.A. Scheufele, 85–92. New York, NY: Oxford University Press.

Hoffman, J. 2019. "How anti-vaccine sentiment took hold in the United States." In *The New York Times*. New York, NY: The New York Times Company.

Holmes, B.J. 2008. "Communicating about emerging infectious disease: The importance of research." *Health, Risk & Society* 10 (4):349–60. doi: 10.1080/13698570802166431.

Horne, Z., D. Powell, J.E. Hummel, and K.J. Holyoak. 2015. "Countering antivaccination attitudes." *Proceedings of the National Academy of Sciences* 112 (33):10321–4.

Hosler, J., and K.B. Boomer. 2011. "Are comic books an effective way to engage nonmajors in learning and appreciating science?" *CBE Life Sciences Education* 10 (3):309–17. doi: 10.1187/cbe.10-07-0090.

Howell, E.L., and D. Brossard. 2021. "(Mis)informed about what? What it means to be a science-literate citizen in a digital world." *Proceedings of the National Academy of Sciences* 118 (15):e1912436117. doi: 10.1073/pnas.1912436117.

Institute, UC Davis One Health. 2021. "Global virome project." Accessed 27 January 2021. www.globalviromeproject.org/.

Jamieson, K.H. 2017. "The need for a science of science communication: Communicating science's values and norms." In *The Oxford Handbook of the Science of Science Communication*, edited by K.H. Jamieson, D. Kahan and D.A. Scheufele, 15–24. New York, NY: Oxford University Press.

Jarrett, C., R. Wilson, M. O'Leary, E. Eckersberger, and H.J. Larson. 2015. "Strategies for addressing vaccine hesitancy—A systematic review." *Vaccine* 33 (34):4180–90.

Johnson, N.F., N. Velásquez, N.J. Restrepo, R. Leahy, N. Gabriel, S. El Oud, M. Zheng, P. Manrique, S. Wuchty, and Y. Lupu. 2020. "The online competition between pro- and anti-vaccination views." *Nature* 582 (7811):230–3. doi: 10.1038/s41586-020-2281-1.

Jones, B.A., D. Grace, R. Kock, S. Alonso, J. Rushton, M.Y. Said, D. McKeever, F. Mutua, J. Young, and J. McDermott. 2013. "Zoonosis emergence linked to agricultural intensification and environmental change." *Proceedings of the National Academy of Sciences* 110 (21):8399–404.

Kahan, D. 2017a. "On the sources of ordinary science knowledge and extraordinary science ignorance." In *The Oxford Handbook of the Science of Science Communication*, edited by K.H. Jamieson, D. Kahan and D.A. Scheufele, 35–50. New York, NY: Oxford University Press.

———. 2017b. "Protecting or polluting the science communication environment? The case of childhood vaccines." In *The Oxford Handbook of the Science of Science Communication*, edited by K.H. Jamieson, D. Kahan and D.A. Scheufele, 421–32. New York, NY: Oxford University Press.

Kahan, D., and A.R. Landrum. 2017. "A tale of two vaccines—and their science communication environments." In *The Oxford Handbook of the Science of Science Communication*, edited by K.H. Jamieson, D. Kahan and D.A. Scheufele, 165–72. New York, NY: Oxford University Press.

Kahan, D.M. 2013. "A risky science communication environment for vaccines." *Science* 342 (6154):53–4.

———. 2015. "What is the 'science of science communication'?" *Journal of Science Communication* 14 (3):1–10.

Kahan, D.M., H. Jenkins-Smith, and D. Braman. 2011. "Cultural cognition of scientific consensus." *Journal of Risk Research* 14 (2):147–74.

Koster, E., and F. Kupper. 2020. "Views of science." In *Science Communication: An Introduction*, edited by F. van Dam, L. de Bakker, A.M. Dijkstra and E.A. Jensen, 17–42. Hackensack, NJ: World Scientific.

Kress, W.J., J.A. Mazet, and P.D. Hebert. 2020. "Opinion: Intercepting pandemics through genomics." *Proceedings of the National Academy of Sciences* 117 (25):13852–5.

Kuhn, T.S. 2012. *The Structure of Scientific Revolutions*. Chicago, IL: The University of Chicago Press.

Kwon, D. 2020. "Science and policy collide during the pandemic." In *The Scientist*. Wilmington, DE: LabX Media Group.

Land-Zandstra, A.M., L. De Bakker, and E.A. Jensen. 2020. "Informal science education." In *Science Communication: An Introduction*, edited by F. van Dam, L. De Bakker, A.M. Dijkstra and E.A. Jensen, 91–118. Hackensack, NJ: World Scientific.

Li, N., N.J. Stroud, and K.H. Jamieson. 2017. "Overcoming false causal attribution: Debunking the MMR-autism association." In *The Oxford Handbook of the Science of Science Communication*, edited by K.H. Jamieson, D. Kahan and D.A. Scheufele, 433–44. New York, NY: Oxford University Press.

Lieu, T.A., G.T. Ray, N.P. Klein, C. Chung, and M. Kulldorff. 2015. "Geographic clusters in underimmunization and vaccine refusal." *Pediatrics* 135 (2):280–9.

Márquez, M.C., and A.M. Porras. 2020. "Science communication in multiple languages is critical to its effectiveness." *Frontiers in Communication* 5 (31). doi: 10.3389/fcomm.2020.00031.

McNeil Jr., D.G. 2019. "Scientists were hunting for the next Ebola. Now the U.S. has cut off their funding." In *The New York Times*. New York, NY: The New York Times Company.

———. 2020. " 'We loved each other': Fauci Recalls Larry Kramer, friend and nemesis." In *The New York Times*. New York, NY: The New York Times Company.

Minkoff, E., and P.J. Baker. 2004. "Biology: Science and ethics." In *Biology Today: An Issues Approach*, edited by E.C. Minkoff and P.J. Baker, 1–32. New York, NY: Garland Publishing.

Monath, T.P., L.H. Kahn, and B. Kaplan. 2010. "One health perspective." *ILAR Journal* 51 (3):193–8.

Morens, D.M., and A.S. Fauci. 2012. "Emerging infectious diseases in 2012: 20 years after the institute of medicine report." *mBio* 3 (6).

Mukherjee, S. 2016. *The Gene: An Intimate History*. New York, NY: Scribner.

National Academies of Sciences, E., and Medicine. 2015. *International Summit on Human Gene Editing: A Global Discussion*. Edited by S. Olson. Washington, DC: The National Academies Press.

NewsHour, PBS. 2020. "Fauci remembers AIDS activist Larry Kramer for 'extraordinary courage'." Accessed 26 January 2021. www.youtube.com/watch?v=72Z0aqHmduQ.

Nisbet, M.C., and D.A. Scheufele. 2009. "What's next for science communication? Promising directions and lingering distractions." *American Journal of Botany* 96 (10):1767–78. doi: 10.3732/ajb.0900041.

Nyhan, B., and J. Reifler. 2015. "Does correcting myths about the flu vaccine work? An experimental evaluation of the effects of corrective information." *Vaccine* 33 (3):459–64.

Nyhan, B., J. Reifler, S. Richey, and G.L. Freed. 2014. "Effective messages in vaccine promotion: A randomized trial." *Pediatrics* 133 (4):e835-e42.

Olson, R. 2009. *Don't be Such a Scientist*. Washington, DC: Island Press.

Patel, M., A.D. Lee, N.S. Clemmons, S.B. Redd, S. Poser, D. Blog, J.R. Zucker, J. Leung, R. Link-Gelles, and H. Pham. 2019. "National update on measles cases and outbreaks—United States, January 1—October 1, 2019." *Morbidity and Mortality Weekly Report* 68 (40):893.

Paterson, P., F. Meurice, L.R. Stanberry, S. Glismann, S.L. Rosenthal, and H.J. Larson. 2016. "Vaccine hesitancy and healthcare providers." *Vaccine* 34 (52):6700–6.

Pew, Research Center. 2020. "Science and scientists held in high esteem across global publics." Accessed 27 January 2021. https://www.pewresearch.org/science/2020/09/29/science-and-scientists-held-in-high-esteem-across-global-publics/ see "Complete Report PDF" on webpage.

Piot, P., H.J. Larson, K.L. O'Brien, J. N'kengasong, E. Ng, S. Sow, and B. Kampmann. 2019. "Immunization: Vital progress, unfinished agenda." *Nature* 575 (7781):119–29.

Planetary Science Division, N.S.M.D. 2021. "NASA science solar system exploration people Carl Sagan (1934–1996)." Accessed 26 January 2021. https://solarsystem.nasa.gov/people/660/carl-sagan-1934-1996/.

Ravi, S.J., K.L. Warmbrod, L. Mullen, D. Meyer, E. Cameron, J. Bell, P. Bapat, M. Paterra, C. Machalaba, and I. Nath. 2020. "The value proposition of the Global Health Security Index." *BMJ Global Health* 5 (10):e003648.

Rensberger, B. 2009. "Science journalism: Too close for comfort." *Nature* 459 (7250):1055–6. doi: 10.1038/4591055a.

Roozenbeek, J., and S. van der Linden. 2019. "Fake news game confers psychological resistance against online misinformation." *Palgrave Communications* 5 (1):1–10.

Ruggeri, K., S. van der Linden, C. Wang, F. Papa, J. Riesch, and J. Green. 2020. "Standards for evidence in policy decision-making." *PsyARXiv Preprint*. Accessed 26 January 2021. https://doi.org/10.31234/osf.io/fjwvk.

Schafer, M.S. 2017. "How changing media structures are affecting science news coverage." In *The Oxford Handbook of the Science of Science Communication*, edited by K.H. Jamieson, D. Kahan and D.A. Scheufele, 51–60. New York, NY: Oxford University Press.

Scheufele, D.A. 2013. "Communicating science in social settings." *Proceedings of the National Academy of Sciences* 110 (Supplement 3):14040–7.

ScienceCounts. 2015. "ScienceCounts' benchmark study on public attitudes of science." Accessed 27 January 2021. https://www.sciencecounts.org/wp-content/uploads/2019/02/ReportBenchmark.pdf. See also https://sciencecounts.org/research/.

———. 2017. "A closer look at public trust in scientists." Accessed 27 January 2021. https://www.sciencecounts.org/wp-content/uploads/2019/02/TrustinScientistsFinal.pdf. See also https://sciencecounts.org/research/.

Sciences, National Academy of. 2014. *The Science of Science Communication II: Summary of a Colloquium*. Washington, DC: The National Academies Press.

———. 2018. *The Science of Science Communication III: Inspiring Novel Collaborations and Building Capacity: Proceedings of a Colloquium*. Edited by S. Olson. Washington, DC: The National Academies Press.

Scientists, Union of Concerned. 2021. "About/history." Accessed 26 January 2021. www.ucsusa.org/about/history.

Smith, T.C. 2017. "Vaccine rejection and hesitancy: A review and call to action." *Open Forum Infectious Diseases* 4 (3): ofx146. doi: 10.1093/ofid/ofx146

Strebel, P.M., M.J. Papania, P.A. Gastanaduy, and J.L. Goodson. 2017. "Measles vaccines." In *Vaccines E-Book*, edited by S.A. Plotkin, W. Orenstein, P.A. Offit and K.M. Edwards, 579–618.e21. Saint Louis, MO: Elsevier.

Stroud, N.J. 2017. "Understanding and overcoming selective exposure and judgment when communicating about science." In *The Oxford Handbook of the Science of Science Communication*, edited by K.H. Jamieson, D. Kahan and D.A. Scheufele, 377–88. New York, NY: Oxford University Press.

The Regents of the University of California, D.C. 2021. "UC Davis school of veterinary medicine/programs&projects/predict." Accessed 27 January 2021. https://ohi.vetmed.ucdavis.edu/programs-projects/predict-project.

Tyson, N.D. 2013. "'Tweet' from Neil deGrasse Tyson." Accessed 27 January 2021. https://twitter.com/neiltyson/status/345551599382446081?lang=en.

Vaidyanathan, G. 2020. "News feature: Finding a vaccine for misinformation." *Proceedings of the National Academy of Sciences* 117 (32):18902–5.

Verhoeff, R., and F. Kupper. 2020. "Science in dialogue." In *Science Communication: An Introduction*, edited by F. Van Dam, L. De Bakker, A.M. Dijkstra and E.A. Jensen, 65–90. Hackensack, NJ: World Scientific.

Villa, V. 2021. "5 facts about vaccines in the U.S." *Pew Research Center*. Accessed 27 January 2021. www.pewresearch.org/fact-tank/2019/03/19/5-facts-about-vaccines-in-the-u-s/.

Wadman, M. 2020. "Antivaccine forces gaining online." *Science* 368 (6492):699. doi: 10.1126/science.368.6492.699.

Wolfe, N.D., C.P. Dunavan, and J. Diamond. 2007. "Origins of major human infectious diseases." *Nature* 447 (7142):279–83.

Yeo, S.K., and D. Brossard. 2017. "The (changing) nature of scientist-media interactions: A cross-national analysis." In *The Oxford Handbook of the Science of Science Communication*, edited by K.H. Jamieson, D. Kahan and D.A. Scheufele, 261–72. New York, NY: Oxford University Press.

Zanatta, A., F. Zampieri, C. Basso, and G. Thiene. 2017. "Galileo Galilei: Science vs. faith." *Global Cardiology Science and Practice* 2017 (2):10. doi: 10.21542/gcsp.2017.10.

Zinsstag, J., L. Crump, E. Schelling, J. Hattendorf, Y.O. Maidane, K.O. Ali, A. Muhummed, A.A. Umer, F. Aliyi, and F. Nooh. 2018. "Climate change and one health." *FEMS Microbiology Letters* 365 (11):fny085.

Index

Note: Page numbers in *italics* indicate a figure and page numbers in **bold** indicate a table on the corresponding page.

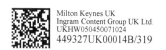